WELL ADVISED ™

A PRACTICAL GUIDE TO
EVERYDAY HEALTH DECISIONS

WELL
ADVISED™

With 130 illustrations and 25 color photographs

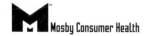 Mosby Consumer Health

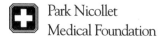 Park Nicollet
Medical Foundation

The material in this publication is for general information only and is not intended to provide specific advice or recommendations for any individual. Your doctor or other health professional must be consulted for advise with regard to your individual situation.

Mosby Consumer Health
11830 Westline Industrial Drive
St. Louis, MO 63146
(800) 433-3803

Park Nicollet Medical Foundation
3800 Park Nicollet Boulevard
Minneapolis, MN 55416
(800) 372-7776

International Standard Book Number ISBN 1-56066-439-8

95 96 97 98 99 / 9 8 7 6 5 4 3 2 1

Printed in Canada

INTRODUCTION

Well Advised™: A Practical Guide to Everyday Medical Decisions comes at a time when the field of health care is undergoing tremendous change. Almost everyone agrees, however, that affordable, easily available, high quality health care is a priority. Yet, to achieve this goal we all must participate in the change. For health care organizations, this means developing medical guidelines and continually measuring the quality of care being delivered. For you, the consumer, it means becoming an active partner in understanding health care options and making informed choices. This guide will help you do just that.

Well Advised™ is based on information gathered from many sources. The Park Nicollet Medical Foundation, a national leader in health care research, developed 100 medical guidelines that served as the core of advice for this book. In addition, the work of quality improvement teams from The Institute for Clinical Systems Integration—including experts from Park Nicollet, Group Health, and the Mayo Clinic—went into developing *Well Advised™*. Nationally published references such as the guidelines from the U.S. Preventive Services Task Force, the Agency for Health Care Policy Research, the U.S. Office of Technology Assessment, and the National Institute of Medicine were also used. The advice of these highly respected sources was reviewed and organized to produce an easy-to-use reference that will help you make truly informed health care choices.

Studies show that when people know more about their health, they make better health decisions. They know which problems are serious and require a doctor's attention and which they can treat at home with self-care techniques. Up-to-date, reliable health information also influences how people feel about their experience at the doctor's office. This is important because when patients feel satisfied with the care they get, they are more likely to follow their doctor's instructions. *Well Advised™* was written to give you the kind of information you need to take an active part in your care. The more you know about your health, the more involved you can be in your care and the better the overall result of your health care experience will be.

What Are Health Care Guidelines?

Health care guidelines are summaries of the current best information about how to treat a particular health problem. They tell the health care provider when, how, and why to treat the problem. When doctors and other providers use guidelines consistently, they get better results from the care they give because they know they are making the most effective choices.

Guidelines are developed using the best scientific research. Typically, a guideline is developed by a team of experts who analyze the collected research on a particular topic and recommend the best course of treatment. Since busy health care professionals often struggle to keep up with mountains of new information, guidelines offer a valuable tool by summarizing the most current information and the best way to practice.

Guidelines reduce variation in medical practice. It will never be possible or desirable for a doctor to treat every patient in exactly the same way. The same health problem in two different people will appear slightly differently because of each individual's personal history and characteristics. Too much variation, however, can be inefficient and even harmful. Guidelines help reduce these effects.

Guidelines improve the quality of health care. Guidelines can act as a yardstick to measure how well a treatment is working. Providing feedback to doctors and clinics about what is effective and what's not leads to better care in the end.

Guidelines help doctors and patients share decisions. Medical guidelines provide a basis for discussion between you and your health care provider. In some cases, the available information provides a straightforward argument for or against a certain treatment. But in many cases, the choice is not so clear. In these instances, your opinions and preferences as a patient become especially important in choosing the direction your treatment will take. You and your doctor will have to take into account the medical information as well as your values, beliefs, and preferences in deciding on the best approach for you.

What Sets *Well Advised* Apart from Other Guides?

Well Advised™ differs from other home medical references in several ways:

- Studies show that the overwhelming majority of calls for medical advice deal with 40 common conditions. This manual focuses on answering your questions about these recurring health problems.

- People want clear, simple advice—not boring facts. In this book the discussion of each problem ends with an easy-to-follow decision guide to let you know when to try self-care steps and when to seek medical treatment.

- The advice in *Well Advised*™ is based on proven, scientific evidence drawn from actual clinical experience.

- The illustrations in *Well Advised*™ are valuable visual aids to help you better understand the condition or perform self-care techniques.

- *Well Advised*™ includes 25 color photographs to help you identify common skin problems.

- Throughout the book, real people describe in their own words their health care problems and how they handled them.

How Is This Guide Organized?

Section One of *Well Advised*™ gives advice on handling emergencies and urgent problems. You will need to contact your health care provider in all emergency situations, but the information found here will help you make decisions until you get professional care. It will also help you determine the severity of the problem: whether you need to go to the hospital emergency room or whether an urgent care center will do.

Section Two, "Self-Care for Common Problems," gives you a basic understanding of common health problems emphasizing doctors' advice that you can use at home. For most people, however, the greatest concern is not everyday aches and pains, but chronic health problems. These are covered in Section Three, "Living with Chronic Health Problems."

Section Four, "Preventing Health Problems," discusses the prevention steps you can take to keep yourself healthy. Section Five, "Health Care Consumers and Shared Decisions," reflects the belief that providers and consumers need to be equal partners in the health care team. Ultimately, your knowledge, actions, and beliefs have more to do with your future health than anything the medical system has to offer.

We hope that you will rely on this guide to care for minor problems and make informed health care decisions. But, like any manual of this kind, it should not be considered a substitute for quality medical care from your doctor or other health care provider. Also, consider your own health history and medical condition when reading the advice presented here and check with your own provider if you are not sure the self-care tips apply to you.

TABLE OF CONTENTS

CONTENTS

SECTION ONE
EMERGENCIES AND URGENT CARE

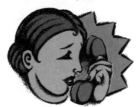

USING THE EMERGENCY ROOM

When you or someone you love is sick, it isn't easy to wait for relief. People often rush to the hospital emergency room with the flu, earaches, sore throats, colds, and the like. Although the emergency room can treat almost anything, some visits may not be covered by your insurance company. The arrival of a hospital bill can be a shock.

Making Sure You're Covered

So how do you get the best possible care while avoiding unnecessary costs? And how do you know if you should use the emergency room?

Life-threatening conditions, brought on by sudden illness or accidental injury, that require immediate treatment to prevent serious harm are always covered. In such cases, you can go right to your insurance plan's hospital emergency room without first speaking to a plan doctor. If your condition is so serious that traveling to a plan health site might endanger your health, go to the nearest hospital.

Some examples of life-threatening conditions that would send you to an emergency room are:

- Chest pain or shortness of breath, which could be symptoms of heart attack (see Chest Pain, p. 85)
- Acute appendicitis or severe abdominal pain (except for constipation or menstrual cramps), especially after an injury (see Abdominal Pain, p. 41)
- Uncontrollable bleeding from a wound (see Cuts, p. 16)
- Loss of consciousness or confusion, especially after a head injury (see Head Injuries—Adult, p. 23, and Child, p. 25)

This list is not complete. Consider the patient's health and past medical problems when weighing the urgency of the situation. When in doubt, the best way to know if you should go to the emergency room is to speak with your doctor first. Emergency room treatment for non-life-threatening conditions is usually covered if a plan doctor approves the visit first.

Many clinics have doctors on call after hours. Often your plan doctor, the on-call doctor, or a clinic nurse can give you advice on how to reduce your discomfort, or how to arrange to see a doctor if necessary. When the clinic is closed, on-call doctors can usually be reached through their answering services at the clinic's regular phone number.

When You Just Can't Wait

Some clinics have urgent care centers with day, evening, and weekend hours to treat patients with non-life-threatening illnesses or injuries that need prompt attention. Even minor broken bones and wounds requiring stitches can—and should—be treated in the clinic or an urgent care center. **You should promptly treat fractures and wounds requiring stitches. When the clinic and urgent care centers are closed, go to the emergency room.** And, often you can use any urgent care center that is covered by your insurance company, whether or not you regularly go to that clinic.

When possible, however, the best bet is to see your regular doctor. He or she can best coordinate your total health care and follow up illnesses and injuries.

Keeping the Costs Down

By using clinic, urgent care center, and emergency room services appropriately, you can get the best care and lower your health care costs. The copayments for emergency room care—if your benefit plan requires them—are usually much higher than the copayments for urgent care center services. Clinic copayments—if your benefit plan requires them—are usually lower still.

The Choice Is Yours

In the end, you are the one who must decide where you will seek treatment and if the extra cost of an emergency room visit that isn't covered is worth it to you. Some situations where emergency room services are covered *only* if first approved by a plan doctor are:

- Earaches, sore throats, colds, flu, upper-respiratory infections, viruses, fever, strep throat, and headaches

- Slight injuries such as bruises and abrasions that do not require stitches

- Abdominal pain from simple constipation or menstrual cramps

- Sprains and cuts that occur during clinic or urgent care center hours

This list is not complete. Consider the patient's health and past medical problems when evaluating the urgency of the situation.

HOW TO USE THE DECISION GUIDES

The **Decision Guides** found throughout this book can help you make decisions about the best course of treatment when you are ill. If you still have doubts after using the guides, seek medical advice.

Decision Guides Are Not for Infants

The decision guides do not apply to infants under 3 months old. Always seek your health care provider's advice if you are concerned that your infant is seriously sick.

The Decision Guide Symbols

The symbols offer a general guide to how and when to seek care:

Use self-care Symptoms can usually be treated at home. If symptoms persist you should call your health care provider for advice.

Call doctor's office for advice Symptoms may be treated at home or they may require a visit to your health care provider. Usually, you and your health care provider need to share additional information about your condition to decide what is best for you.

See doctor Symptoms need to be evaluated by a health care provider. As you call to make an appointment, your provider will help you determine how soon you need to be seen.

Seek help now Symptoms in this category are serious and should usually be seen within less than 2 hours. Depending on your health insurance, you may choose to call your health care provider to determine if you should be seen in the doctor's office, in an urgent care center, or in the emergency room.

Emergency, call 911 Symptoms in this category are life threatening and require immediate medical treatment.

EMERGENCIES AND FIRST AID

Self-care education offers recommendations about caring for illnesses by yourself. *All true emergencies need to be treated by an appropriate medical professional.* The self-care guidelines in this section are only appropriate for use when medical professionals are not immediately available and before you can get to an emergency room. This section offers advice on how to assess the needs of an accident victim, how to offer life support if needed, and when to offer first aid.

Learning first-aid skills is your first step in being prepared to help keep emergency victims alive or knowing how to keep injuries from getting worse. Many communities have American Red Cross agencies that offer first-aid classes. First-aid instruction also is often available through community education programs or local community colleges and universities. These first-aid courses teach you how to identify medical emergencies; understand causes, symptoms, and signs of injuries; and apply first aid. The more you know about first aid, the more likely you are to stay calm when helping yourself or someone suffering from an accident.

Before trying to help someone who is hurt, you should always ask his or her permission or the permission of a guardian. You are legally protected for trying to help someone if you do so in good faith and are not guilty of willful misconduct. Legally, you can assume you have the victim's consent to help if the victim is unconscious or so badly hurt that he or she cannot give permission.

Many diseases can be spread through contact with the blood of an accident victim. These infections do not penetrate intact skin, but you may have cracked or scratched skin that is vulnerable.

Latex gloves offer the best protection if you are giving first aid. Otherwise, keep plastic wrap, several layers of gauze pad, or other barriers between you and the blood of the victim.

Along with first aid advice, this section helps you decide when to go to an urgent care center versus the emergency room. Review this information before an accident occurs so that you are prepared to make the best decision at the time.

FIRST-AID SUPPLIES

Also see Equipping Your Home for Self-Care, p. 40.

First-aid kits should have everything you might need in an emergency. Keep them organized and in an easy to find place in your home and vehicles.

Check your first-aid kits periodically to be sure they are well stocked and up-to-date. Discard and promptly replace any outdated medicine or ointment. Store your first-aid kit on an upper shelf out of reach of small children. Don't store in a hot or cold area, or in a bathroom. You can buy complete first-aid kits from a drug store or medical supply outlet.

Everyday items that can be used in an emergency

- Disposable or regular diapers for compresses, bandages, or padding for splints

- Sanitary napkins (same uses as above)

- Magazines, newspapers, or umbrella for use as a splint for broken bones

- Clean dish towel, scarf, or handkerchief for bandages or slings

- Table leaf or old door for stretchers *Note: Do not move people with head and neck injuries unless they are in a life-threatening situation.*

STOCKING YOUR OWN FIRST-AID KIT

To assemble your own complete first-aid kit, place a copy of this book in a small tote bag or sturdy, easily carried box, along with the following items:

Dressings
- Adhesive bandage strips (assorted sizes)
- Butterfly bandages
- Elastic bandages, 2 or 3 inches wide
- Adhesive dressing tape
- Sterile cotton balls
- Sterile eye patches
- Sterile gauze pads, 4 by 4 inches
- Sterile nonstick pads for use with sterile gauze pads
- Stretchable gauze, one roll
- Triangular bandage for sling or dressing cover

Instruments
- Bulb syringe to rinse eyes or wounds
- Sharp scissors
- Tweezers

Medication
- Antiseptic ointment
- Antihistamine tablets for allergic reactions
- Aspirin or acetaminophen. Do not give aspirin to children under age 16.
- Syrup of ipecac to induce vomiting. Follow directions of poison control center or health care provider.

Miscellaneous items
- Airtight packages of hand wipes
- Candle and waterproof matches
- Instant chemical cold packs
- Cotton swabs
- Disposable latex gloves
- Flashlight—remove batteries to prevent corrosion and/or accidental discharge
- Paper and pen or pencil
- Soap
- Tissues
- Safety pins
- Blanket
- Sterile eye wash and/or plastic cup

Special needs items
- Adrenaline or epinephrine, insulin and sugar, or nitroglycerin

ALLERGIC REACTIONS

For Allergic Reactions, see p. 148.

BITES

For Insect Bites, see p. 29; for Snakebites, see p. 38.

Human Bites

Human bites happen more often than you think and are usually done by children while playing or fighting. Infection often results due to the amount and type of bacteria in the human mouth. If a human bite breaks the skin, thoroughly wash the area, then see your doctor.

One of the most frequent human bites is the result of a person punching someone in the mouth and then discovering that the skin over the knuckles has been broken by the intended victim's teeth.

The possibility of AIDS being spread through the bite of an HIV-infected person is considered extremely unlikely. To date there have been no documented examples of HIV transmission through biting.

SELF-CARE STEPS FOR HUMAN BITES

• Check for bleeding if you have a human bite. If the wound is bleeding, apply direct pressure and try to raise the wound above heart level. Wash it vigorously with mild soap and a wash cloth under running water for at least 5 minutes.

• Check to be sure you've received a tetanus booster within the last 10 years. A booster for tetanus is recommended more often, maybe every 5 years, if you have ever had a serious open wound. Watch the wound site closely for signs of infection, and see your health care provider immediately if you have been bitten hard enough to penetrate the skin or if you have any of the signs or symptoms listed in the Decision Guide for Infected Wounds, p. 28.

Animal Bites

More than 2 million dog bites resulting in puncture wounds or cuts are reported each year. Half of the victims are children. Millions of bites and nips from other animals are believed to go unreported.

Animal bites raise three concerns: bleeding, the possibility of viral infections like rabies, and the possibility of bacterial infections like tetanus. Animal bites that break the skin often cause bacterial skin infections. Cat bites are generally more likely to cause infection than dog bites.

Perhaps the best way to treat an animal bite is in advance, before you are bitten. Avoid wild animals, especially if they let you approach. Don't pester unfamiliar dogs or cats or attempt to pet them if they appear at all unfriendly.

SELF-CARE STEPS FOR ANIMAL BITES

• Wash all animal bites vigorously with soap and under running water for 5 minutes, even if they have not bled. Apply an antiseptic ointment (bacitracin, Neosporin) to shallow puncture wounds, and watch for signs of infection. Deep puncture wounds, especially cat bites, carry a greater risk of infection and should be treated immediately by your health care provider.

• The main carriers of rabies are wild animals—especially skunks, raccoons, bats, and foxes. Rabid animals act strangely, attack without provocation, and may drool or foam at the mouth. If a pet has bitten you, the animal needs to be confined and watched for 10 days to see if it develops rabies symptoms.

• It is very important to catch and confine any wild animal that has bitten you, so it can be evaluated for rabies. (Call the animal control office, police or sheriff's department for help with animals.) Capture the animal alive if you can safely do so without risking further injury or, if necessary, kill the animal but do not damage its head. Save the carcass in the refrigerator (or freezer) until it can be turned over to health department officials for examination. For information after hours, check to see if there is a rabies hotline in your area.

Call your health care provider if:

• Any wild animal bites you.

• A strange dog or any cat bites you.

• The animal owner has no vaccination records.

• You are concerned that the animal is ill, or if the bite was not provoked.

• Your tetanus shots aren't up-to-date (every 10 years, or every 5 years if you have ever had a serious open wound).

• Any sign of infection appears (see Decision Guide for Infected Wounds, p. 28).

• The bite is severe, especially on the face or hand.

BURNS

For Chemical Burns, see p. 9; for Electrical Burns, see p. 18.

Burns occur when the skin touches hot surfaces, liquids, steam, or flame (also see Chemical Burns, p. 9, and Electrical Burns, p. 18). Skin burns are graded by degree. The higher the number, the more severe the burn. **First-degree** burns are slight burns affecting the top portion of the skin. Symptoms include redness, pain, and minor swelling.

Second-degree burns affect the top layer of skin and the second layer. These burns cause redness, pain, swelling, and some blisters. Although second-degree burns are probably the most painful burns, most can be treated successfully at home if only a small amount of skin is burned.

Third-degree burns destroy all skin layers and may penetrate deep below the surface of the skin. The damaged skin may be red, white, or charred black. Because there is a lot of nerve damage, there may be no pain and little bleeding. All third-degree burns should be seen by your doctor immediately. Large-area burns, burns that result in a lot of blistering, or serious burns on the hand or face should also be seen.

In **severe burns**, the wound will weep or ooze large amounts of plasma—the clear liquid portion of blood—from damaged blood vessels in the wound area.

DECISION GUIDE FOR BURNS

SYMPTOMS/SIGNS	ACTION
First-degree burn	▨
Second-degree burn	☎
No tetanus booster received within last 10 years or more recently if victim has ever had a serious open wound	☎
Third-degree burn (see Shock, p. 36)	🏢

▨ Use self-care   🏢 Seek help now

☎ Call doctor's office for advice   *For more about the symbols, see p. 2.*

SELF-CARE STEPS FOR BURNS

• For fast pain relief, soak a small-area burn in cold water or apply cold, wet compresses. Do not use ice water or snow, unless that is the only source of cold available. The wet, cooling action stops the burning process below the skin surface by dissipating the heat that remains after the initial burn.

For minor burns: soak burned area in cold water, use bacitracin to prevent dehydration, apply a light gauze bandage, and tape where skin is not burned.

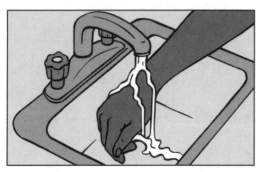

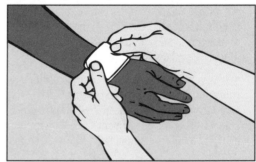

SELF-CARE STEPS FOR SEVERE BURNS

• If the victim's clothes are on fire, smother the flames with a blanket, towel, rug, or coat. Wrap it over the flames, pressing down to keep air from reaching the fire. The victim may struggle or attempt to run. Get the victim on the floor so the burning surface is uppermost and flames can rise away from the body.

• Pull away any bits of clothing that may be smoldering. Leave any material that is burnt but extinguished and sticking to the skin. Solvents stocked by hospital emergency rooms can safely remove these bits.

• **Call 911, or immediately drive the victim to a health care provider if the area of the burn is not too large** (the victim should not drive).

Cover the burn with a clean, dry dressing that covers the entire burn area. Do not apply butter, first-aid creams, or antiseptics to the wound. Do not rupture blisters that form on the burn.

• Treat the victim for shock (see p. 36) if there is a delay in getting to a hospital. Cover the victim with a blanket and raise his or her feet 8 to 12 inches. **Do not elevate the victim's feet if you suspect head, neck, back, or leg injuries.**

• If conscious and showing no signs of vomiting, the victim should be encouraged to drink tepid water to replace fluids and salts lost in weeping plasma.

• Check to see whether the victim has had a tetanus shot within the past 10 years or more recently if he or she has ever had a serious open wound.

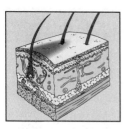

First-Degree Burn

Minor burns injure the epidermis, or outside skin layer. The skin will be red, dry, or swollen. These burns may peel and are usually painful. Examples include mild sunburns or slight scaldings. Medical attention is not needed unless a larger area of skin is damaged. Such burns usually heal within 5 to 6 days without permanent scars.

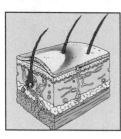

Second-Degree Partial-Thickness Burn

Some of the skin layers beneath the surface are injured by partial-thickness burns. These burns are marked by blisters, local swelling, clear fluid discharge, and mottled skin. The pain may be severe. If the burn covers an area larger than a square inch, get medical attention. Partial-thickness burns can be fatal if more than 50 percent of the body is involved. Healing takes 3 to 4 weeks and may leave scars.

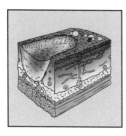

Third-Degree Full-Thickness Burn

Full-thickness burns destroy all of the skin layers and any or all of the nerves, muscles, bones, or fat underneath. These burns have a charred appearance. The tissues surrounding or beneath the burn may be white or look waxy. Full-thickness burns are either very painful or painless, depending upon nerve damage. Medical attention is crucial. Even if the burn is in one spot, specialist treatment and skin grafts will be necessary. Scars may occur, depending upon the severity of the burn.

CARBON MONOXIDE POISONING

Carbon monoxide is a colorless, odorless gas made when carbon or carbon-containing materials (such as gasoline, kerosene, or natural gas and wood) are burned. Poisoning may occur from exposure to improperly vented gas appliances (such as a furnace, hot-water heater, or oven), automobile exhaust, or smoke inhalation from a fire.

Unconsciousness resulting from carbon monoxide poisoning is a life-threatening emergency. If you suspect carbon monoxide poisoning, **call 911** *or* **take the victim to a hospital right away.** Carbon monoxide can cause death by reducing the blood's oxygen-carrying capacity and depriving the tissues of necessary oxygen.

Carbon monoxide does not change the color of blood, so the victim's skin color looks normal. It does not smell, so the victim may not be aware of being exposed to it until he or she is ill.

Carbon monoxide poisoning should be suspected in situations where gas cannot escape, such as a car with a running engine or a fire in a poorly ventilated area. Symptoms include severe headache, confusion, agitation, tiredness, stupor, or coma.

Many gas and electric utilities offer inexpensive carbon monoxide detectors to their customers or will promptly check your house if you suspect a gas leak or carbon monoxide poisoning. Check to see if your local utility provides this service.

SELF-CARE STEPS FOR CARBON MONOXIDE POISONING

• Do not remain in the room if carbon monoxide poisoning is suspected. Move the victim as quickly as possible into fresh air before beginning first aid.

• Check for breathing and pulse. If the victim is not breathing, call 911. Start mouth-to-mouth breathing (see p. 12 for adults and older children; p. 15 for children under 8 years old) and continue until the victim starts breathing or trained medical assistance arrives.

• If pulse is absent, begin massaging the heart (see p. 12 for adults and older children; p. 15 for children under 8 years old) and continue until trained medical assistance arrives.

CHEMICAL BURNS

Chemical burns are caused by being doused or splashed with a harsh acid or alkaline chemical. These chemicals can burn the skin in exactly the same way as fire. Chemical burns are a serious medical problem.

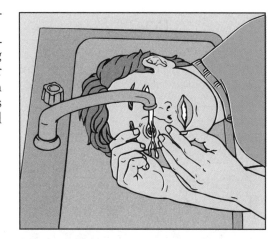

Flush eye with cool, clean water for at least 20 to 30 minutes.

SELF-CARE STEPS FOR CHEMICAL BURNS

Skin Burns

• Flush the burned area with a gentle, constant spray of water for at least 10 minutes using a hose, bucket, or shower. Remove all clothing on the burned area and keep flushing until you are certain all the chemical has been washed away.

• After flushing, call the local poison control center or your health care provider for more instructions. Dry the wound site and cover with a clean cloth or dressing.

• Do not apply first-aid ointments, antiseptics, or home remedies to chemical burns. Cool, wet dressings work best to relieve pain.

Eye Burns

• Speed in removing a chemical from the eye is vital. Before calling your health care provider, flush the eye right away with a constant stream of cool, clean water for at least 20 to 30 minutes. A stream of water can't harm the eye and thorough washing can reduce the risk of permanent eye damage. Use milk if water is unavailable. Do not bandage the eye before seeing a health care provider.

• To flush the eyes, hold the victim's head under a faucet or use a pitcher of water, a plastic squirt bottle, a drinking fountain, or shower spray. Hold the eyelids open for proper flushing. Make sure the water runs from the inside corner of the eye (near the nose) outward, so that the contaminated water doesn't flow into the unaffected eye.

• If both eyes are affected, let water flow over both or quickly alternate flushing each eye. Make sure water reaches all parts of the eye by lifting and separating the eyelids. Another method is to submerge the top half of the victim's face in a large bowl or sink. Have the victim open both eyes and move the eyelids up and down. **This technique should not be used with young children who are upset or who cannot hold their breath.**

• Advise the victim not to rub his or her eyes. After rinsing the eye, seek immediate medical care at the nearest hospital emergency room. Bring the chemical container with you for analysis.

CHOKING

Choking occurs when a piece of food or other object becomes lodged in the throat, blocking air flow. Choking vic-tims may react by coughing hard in an effort to dislodge the object. A person whose airway is completely blocked is unable to speak, breathe, or cough, and may clutch his or her throat.

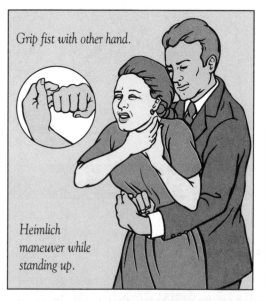

Grip fist with other hand.

Heimlich maneuver while standing up.

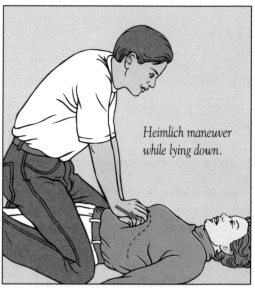

Heimlich maneuver while lying down.

SELF-CARE STEPS FOR CHOKING

Choking is life threatening and requires immediate action. If the victim can speak, cough, or breathe, this means air is still passing through the airway. Do not interfere in any way with the victim's efforts to expel the object. Reassure the victim, and advise him or her to breathe deeply and slowly. This will help relax the muscles surrounding the windpipe.

Heimlich Maneuver for Adults or Children
When the Victim Is Standing or Sitting
If the victim is unable to breathe or make sounds, have someone call 911. Meanwhile, perform the Heimlich maneuver:

• Stand behind the choking victim and wrap your arms around the victim's midsection. Place the thumb side of your fist against the victim's stomach slightly above the navel.

• Grip your fist with your other hand and press the doubled fist into the victim's abdomen with a quick upward thrust. Repeat the thrusts until the object is expelled from the airway or the victim loses consciousness.

• Do not squeeze the victim's ribs with your arms. Use only your fist in the abdomen. Each thrust should be a separate and distinct movement.

When the Victim Is Lying Down
• If the victim is lying down and still conscious, turn him or her onto the back.

• Kneel and straddle the victim, placing the heel of your hand on the victim's stomach above the navel and below the ribs. Place your other hand over the fist.

• Keeping your elbows straight, give four quick, strong, downward thrusts toward the chest.

• Repeat this procedure as needed until the object is cleared from the airway or the victim loses consciousness.

SELF-CARE STEPS FOR CHOKING

Self-Application

The Heimlich maneuver can also be self-applied if no one else is around.

• Make a fist and place the thumb side on the abdomen above your navel.

• Grasp the fist with the other hand. Press inward and upward with a quick motion.

• If this is unsuccessful, press your upper abdomen over any firm surface such as the side of a table or the back of a chair. Repeat these single thrusts until the object is cleared from your airway.

Heimlich Maneuver for Infants—*small enough to be supported on your forearm or up to 1 year old*

• Ask someone to call 911 immediately. Meanwhile, rest victim face down on your forearm. Support the infant's head by firmly holding the jaw.

• Give four quick back blows between the shoulder blades with the heel of your hand. If this is unsuccessful, perform the Heimlich maneuver as described below.

• Place two fingers 1 fingerwidth below the infant's nipples in the center of the chest on the breastbone, avoiding the tip of the breastbone.

• Push forward and downward. These thrusts should be more gentle than those used on an adult. Repeat both procedures if necessary.

If the Heimlich maneuver is not successful, follow CPR instructions for blocked airway (p. 15).

Call your health care provider after a rescue using the Heimlich maneuver. Some internal injuries can result from the thrusting motion; however, the risk of injury is reduced by correctly positioning your hands.

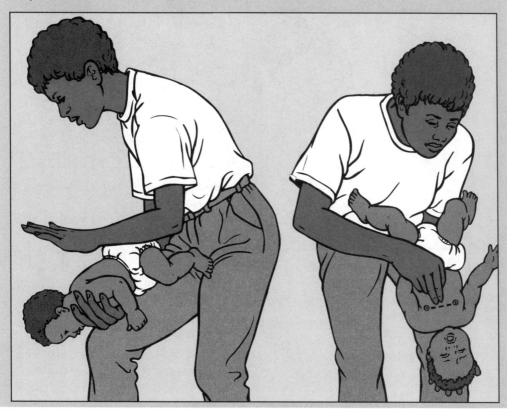

CARDIOPULMONARY RESUSCITATION (CPR)

This is meant to be a review and is not intended to replace an American Heart Association-certified CPR class.

Cardiopulmonary resuscitation (CPR) is a basic life-support technique that is used when the victim is not breathing and the heart may have stopped. CPR allows you to manually perform the functions of the heart and lungs which send blood and oxygen to all parts of the body.

All the body's cells, especially the brain cells, need a steady supply of oxygen. CPR opens and clears the victim's airway and restores breathing and blood circulation through mouth-to-mouth breathing and repeated pressure on the chest.

SELF-CARE STEPS FOR CPR

Adults and Children Age 8 or Older
Check for consciousness. Gently shake the victim and shout, "Are you OK?" If there is no response or the victim is not breathing, shout for help and ask someone to **call 911 immediately.** The order of action to take in an emergency can be remembered as the ABCs—**Airway, Breathing, and Circulation.**

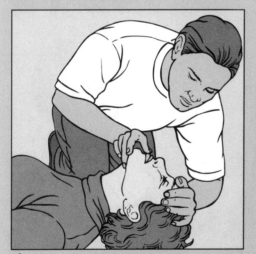

Airway: *Open the Airway (Head Tilt/Chin Lift)*
• Tilt the victim's head back if no neck/spinal injuries are suspected.

• Place one hand on the forehead and apply firm, backward pressure to tilt the head back.

• Push down on the forehead and lift the victim's chin.

• Place two fingers of your other hand on the bony part of the victim's chin. Pull the victim's chin forward and support the jaw, helping to tilt the head back.

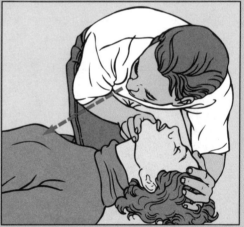

Breathing: *Check Breathing/Perform Rescue Breathing*
Place your ear over the victim's mouth and nose while keeping up an open airway. Look for the chest to rise and fall; listen for air escaping during exhalation; and feel for the flow of air. Watch for 5 seconds. If there is no sign of breathing, perform rescue breathing as follows:

• Keep the airway open by using the head tilt/chin lift maneuver described above. Gently pinch the victim's nose shut using the thumb and index finger of the hand on the forehead.

CONTINUED SELF-CARE STEPS FOR CPR

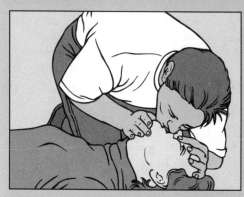

- Take a deep breath and seal your lips tightly around the victim's mouth.

- Give two full breaths—1¹/₂ to 2 seconds per breath, 10 to 12 breaths per minute. Take a breath for yourself after each two breaths for the victim. Watch for the victim's chest to rise with each breath. Let the victim's chest fall between breaths.

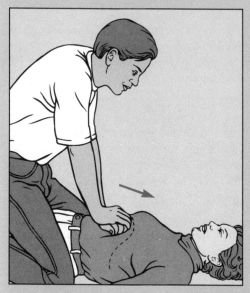

Clearing a Blocked Airway

If the victim's chest doesn't rise during rescue breathing, the airway is blocked. Retilt the victim's head and try again. If the airway is still blocked, perform the Heimlich maneuver as follows:

- Kneel and straddle the victim, placing the heel of your hand on the victim's stomach above the navel and below the ribs.

- Place your other hand over your fist. Keeping your elbows straight, give four quick, downward thrusts toward the chest.

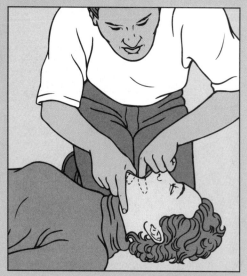

- Open the victim's mouth by grasping both the tongue and lower jaw between the thumb and fingers and lift. This will draw the tongue away from the back of the throat and away from any object that might be lodged there. Look to see if an object is visible in the back of the throat.

- Next, perform the **finger-sweep maneuver** as follows: Insert the index finger of the other hand down along the inside of the cheek and deeply into the throat to the base of the tongue. Use a hooking action to dislodge the object and move it into the mouth so that it can be removed.

- Attempt rescue breathing again. If you are still unable to breathe air into the victim's lungs, reposition the head and try again. Repeat the sequence of Heimlich maneuver, finger sweep, and rescue breathing. Perform this cycle until the object is dislodged, and you are able to continue rescue breathing.

Continued on next page

CONTINUED SELF-CARE STEPS FOR CPR

*C*irculation: *Check for Pulse*

While keeping the head tilted, move two fingers from the Adam's apple to the side of the neck between the windpipe and the neck muscles. Press down gently and gradually for 5 to 10 seconds. A pulse shows that the heart is beating.

Don't rock back and forth or pause between compressions. Lock your arms straight and press hard on the breastbone to $1\frac{1}{2}$ to 2 inches or one-third of the chest depth.

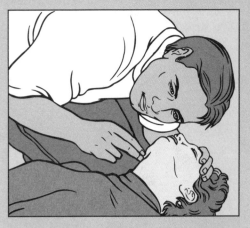

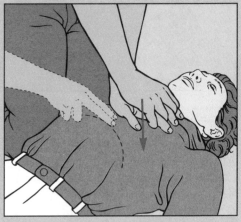

If the victim has a pulse but is not breathing, continue rescue breathing at a rate of 10 to 12 times per minute, or once every 5 or 6 seconds. If the victim has no pulse and is not breathing, begin CPR.

• Find the notch where the victim's ribs meet the breastbone in the center of the chest. Place the heel of your hand 2 fingerwidths above the notch. Place your other hand on top of this hand, interlocking your fingers.

• Lean forward until your shoulders are directly over your hands. Your body weight falling forward provides the force to depress the breastbone.

• Do 15 chest compressions (at a rate of 80 to 100 per minute), continuing to lean over the victim so your shoulders are over your hands.

• Count out loud "one and, two and, three and, four and," as you push straight down. Allow the chest to return to its normal position after each compression. Do not lift your hands from the chest or change position, or correct hand position may be lost.

• Open the airway again using the head tilt/chin lift and give two slow rescue breaths. Watch for the chest to rise. Repeat this sequence of 15 compressions and two breaths for four cycles. Recheck for pulse.

• When the victim is breathing and has a pulse, stop performing CPR. If the victim has a pulse but is not breathing, continue rescue breathing. Recheck the pulse every 60 seconds. Start CPR again if pulse stops. If the victim has no pulse and is not breathing, repeat sequence of 1˜ compressions and two breaths, checking fo pulse every four cycles. Continue until the victim revives or help arrives.

SELF-CARE STEPS—CPR FOR CHILDREN

Children under 8 Years Old

Shout for help and ask someone to **call 911 immediately**. Then provide the basic ABCs (*Airway, Breathing, Circulation*) of life support.

Airway: *Open the Airway*

If no neck/spinal injuries are suspected, open the airway by placing one hand on the child's forehead and tilting the head back into a neutral position. Place the fingers of your other hand under the bony part of the lower jaw at the chin and lift upward and outward.

Breathing: *Check Breathing/Perform Rescue Breathing*

• After the airway is opened, check if the child is breathing. Look for a rise and fall of the chest and abdomen; listen for exhaled air; and feel for exhaled air flow at the mouth.

• If no spontaneous breathing is detected, begin rescue breathing while keeping the chin lifted. If the victim is under 1 year old, place your mouth over the infant's mouth and nose. If the victim is 1 to 8 years old, make a mouth-to-mouth seal and pinch the victim's nose tightly with the thumb and forefinger of the hand maintaining head tilt.

• Give two slow breaths (1 to 1^1/$_2$ seconds per breath) to the victim. Pause to take a breath after the first breath. If the air enters freely and the chest rises, the airway is clear. If air does not enter freely or if the chest does not rise, either the airway is blocked or more breath pressure is necessary.

Improper opening of the airway is the most common cause of airway blocks. Reattempt to open the airway and try rescue breathing again. If you suspect an object is blocking the airway, see Choking (p. 10). If a child loses consciousness or has more difficulty breathing, have someone **call 911** immediately and perform the Heimlich maneuver (see p. 10 for children; p. 11 for infants).

Circulation: *Check for Pulse*

Spend only a few seconds trying to get a pulse in a nonbreathing infant before starting chest compressions.

• In infants under 1 year old, gently press your index and middle fingers on the inside of the upper arm, between the infant's elbow and shoulder. In children 1 to 8 years old, find the Adam's apple with two or three fingers. Slide your fingers into the groove on the side of the neck between the windpipe and neck muscles.

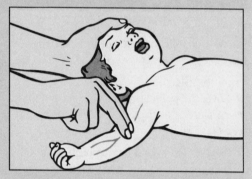

• If a pulse is present but the child is not breathing, do rescue breathing at a rate of 20 breaths per minute (once every 3 seconds) until spontaneous breathing resumes. After giving 20 breaths, call 911.

• If pulse is nonexistent, do chest compressions as follows: Use one hand to maintain infant's head position. Use the other hand to compress the chest. Place the index finger just below the level of the infant's nipples. Place the middle fingers on the breastbone next to the index finger. Using two or three fingers, compress the breastbone by about one-third to one-half the depth of the chest—about ^{1}/$_2$ to 1 inch. Do compressions at a rate of at least 100 per minute. Coordinate with rescue breathing by doing five compressions to each breath. Continue until medical help arrives. If the infant starts breathing, place the victim in the recovery position (on one side with the arm supporting the head).

Signs of infection usually don't appear until at least 24 hours after the injury. Bacteria need time to grow and multiply. If you have fever, swelling, redness or a red streak, increased pain, or pus oozing from the wound, call your doctor.

Family Practitioner

CUTS

For Puncture Wounds, see p. 34.

Simple cuts can become not-so-simple infections, so it is important to know how to treat them properly.

Minor cuts damage only the skin and the fatty tissue beneath it. They usually heal without permanent damage. More serious cuts may damage muscles, tendons, blood vessels, ligaments, or nerves, and these cuts should be examined by a doctor.

The three major concerns in treating a cut are:

- To stop the bleeding, apply direct pressure to the wound

- To avoid infection, clean the wound thoroughly

- To promote healing, bring the edges of the skin together with tape or stitches

SELF-CARE STEPS FOR CUTS

The next time you get caught on a nail, sliced by a knife, or even cut by a piece of paper, follow these steps:

Stop the Bleeding
- Cover the wound with a gauze pad or a thick, clean piece of cloth. Use your hand if nothing else is available.

- Press on the wound hard enough to stop the bleeding. Don't let up on the pressure even to change cloths. Just add a clean cloth over the original one.

- Raise the wound above heart level, unless this movement would cause pain.

- Get medical help immediately if blood spurts from a wound or bleeding does not stop after several minutes of pressure.

Clean the Wound
- Wash the cut with soap and water or use hydrogen peroxide (3 percent solution). Don't use Mercurochrome, Merthiolate, or iodine. They are not necessary and can be very painful.

- Make sure no dirt, glass, or foreign material remains in the wound.

Bandage the Wound
- Bandage a cut (rather than seeing a doctor for stitches) when its edges tend to fall together and when the cut is not very deep.

- Use "butterfly bandages," strips of sterile paper tape, or adhesive strip bandages. Change them daily.

- Apply the bandage crosswise, not lengthwise. This will bring the edges of the wound into firm contact and promote healing.

Are Stitches Needed?
See a doctor for stitches as soon as possible if:

- The wound is deep and gapes widely, is very dirty or irregular, or can't be held together with a bandage.

- A deep cut is located on an elbow, knee, finger or other area that bends.

- The cut is on the finger or thumb joint, palm of the hand, face, or other area on which you would like to avoid scars.

- The cut damages bones or muscles or feels numb.

- The victim is a young child who is likely to pull off the bandage.

- Bleeding cannot be controlled after applying pressure for 20 minutes.

- The cut was caused by an obviously dirty object or a foreign object is embedded in the wound.

- The victim has not had a tetanus booster within the last 10 years (or more recently if he or she has ever had a serious open wound).

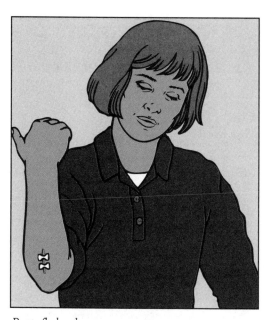

Butterfly bandages

SYMPTOMS/SIGNS	ACTION
Bleeding stops within 10 minutes with direct pressure	
Cut is shallow	
Cut doesn't heal in 10 to 14 days	
No tetanus booster in the last 10 years or more recently if the victim has ever had a serious open wound	
Cut is deep or irregular or the edges of the wound cannot easily be held together with a bandage	
Signs of infection (p. 28)	
Cut is deep and located on the face, chest, abdomen, back, palm, finger, knee, or elbow	
More than 2 to 3 tablespoons of blood lost in 24 hours	
Numbness or weakness	
Wound spurts or gushes blood	
Unable to move fingers or toes normally	
Signs of shock (p. 36)	

These days it's a good idea to have a couple pairs of rubber gloves in your medicine cabinet. Unfortunately, we all must be aware of the risk posed by AIDS, which can be spread by infected blood. If you're giving first aid to someone with a bleeding wound, wear gloves. Medical professionals do.

Infectious Disease Nurse

 Use self-care

 Call doctor's office for advice

See doctor

Seek help now

 Emergency, call 911

For more about the symbols, see p. 2.

DROWNING

See Near Drowning, p. 32.

ELECTRICAL BURNS

Electrical burns are serious medical emergencies. These burns are often deep, and, although it may not look threatening, a small skin burn can indicate extensive internal damage. Electricity can also cause the heart to stop beating or to beat unevenly.

Never approach the victim of an electrical injury until you are certain the power has been shut off. If possible, turn off the electric current by flipping the main breaker or removing the fuse.

Do not touch someone who is being electrocuted, and do not get within 20 yards of a high-voltage electrocution victim. This electricity can leap across gaps and strike you. Don't try to rescue the victim until the current has been shut off. The victim of a lightning strike can be approached right away. Unless the victim is in immediate danger, do not try to move him or her.

FISHHOOK WOUNDS

A fishhook caught in the body is a common injury. The biggest problem, of course, is the barb on most fishhooks. Although fish seem to be able to get loose quite easily, children—and adults—may stay hooked.

When only the point of the fishhook has entered the skin, the fishhook can easily be removed by simply backing the fishhook out the way it went in. If the fishhook is so deeply embedded that the barb has entered the skin, there are two options:

SELF-CARE STEPS FOR ELECTRICAL BURNS

• **Call 911** and report a medical emergency.

• When the victim is no longer touching a live wire, check to see that he or she is breathing and has a heartbeat. If the victim has stopped breathing, **call 911** *before* beginning CPR immediately. If the victim's heart has stopped, begin external heart massage. (For CPR and external heart massage for adults and older children, see p. 12; for children under 8 years old, see p. 15.)

• Use cool water to soothe burned area and avoid more tissue damage.

• Cover burned area with dry, sterile dressings.

• To prevent shock, lay the victim on a flat surface and raise his or her feet 8 to 12 inches. **Do not raise the victim's feet if you suspect head, neck, back, or leg injuries.** Cover the victim with a blanket or coat to maintain body temperature. Stay with the victim until professional medical assistance arrives.

• If medical care is nearby, take the victim to a health care provider to get the hook removed. A local anesthetic may be administered to the area around the hook before it is removed.

• If the victim is in a remote area far from medical care, the fishhook can be removed by using either pliers or fishline, as described on the next page. If not removed easily, medical care should be sought. **No attempt should be made to remove a fishhook embedded in the eye. Seek medical attention immediately!**

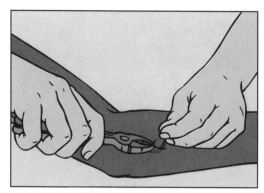

Pliers method

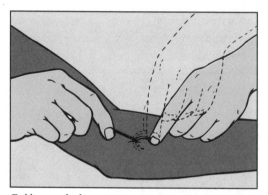

Fishline method

DECISION GUIDE FOR FISHHOOK WOUNDS

SYMPTOMS/SIGNS	ACTION
Barb not embedded	
Hook with barb embedded, not easily removed	
Signs of infection (p. 28)	
Stitches needed	
No tetanus shot within last 10 years (or more recently if victim has ever had a serious open wound)	
Hook embedded in eye or near major artery	

 Use self-care

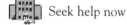 See doctor

Seek help now

For more about the symbols, see p. 2.

SELF-CARE STEPS FOR FISHHOOK WOUNDS

Use these methods only if you don't have access to a doctor within 24 hours.

Pliers Method
• Before beginning this method, check to be certain you have pliers with tempered jaws that can cut through the hook. Cut through an extra hook to ensure that the pliers work well enough. Use ice, cold water, or hard pressure to temporarily numb the area before beginning.

• Gently push the embedded hook farther into the skin until the point and barb come out through the skin. Using the pliers, cut off the barb and back the hook out the way it entered or cut off the other end of the hook and pull it through. Although this method can be painful, it works if the proper pliers are available and the barb is not too deeply embedded to be pushed through to the surface of the skin.

Fishline Method
• Loop or tie a piece of fishline to the embedded hook near the skin surface. Immobilize the area where the hook is embedded and use ice, cold water or hard pressure to temporarily numb the skin.

• With one hand, press down about $1/8$ inch on the eye of the hook to disengage the barb. While still pressing the hook down, jerk the line parallel to the skin surface so the hook shaft leads the barb out of the skin.

After the hook has been removed by either method, wash the wound thoroughly with mild soap and running water if possible. Cover the wound with an adhesive bandage and seek medical follow-up care (see Decision Guide for Infected Wounds, p. 28).

FRACTURES

A broken or cracked bone is a fracture. There are two types of fractures: open or closed. A closed fracture means the bone isn't poking through the skin. Open (or compound) fractures are more dangerous and may involve severe bleeding. These fractures also are more likely to get infected.

Bone fragments in many fractures are still aligned, and "setting" is not required. A fracture that injures nearby nerves or arteries may result in a limb that is cold, blue, or numb. It may also result in an inability to use the limb. Fractures of the pelvis or thigh may be particularly dangerous.

A crooked limb, a lot of swelling or discoloration, and an inability to bear weight after an injury or fall are obvious reasons to check for a fracture. Call your health care provider if pain prevents any use of the injured limb. When great force is involved in an injury, such as in an automobile accident or a fall from a roof, the possibility of a broken bone increases.

A fracture may show one or both of the following symptoms:

- Pain with motion or pressure
- A grating sensation of bone-ends rubbing together

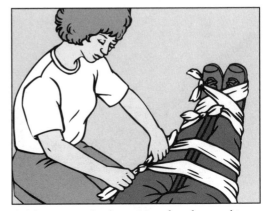

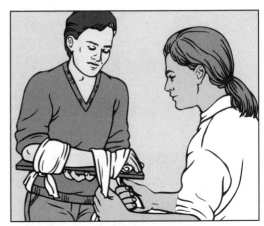

Applying a rigid splint—Use a board or anything stiff to immobilize a broken limb. Take care not to cut off circulation by tying too tight. Check for feeling, warmth, and color.

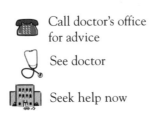

📞 Call doctor's office for advice

🩺 See doctor

🏥 Seek help now

For more about the symbols, see p. 2.

DECISION GUIDE FOR FRACTURES

SYMPTOMS/SIGNS	ACTION
Suspected fracture	📞
Limb is crooked	🩺
Unable to use limb or bear weight	🩺
Limb or portion of limb is cool, blue, or numb	🏥

SELF-CARE STEPS FOR FRACTURES

Limb Fractures

• Apply ice packs to the injury. For open fractures, use clean, preferably white, wrappings. Immediately applying cold will help decrease swelling and inflammation. If a broken bone is suspected, protect and rest the injured limb immediately. To rest a bone effectively, immobilize the joint above and below the suspected fracture.

• Splints are used to immobilize a suspected fracture to prevent further injury until treatment is completed (this also applies to ribs or collarbones). A fracture can be immobilized by wrapping something around the injured limb or fixing the limb to some other part of the victim's body. It is best to immobilize the joint above and below the injured area. Magazines, cardboard, or rolled newspaper can be used as a splint. Do not wrap too tightly or circulation will be cut off. A limb that cannot be used at all is probably broken and should be seen by a doctor.

• Minutes and hours are not crucial unless the limb is crooked, arteries or nerves are injured, or the injury is causing great pain. A fractured limb that is protected and rested is likely to mend well, even if casting or splinting is delayed.

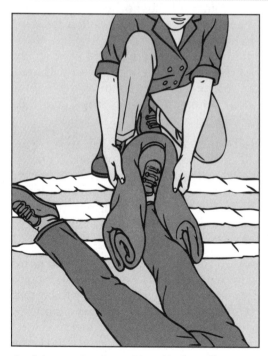 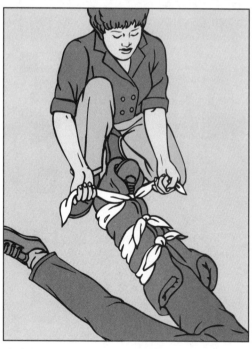

Applying a soft splint—Use a blanket, pillow, or any soft object to support the injured area. Check for feeling, warmth, and color after tying bandages.

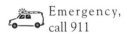

Use self-care

Call doctor's office for advice

Seek help now

Emergency, call 911

For more about the symbols, see p. 2.

FROSTBITE/HYPOTHERMIA

Many of us live in regions where winter brings the threat of frostbite and hypothermia (the loss of vital body heat). Fortunately, most cold weather risks are easily managed by using good judgment and the proper clothing.

Frostbite

Frostbite occurs when the skin and tissues below freeze after exposure to very cold temperatures. Hands, feet, nose, and ears are the areas most commonly affected.

DECISION GUIDE FOR FROSTBITE/HYPOTHERMIA

SYMPTOMS/SIGNS	ACTION
Numb skin	Use self-care
Blistered skin	Call doctor's office for advice
Headache	Call doctor's office for advice
Nausea, dizziness, vomiting, or uncontrollable shivering	Call doctor's office for advice
Pale, cold, clammy skin or cold, white, or grayish-yellow skin	Seek help now
Rapid pulse and breathing	Seek help now
Unconsciousness	Emergency, call 911
Stiff muscles and bluish skin	Emergency, call 911
Confusion, slurred speech	Emergency, call 911

Frostbitten areas are cold, white, or grayish-yellow, and hard to the touch. The area may feel very cold and numb, or there may be pain, tingling, or stinging. As the area thaws, it becomes red and painful.

If you suspect frostbite, get out of the cold immediately. Warm the affected area by putting it in barely warm, **not hot**, water (100° F). **Do not rub the frostbitten area.**

Seek medical help immediately if the frostbitten area remains numb after you've tried to warm it.

Hypothermia

Hypothermia happens when the body's core temperature drops through exposure to cool and/or damp conditions. The symptoms of hypothermia include uncontrollable shivering; cold, pale skin; slurred speech; memory lapses; fumbling, stumbling or staggering; and abnormally slow breathing. The victim may feel tired or apathetic. The condition becomes grave when shivering stops, muscles become stiff, and skin turns bluish.

To treat hypothermia, get the victim out of the cold and remove any damp or wet clothing. Dress the victim in warm, dry clothing and wrap in blankets. Or put the victim in a bath of warm water. Give warm, nonalcoholic drinks like coffee, tea, hot cider, or cocoa.

Call the doctor's office for advice if the symptoms are only shivering and cold, pale skin. The doctor or nurse will be able to tell you whether a trip to the clinic or hospital is necessary. If the victim develops other symptoms of hypothermia, get medical help as soon as possible.

HEAD INJURIES

In Adults

Traffic or work accidents, falls, and fights can cause head injuries. Although most are minor, any head injury poses the threat of a more serious problem. Head injuries can range from a concussion, which usually is not serious, to bleeding inside the head that can be life threatening.

A **concussion** is a brief loss of consciousness due to a blow to the head. The most common symptom is a constant headache that may get worse, sometimes accompanied by vomiting. Other symptoms can include blurred vision, sleepiness, and memory problems. Sometimes the symptoms may seem like those of a stroke. Athletes who have had a head injury should not return to their sport without a medical evaluation. People taking anticoagulants (drugs to prevent blood clotting) need to take special precautions to prevent falls because they could bleed more easily from a blow to the head. In older people, a fall—even without a direct blow to the head—can cause life-threatening head injury complications.

Cerebral hemorrhages caused by broken blood vessels in the brain are more serious than concussions. Symptoms include headaches and repeated vomiting that can lead to confusion, weakness, and difficulty staying awake or being awakened.

Call 911 if a head injury results in loss of consciousness, breathing difficulty, or a neck injury. Every person with a head injury that isn't bleeding should be watched for 24 hours for symptoms. In the absence of nausea, vomiting, or other symptoms, careful observation is the best way to monitor a head injury.

DECISION GUIDE FOR HEAD INJURIES IN ADULTS

SYMPTOMS/SIGNS	ACTION
Bleeding from the scalp lasts more than 10 minutes with pressure	
Person appears dazed or confused or is hard to awaken	
Person has difficulty walking or talking	
Headaches increase in severity	
Vomiting persists	
Person has blurred vision or unequal pupils	
Person has severe headache or neck pain	
Breathing is difficult	
Bloody drainage occurs from the person's nostrils or ears	
Person's temperature rises above 100° F	
Person loses consciousness	
Seizures occur	

In head injury cases, the eyes should be examined to see if the pupils are constricting evenly. This can be done at home by shining a flashlight in the eyes to see if both pupils become smaller, even when the light is only in one eye. Unequal pupil size can be a symptom of internal bleeding. It requires immediate medical attention.

Urgent Care Physician

 See doctor

Seek help now

Emergency, call 911

For more about the symbols, see p. 2.

ACCIDENT PREVENTION

Adults

• Wear a helmet when riding bikes, horses, or motorcycles, or when using in-line skates.

• Use seat belts in automobiles.

• Wear hard hats at industrial sites.

• Never dive into shallow water.

Children

• Childproof your home.

• Be very careful when picking up and carrying infants.

• Do not use baby walkers and never leave infants alone on beds, changing tables, or other high places.

• Supervise outside play.

• Teach safety in crossing streets.

• Have children wear a helmet when biking, riding horses, or wearing in-line skates.

• Use seat belts and car safety seats in vehicles.

• Teach children not to dive into shallow water.

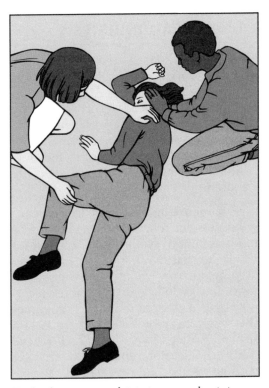

For head, spine, or neck injuries, move the victim only if it is absolutely necessary. Immobilize the head. Stay with the victim until help arrives, making sure airway is not blocked.

SELF-CARE STEPS FOR NECK AND SPINAL INJURIES

• First, call 911 and then stay with the victim. Do not move the victim if you suspect head, neck, or spinal injuries unless the victim is in immediate danger from fire, drowning, explosion, or gas. If possible, wait for professional help. Neck and spinal injuries may result in permanent paralysis if not carefully treated. This type of injury should be immobilized with a board or similar rigid support before moving the victim.

• If the victim has to be moved for safety reasons, immobilize the head and neck first, using a backboard, table leaf, or door, or using several people moving as a team to support the head and neck and keep them level with the back.

• When a board or other flat, rigid surface is used, it should extend from the head to the buttocks.

In Children

Over 200,000 children are admitted to hospitals yearly with head injuries. Children's large head-to-body ratios and not fully developed brains and muscles put them at great risk for head injuries. Children's head injuries require prompt attention because they can be life threatening and can affect growth and development.

Quick action is required if a head injury results in unconsciousness, breathing difficulty, or a neck injury. Head injuries may also create a lot of bleeding from the scalp, which is not *necessarily* serious. Even without these symptoms, watch the child closely for a 24-hour period since some symptoms may develop over time. Careful observation, which in most cases can be done at home, is the best way to diagnose a head injury (see definitions of concussion, p. 23, and cerebral hemorrhage, p. 23).

For more about the symbols, see p. 2.

 Call doctor's office for advice

 See doctor

 Seek help now

 Emergency, call 911

DECISION GUIDE FOR HEAD INJURIES IN CHILDREN

SYMPTOMS/SIGNS	ACTION
Child doesn't lose consciousness but appears dazed	
Bleeding from scalp lasts more than 10 minutes with pressure	
Difficulty walking or talking	
Confusion (disorientation)	
Headaches increase in severity	
Vomiting occurs three or more times	
Blurred vision or unequal pupils	
Bloody drainage from nostrils or ears	
Severe headache or neck pain	
Child is difficult to awaken or loses consciousness	
Seizures	

We were really frightened to see our baby fall from his crib. Fortunately, the nurse telephone care service told us just what to do. After he stopped crying, regained his normal color, and didn't vomit, we were hopeful that he hadn't injured his head. We woke him throughout the night to be sure he was OK.

Jennifer and John

SELF-CARE STEPS FOR HEAD INJURIES

- If the head is bleeding, apply pressure to control bleeding.
- Clean and bandage the wound; apply an ice bag for swelling.
- Check to see if the victim's pupils are equal in size.
- Check skin color every few hours. Wake a child every 2 hours to observe breathing and to be assured of consciousness. Wake an adult every few hours to check breathing and level of consciousness.
- Question an adult about name, age, and address to check his or her level of confusion.
- Don't give any medicine without talking with your doctor.
- Limit activity for 24 hours after the injury.

HEART ATTACK

See Chest Pain, p. 85.

HEAT-RELATED PROBLEMS

Many of us live in regions where sunburn, heat exhaustion, and heat stroke are summer health risks. If you live in a hot region, the weather can affect your health all year round.

Sunburn

See Sunburn, p. 171.

Heat Exhaustion

Heat exhaustion typically occurs when people work or exercise in hot, humid conditions. The symptoms are cool, pale, and clammy skin; heavy sweating; dilated pupils; headache; nausea; dizziness; vomiting; faintness; and rapid pulse and breathing.

When heat exhaustion strikes, have the victim lie on his or her back in a cool, quiet place with the feet slightly raised. The person should drink half a glass of cold water every 15 minutes and eat salty snacks like salted crackers, pretzels, or nuts.

Call the doctor's office for advice if you don't notice an improvement within a half hour. Also stay alert to signs of heat stroke.

Heat Stroke

Heat stroke is life threatening. It requires immediate medical attention. In heat stroke, the mechanism that regulates the body's temperature stops working and body temperature rises rapidly to 104° F or higher. A heat stroke victim's skin is bright red, dry, and hot. There is a strong, rapid pulse. The victim may be confused or unconscious.

Call for an ambulance immediately if someone is suffering from heat stroke. While waiting for help, put the victim into a tub of cool water or wrap him or her in wet sheets, and fan the body with your hands or an electric fan. Give the victim water if he or she is able to drink.

DECISION GUIDE FOR HEAT-RELATED PROBLEMS

SYMPTOMS/SIGNS	ACTION
Headache	🩹
Heavy sweating	🩹
Mild sunburn	🩹
Nausea, dizziness, vomiting	🩺
Blistered skin	🩺
Bright red, dry, hot skin (can be a sign of heat stroke, which requires immediate attention)	🏥
Unconsciousness	🚑
Stiff muscles and bluish skin	🚑
Confusion, slurred speech	🚑
Rapid pulse and breathing	🚑

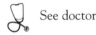 Use self-care

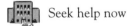 See doctor

Seek help now

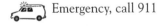 Emergency, call 911

For more about the symbols, see p. 2.

HYPERVENTILATION

Hyperventilation means breathing faster and more deeply than normal due to anxiety or stress. Breathing too quickly causes the carbon dioxide levels in the blood to fall quickly. Hyperventilation is usually caused by anxiety, but injury or illness can also be the cause.

The victim feels there is not enough air getting into the lungs and may complain of light-headedness. Feeling the need for more air, the victim breathes faster and makes the symptoms worse.

These symptoms may accompany hyperventilation:

- Rapid breathing
- Difficulty getting a deep, satisfying breath
- Light-headedness
- Numbness or tingling in the hands and feet and around the mouth
- Muscle twitching
- Convulsions or fainting

Rapid breathing, shortness of breath, or light-headedness may also be signs of other, more serious conditions.

Hyperventilation may also be linked to emotional problems, such as a panic attack. A **panic attack** is defined as a brief period of intense fear or discomfort in which symptoms such as dizziness, sweating, or palpitations occur.

Hyperventilation symptoms usually occur because too much carbon dioxide is given off during rapid breathing. Slowing down the victim's breathing will restore the normal balance in the blood, and the symptoms should disappear.

SELF-CARE STEPS FOR HYPERVENTILATION

- Encourage the victim to breathe more slowly and calmly. Reassure and calm the victim by talking to him or her. The anxiety that can cause hyperventilation can bring on greater anxiety, leading to a cycle that needs to be broken.

- If you are unable to calm the victim and slow his or her breathing, or if the victim faints, bring the victim to the nearest hospital or call 911.

- If the victim is prone to hyperventilation, learning deep-breathing exercises, such as those taught in yoga, may also be helpful. Because hyperventilation is caused by breathing too deeply and rapidly, it is recommended that the victim simply close his or her mouth and slow down the breathing rate. Tell the victim to hold his or her breath and silently count "one-one-thousand, two-one-thousand, three-one-thousand." Then the victim should take a shallow breath (mouth still closed) and repeat this. Within several moments, the symptoms should begin to disappear.

INFECTED WOUNDS

All wounds—from paper cuts to gunshot wounds—share a danger of infection. Bacterial infection usually occurs within 24 hours but can take up to 3 to 4 days to develop. A prolonged increase in pain, redness, or swelling around a wound is cause for concern.

If a wound results from a dirty object such as a rusty nail or shovel point, a tetanus shot should be given to prevent this disease. A tetanus shot is needed every 10 years and more often if the victim has ever had a serious open wound.

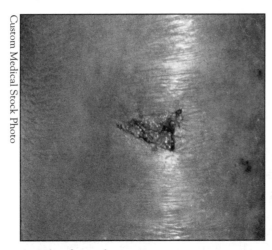

Custom Medical Stock Photo

An infected wound.

SYMPTOMS/SIGNS	ACTION
Increased pain at the wound site	
Redness or swelling around the wound	
Swollen lymph nodes (see Swollen Glands in Children, p. 76)	
Fever over 100.5° F	
Red streaks spreading from the wound site toward the heart	
Pus draining from the wound	

  Call doctor's office for advice

  See doctor

For more about the symbols, see p. 2.

SELF-CARE STEPS FOR INFECTED WOUNDS

• Apply pressure to the wound and raise it above the level of the heart.

• Carefully wash the wound with soap and warm water immediately. Remove all dirt and debris. Washing a wound early will reduce the number of germs in and around a wound, so the body's natural defenses can stop infection.

• After cleaning, leave the wound open to the air unless it will get dirty easily or oozes blood. If necessary, cover the wound with a dressing or bandage. Change the bandage daily, checking

for signs of infection. An antibiotic ointment can be used around the wound to keep the bandage from sticking to the wound.

• Depending on the situation, the health care provider may recommend treatment ranging from soaking the wound daily in warm water to draining the wound with a needle or scalpel and prescribing antibiotics.

INSECT BITES

For tick bites, see Lyme Disease/Deer Ticks, p. 163.

Most bug bites are harmless. But some insect bites can be very dangerous, even fatal.

Here's how to tell the difference between a bite that's a bother and one that's a serious medical problem. The reaction to minor bites is local, confined to the area around the bite itself.

Dangerous, life-threatening reactions to insect bites occur throughout the body. The reaction appears on a part of the body separate from the sting site. Generalized reactions include hives or swelling all over the body, shortness of breath, wheezing, swelling of the throat that causes difficulty swallowing, nausea, stomach cramping, vomiting, loss of bowel and bladder control, weakness, dizziness or fainting, drop in blood pressure, shock, or unconsciousness. If the victim experiences a generalized reaction to an insect bite, make a beeline for the doctor's office or hospital or **call 911.**

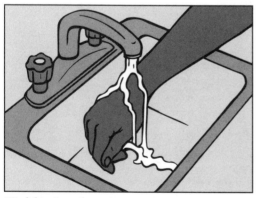

Wash bite in cool running water.

DECISION GUIDE FOR INSECT BITES

SYMPTOMS/SIGNS	ACTION
Throbbing pain	🩹
Burning, redness	🩹
Pain doesn't subside within 48 hours	☎
An unusual rash	☎
Signs of infection (p. 28) or fever over 101° F	☎
Bite by a brown house spider or black widow spider (most common in the South)	🩺
Nausea, vomiting, loss of bowel and bladder control	🏥
Dizziness or fainting, shortness of breath, swelling of throat, difficulty swallowing	🚐
Hives or swelling all over the body	🚐

🩹 Use self-care

☎ Call doctor's office for advice

🩺 See doctor

🏥 Seek help now

🚐 Emergency, call 911

For more about the symbols, see p. 2.

Scratching an insect bite can lead to infection. An ice cube will help calm a painful insect bite. Calamine lotion, hydrocortisone cream, or an appropriate dose of Benadryl can help relieve an itchy bite.

Pediatrics Nurse

Allergic to Bees?

People who are allergic to bee stings need to know about effective treatment methods. Anyone who has had an allergic reaction to an insect sting should follow the suggestions below:

- Carry a bee sting kit at all times. A health care provider can prescribe one. These kits contain injectable adrenaline that can be lifesaving.

- Carry a card or wear a bracelet that alerts others to the condition.

- Ask the health care provider if venom desensitization injections will help. This series of injections can reduce the reaction to bee, wasp, hornet, or yellow jacket stings for some allergic people.

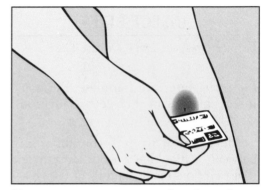

To remove a stinger, scrape it gently with a credit card, fingernail, knife blade, or other rigid object. Do not squeeze with your fingers or tweezers because this can inject more venom into the skin.

MARINE-LIFE STINGS

Stings from some types of marine life are poisonous. Jellyfish and Portuguese man-of-war stings are the most common marine-life stings encountered by swimmers, divers, and beachcombers.

SELF-CARE STEPS FOR INSECT BITES

Bees, mosquitoes, flies, chiggers, ticks, gnats, and other insects can all produce painful stings or bites. Here's what to do for local insect stings and bites:

- Remove the stinger when stung by a bee. Scrape over the stinger (which looks like a splinter) with a credit card, fingernail, knife blade, or other rigid object. Do not remove it with your fingers or tweezers because you may inject more venom into the skin.

- Apply cold quickly. Cool compresses or ice packs will help relieve the pain and prevent swelling from most bug bites. The longer you wait to apply a cold treatment, the worse the local reaction will be. Apply cold packs for no more than 20 minutes at a time to avoid frostbite.

- Wash all insect bites. The site of the bite and the surrounding area should be thoroughly washed with soap and water.

- Don't scratch that itch. Apply calamine lotion or hydrocortisone cream. Take Benadryl (an antihistamine) if itching or more local swelling occurs. Benadryl will help reduce late-appearing symptoms but is not an effective emergency treatment.

Preventing Insect Bites

Avoid perfumes, aftershave, scented hair sprays, and scented deodorants. Wear insect repellent, light-colored clothing, long-sleeved tops, long pants, socks, and shoes. Floral patterns attract bees; so do food, beverages, and garbage cans. If a bee comes near you, avoid sudden movements. Stay still or move away slowly.

Symptoms of marine-life stings may include:

- Skin rash
- Muscle cramps
- Severe burning pain
- Nausea and vomiting
- Difficulty in breathing
- Shock due to severe allergic reaction

Jellyfish deliver their venom through stinging cells on their tentacles. These stings produce a mild burning and stinging sensation and develop long, whiplike marks. In most cases, these stings can be treated at home. If the reaction is severe, however, call your health care provider immediately.

Floating colonies of Portuguese man-of-war are easily spotted, but their transparent tentacles can trail invisibly for up to 60 feet. The pain and burning from these stings can be far more severe than those of jellyfish stings and may cause breathlessness, stomach cramps, nausea, and shock.

DECISION GUIDE FOR MARINE-LIFE STINGS

SYMPTOMS/SIGNS	ACTION
Mild burning and stinging sensation	Use self-care
Severe reaction to sting	See doctor
Signs of shock (p. 36)	Emergency, call 911

For more about the symbols, see p. 2.

SELF-CARE STEPS FOR MARINE-LIFE STINGS

- Be careful around pieces of tentacle. They can still sting even after the tentacle is removed from the body of the jellyfish. Carefully remove any embedded tentacles using tweezers, pliers, or forceps (or wrap cloth around your hands). **Never rub tentacles off!** This will activate more stinging cells.

- Try to find out what caused the sting. If you can do so quickly and without endangering yourself, capture or kill the creature and have it identified.

- If the sting is not bleeding severely, clean the wound and rinse with sea water or salt water. Marine-life stings need to be thoroughly cleaned to remove contaminants such as sand, spines, bristles, shell fragments, and coral. If the sting is bleeding heavily, cover it with a towel and apply direct pressure.

- Wash the sting area with sea water or salt water to deactivate the stinging cells, apply vinegar, and place ice wrapped in cloth or a cold compress on the sting. Be careful not to touch the area with an unprotected hand.

- After washing, apply a thick (heavy enough to stick on) paste of baking soda or a vinegar solution ($1/3$ cup vinegar to $2/3$ cup water). Scrape off the paste after half an hour and reapply the solution. **Don't rub the wound or rinse it with fresh water,** since this may discharge inactivated cells. If a significant reaction or signs of shock occur, **call 911.**

- Do not raise a venomous bite above the level of the victim's heart or give the victim aspirin, stimulants, or pain medication unless instructed to do so by your health care provider.

- To slow the rate at which the venom spreads in the victim's body, do not allow the sting victim to exercise. If necessary, carry the victim to safety. Remove any rings or other constricting items as a precaution in case the injured area swells. If pain persists, call your health care provider.

NEAR DROWNING

Drowning is the fourth leading cause of accidental death in the United States. Drowning can occur whether or not the lungs fill with water. The key factor is how much oxygen continues to reach the victim's brain.

Near drowning is the aftereffect of prolonged submersion in water. Submersion causes spasms that keep oxygen from reaching the lungs, while water in the lungs disrupts blood circulation and can lead to brain injury.

The near-drowning victim may be awake, semiconscious, or unconscious, with little or no breathing or heartbeat. Vomiting, cold skin, and bluish-white paleness are common signs.

Near drowning is a very upsetting experience. Stay with a recovering near-drowning victim to provide support and reassurance. Any near-drowning victim should be taken to the nearest hospital for intensive care, even if the victim has regained consciousness. Complications or death due to heart-rhythm disturbances may occur as long as 24 to 48 hours after the accident.

POISONING

Poison can enter the body in many ways, including swallowing, breathing in, injection, or skin contact. Suspect poisoning if someone suddenly becomes ill for no apparent reason, acts strangely, or is found near a toxic substance.

Different poisons affect body functions differently. Some poisons interfere with the blood's ability to carry oxygen, while others burn and irritate the digestive tract and respiratory system.

SELF-CARE STEPS FOR NEAR DROWNING

Rescue the near-drowning victim if you can do so without endangering yourself. If head and spinal injuries are suspected, see below. Immediately establish an airway and begin artificial respiration (CPR) if necessary, even before the person is removed from the water.

How to Perform CPR

• Look, listen, and feel for breathing. Look to see if the victim's chest is rising and falling.

• If the victim is not breathing, see CPR for adults and older children (p. 12) or for children under 8 years old (p. 15).

• Stay with the victim and have someone **call 911** for emergency medical help. Check for pulse by moving two fingers along the victim's throat to the Adam's apple. Then move fingers off to the side of victim's throat between the windpipe and the muscles at the side of the neck. Firmly press down until you feel a pulse (as detailed on p. 14 for adult victims and p. 15 for children).

• A pulse indicates the heart is beating. If there is no heartbeat, begin external cardiac massage. Hypothermia—the lowering of body temperature—often afflicts near-drowning victims, especially when incidents involve submersion in icy water; therefore, **it is extremely important that CPR be continued until medical help arrives.** Complete recovery has been reported after prolonged resuscitation of hypothermia victims.

Head and Spinal Injuries

These injuries are often caused by diving accidents. If the victim is floating face down, gently turn the victim over, supporting the victim's head and neck to keep them level with the back. Do not remove the victim from the water; instead keep the victim floating on his or her back. Basic CPR rules apply to victims of head and spinal injuries.

If possible, wait for professional assistance. If the victim has to be moved, follow the instructions for neck and spinal injuries (p. 24).

Poisoning symptoms include:

- Fever
- Chills
- Loss of appetite
- Headache or irritability
- Dizziness, weakness, or drowsiness
- Pain in swallowing or more saliva
- Abdominal pain, vomiting, diarrhea, or nausea
- Skin rash or chemical burns around the nose or mouth
- Seizures, stupor, or unconsciousness
- Double vision or blurred vision
- Muscle twitching

Poison Fumes

Many substances or combinations of substances can produce fumes that can be especially toxic in a closed area (see Carbon Monoxide Poisoning, p. 8). Remove victim from the area before starting treatment.

Take a few deep breaths of fresh air, then hold your breath before entering the area. Drag or pull the victim to fresh air. If possible, quickly shut off any open source of fumes. Do not flip a switch or light a match; either action could produce a spark or a flame and cause an explosion.

SELF-CARE STEPS FOR POISONING

Poisoning is a life-threatening situation. If you suspect poisoning, even if there are no symptoms, call a poison control center, 911, hospital emergency room, or your health care provider immediately. Be prepared to provide the following information:

- Information from the label of the substance container (keep the original container)
- The victim's age
- Name of the poison and how much was swallowed
- When the poison was swallowed
- Whether or not the victim has vomited
- How long it will take to get the victim to a hospital

If the victim is unconscious, keep the airway open. Be prepared to begin artificial respiration (for CPR for adults and older children, see p. 12; for children under 8 years old, see p. 15), if necessary. Do not induce vomiting unless told to do so.

Signs and symptoms of poisoning can vary widely, depending on the type of poison involved, the size and general health of the victim, and how much time has elapsed. Symptoms can also take time to develop. Do not wait for them to become obvious. **Seek immediate medical attention if you suspect poisoning has occurred.**

If you have been told to induce vomiting, use syrup of ipecac, if available. Follow the directions on the label, and do not attempt to give it to a victim who is not alert enough to swallow it. Save a sample of vomit and the poison container for analysis. **Do not induce vomiting if you are unsure what poison is involved.**

For Poison Fumes

- Check breathing and pulse (see p. 14 for adults and older children; p. 15 for children under 8 years old). If the victim is not breathing, have someone call 911 and begin CPR (p. 12 for adults and older children; p. 15 for children under 8 years old). Continue until medical help arrives. If the victim is conscious and breathing, cover him or her with a blanket and check on breathing until help arrives.

A puncture wound from a dirty nail or an animal's tooth is more likely to get infected because dirt and germs are carried deep into the tissues. So, for puncture wounds, we may give antibiotics and a tetanus booster.

Urgent Care Specialist

PUNCTURE WOUNDS

For Cuts, see p. 16; for Bites, see p. 4.

A puncture wound is a small, but deep hole produced by a sharp object such as a pin, nail, tack, needle, tooth, or fang. These wounds are often deep and narrow, with little bleeding. Puncture wounds often become infected because they are difficult to clean and germs are not washed out by the flow of blood.

Infections from puncture wounds deep in the hand (not the fingers) are hard to treat and may lead to loss of hand functions. Call your health care provider if you receive a deep puncture wound in the hand.

Deep puncture wounds in a joint such as the knee or ankle should be seen by your health care provider. Puncture wounds caused by stepping on a nail are often contaminated by dirt or pieces of shoe or sock carried into the wound by the nail. This type of wound also should be seen by your health care provider. Check to be sure the victim has had a tetanus shot within the last 10 years or more recently if he or she has ever had a serious open wound.

DECISION GUIDE FOR PUNCTURE WOUNDS

SYMPTOMS/SIGNS	ACTION
Minor puncture wound	🩹
Signs of infection (p. 28)	☎
No tetanus shot within last 10 years or more recently if victim has ever had a serious open wound	🩺
Animal or human bite (see Bites, p. 4)	🩺
Possible foreign object in wound	🩺
Wound bleeds heavily or sprays	🏥

🩹 Use self-care		🩺 See doctor	
☎ Call doctor's office for advice		🏥 Seek help now	

For more about the symbols, see p. 2.

SELF-CARE STEPS FOR PUNCTURE WOUNDS

• Allow the wound to bleed freely unless a lot of blood has been lost or the blood is spraying out. Bleeding will cleanse the wound and help prevent infection. After several minutes, stop the bleeding by applying pressure to the wound and raising it above the level of the heart.

• Next, clean the area around the wound with soap and warm water. For the next 4 or 5 days, soak the wound in warm water for 15 minutes several times a day. This will clean the wound

from the inside. Cover the wound with a sterile or clean dressing and tape in place.

• Do not tape the wound closed or apply antibiotic ointment. Sealing off the wound can increase the risk of infection. Signs of infection usually take more than 24 hours to develop. Call your health care provider if redness, swelling, or pus appears around the wound; if the victim has pain or a fever; or if the wound doesn't heal within 2 weeks.

SCRAPES AND ABRASIONS

Scrapes or abrasions occur when one or more layers of skin are torn or scraped off. They happen so often they may seem unimportant, but they should be treated to reduce the chance of infection or scarring.

Scrapes are usually caused by falls onto the hands, knees, or elbows. This exposes millions of nerve endings, all of which carry pain impulses to the brain. Because scrapes can affect so many nerve endings, they are usually much more painful than cuts.

Although most abrasions and scrapes can be treated at home, you should call your health care provider if they become infected (see Decision Guide for Infected Wounds, p. 28).

Carefully remove any dirt or particles from a scrape.

DECISION GUIDE FOR SCRAPES AND ABRASIONS

SYMPTOMS/SIGNS	ACTION
Minor scrape	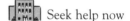
Signs of infection (p. 28)	
Scrape cannot be adequately cleaned or debris may be in the wound	
Bleeding cannot be controlled	

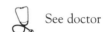 Use self-care

See doctor

Seek help now

For more about the symbols, see p. 2.

SELF-CARE STEPS FOR SCRAPES AND ABRASIONS

• It is important to carefully clean scrapes to help prevent infection. Carefully remove all dirt and debris. Use soap and warm water or hydrogen peroxide to thoroughly scrub the wound for no less than a minute or two. If you don't wash the wound for a full minute, you are not cleaning it well enough.

• Next, apply direct pressure to the wound, using gauze or a clean cloth to hold on the wound and stop the flow of blood. If the gauze or cloth becomes soaked with blood, do not remove it. Instead, place another clean layer of cloth or gauze directly on top and reapply pressure. Because blood takes a while to clot, you may have to apply pressure for 5 to 10 minutes. Raising the wound above the level of the heart will also help reduce the blood flow. If you cannot control the bleeding, see your health care provider.

• On the scalp or a fingertip, you may apply an ice pack wrapped in a towel to constrict the blood vessels and stop the bleeding. Apply the ice pack for no more than 15 minutes or until the wound begins to feel numb. After a 10-minute rest, the ice pack may be reapplied. This 15 minutes on, 10 minutes off procedure can be repeated several times.

• Within 24 hours, remove the bandage and wash the area with mild soap and running water. The wound should be washed daily with plain tap water and soap. Change bandages two to three times daily. Watch for signs of infection.

SHOCK

Shock occurs when the heart and blood vessels can't send enough oxygen to every part of the body. It happens when blood flow to the body—and thus oxygen—is reduced. Without oxygen, the brain, heart, kidneys, and other organs will begin to slow their functions and ultimately die.

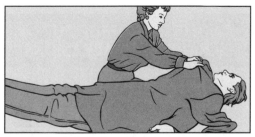

Lay the shock victim flat with feet raised and cover to keep warm.

Shock is a life-threatening condition that requires immediate medical treatment. Any serious injury or illness such as blood loss, heart failure, severe infection, burns, or breathing trouble can result in shock. Shock does not spontaneously improve. It typically goes from bad to worse. Without treatment, the shock victim will die.

Shock may produce these symptoms:

- Shallow breathing
- Rapid and weak pulse
- Nausea and vomiting
- Pale, clammy skin
- Shivering and coldness in limbs
- Confusion
- Bluish tint to skin

SELF-CARE STEPS FOR SHOCK

- **Call 911** and state that you have a medical emergency. People in shock need to go directly to a hospital emergency room as soon as possible. The following suggestions for action are things you can do until the ambulance arrives.

- If you suspect the victim has neck or back injuries, see below. Try to find the cause of shock and check for a medical alert tag. Make sure the victim has an open airway and is breathing. If necessary, begin rescue breathing or CPR (p. 12 for adults and older children; p. 15 for children under 8 years old).

- Stop any bleeding. Lay the victim flat and raise the feet 8 to 12 inches, using any available materials for support. **Do not raise feet if you suspect any head, neck, back, or leg injuries** or if the victim is having trouble breathing. **Do not place pillows under the victim's head.**

- Give first aid for the underlying illness or injury, if possible. Cover the victim with a blanket or coat for warmth. Do not apply direct heat. If the victim is drooling or vomits, turn the head to one side so fluids can drain. Check the victim's breathing and pulse until trained medical help arrives.

Shock Victim with Possible Spinal Injury

- Do not move a shock victim who may have a neck or back injury. Keep the victim in the same position unless he or she is in immediate danger. Cover the victim with a coat or blanket to help keep warm. Do not apply direct heat.

- Try to find the cause of shock and check for a medical alert tag or card. Make sure the victim has an open airway and is breathing. If necessary, begin rescue breathing or CPR (p. 12 for adults and older children; p. 15 for children under 8 years old).

- If the victim vomits or is drooling, protect the airway by rolling the victim onto one side while carefully supporting head and neck. Enlist others' help to gently roll the victim. Begin CPR if needed. Continue to check the victim's breathing and pulse until medical help arrives.

SMASHED FINGER

A finger smashed in a car door or with a hammer is a common injury, especially among children. When these injuries involve only the end segment of the finger and not a deep or bad cut, they can often be treated successfully at home.

Fractures of the bone in the end segment of the finger are often left untreated. However, some fractures need to be splinted.

Blood often pools under the fingernail of the smashed finger, causing severe throbbing pain due to the pressure under the nail. A health care provider can relieve this pressure by draining the blue-black blood that is visible through the nail. If the blood is under more than one-third of the nail, see your health care provider.

Often the fingernail is partly pulled off during the accident. **Do not remove the nail.** See your health care provider, who may be able to fix the nail.

DECISION GUIDE FOR SMASHED FINGER

SYMPTOMS/SIGNS	ACTION
Minor discomfort	🩹
Bone fracture suspected (see Fractures, p. 20)	☎
Numbness in the finger	🩺
Nail completely pulled off (bring nail to doctor)	🩺
Finger badly cut (see Cuts, p. 16)	🏥
Unable to move finger in a normal fashion	🏥

🩹	Use self-care	🩺	See doctor
☎	Call doctor's office for advice	🏥	Seek help now

For more about the symbols, see p. 2.

SELF-CARE STEPS FOR SMASHED FINGER

- If the victim can move the smashed finger easily and the injury does not involve the nail bed, apply an ice pack to reduce swelling and use acetaminophen (Tylenol) or a similar nonprescriptive pain reliever.

- If the finger is bleeding, apply pressure on the wound and elevate above the heart until bleeding stops. Wash the wound with soap and water, and watch for any signs of infection. If you suspect a possible bone fracture or the smashed finger involves a deep or serious cut, seek medical attention immediately.

SNAKEBITES

Most snakes you encounter are harmless, but to be safe avoid all snakes. Don't risk a snakebite by approaching or handling them. Your best defense is to leave snakes alone. Learn to identify snakes in your area, and find out if any are poisonous.

There are four kinds of poisonous snakes in North America: the copperhead, coral snake, cottonmouth (also called a water moccasin), and rattlesnake. Coral snakes are found mainly in the southeastern United States. Cottonmouth and copperhead snakes live mainly in the southeast and south-central United States. Rattlesnakes are found all over the country.

Snakebites from poisonous snakes are rarely fatal when medical assistance is quickly provided. However, anyone bitten by a poisonous snake needs immediate medical attention.

If you are bitten by a snake, try to kill it without deforming its head and bring it with you when you seek medical attention. If you are unable to kill the snake, remember what it looked like. The rattlesnake, copperhead, and cottonmouth all share these characteristics:

- Slitlike eyes
- Fangs
- Poison sack located behind eyes

The coral snake has rounded eyes, and distinctive yellow, red, and black rings. The coral snake also has fangs and a black nose.

PREVENTING SNAKEBITES

- When hiking, wear long pants and boots to protect your feet and ankles.
- Walk on clear paths and carry a walking stick.
- Never reach into an area like a hole or cave without first looking into it. Be cautious when looking.
- Stop walking if you see a snake. Quickly move away at least 20 feet back along the path you just walked. Watch for other snakes in the same area.

SELF-CARE STEPS FOR SNAKEBITES

- Don't panic! Venom will spread more rapidly through the body if the victim runs or becomes excited. Before giving first aid, identify the snake. Do not use ice on the bite as this may result in extensive tissue damage.

- If the bite involves a coral snake, elevate and immobilize the bitten area and go to the nearest emergency facility.

- If the bite involves another poisonous snake, within 30 minutes place a light tourniquet (constricting band of any sort) 3 to 4 inches above the bite, closer to the torso. Do not cut off the circulation. You should be able to slip a finger beneath the band.

- Avoid manipulation of the bitten area and do not allow alcohol or stimulants. Do not use a snakebite kit to suction venom unless medical treatment is more than 1 hour away. If you need to use the kit, make an incision over the bite, 1/4 inch long by 1/8 inch deep, being careful not to cut deeper than the skin. Place suction cups over the wound and draw out body fluids containing venom. **Do not suction by mouth.**

- For a nonpoisonous snakebite, keep the bite below the level of the heart. Clean the area thoroughly with soap and water, and place a bandage over the wound. Seek medical help promptly.

SECTION TWO
SELF-CARE FOR COMMON PROBLEMS

MEDICAL SELF-CARE

The more you know about common health problems, the more likely you will be to use the health care system well. Even though your doctor's office probably tries to give good customer service—with friendly staff and compassionate care—the fact remains, most people don't want to go to the doctor. It's no fun being sick, and it's inconvenient and often uncomfortable to go to the doctor's office for treatment. That—along with cost and time—is why it is important to know when you or a family member has symptoms that can be cared for at home and when symptoms are serious enough to be seen by a health care provider.

Studies show that when patients read self-care information, they make better choices about when they need to see a doctor. This means that for serious problems, they are more likely to get care when they need it. For problems that do not require a visit to the doctor's office, educated patients are more likely to use the right home remedies. Follow-up telephone interviews with patients who know about self-care show that 80 percent continue to refer to self-care materials when necessary.

To help you make decisions about how to relieve symptoms, we offer self-care tips whenever possible. For some health problems, only a few self-care remedies are suggested. This is because we try to recommend only remedies that have been proven effective. It is better to do nothing and be wrong than to do something and be wrong. After all, the medical credo is: "First, do no harm."

For a quick review of symptoms, check the Decision Guide at the end of each medical topic. You will see that for many symptoms, we recommend that you call your doctor's office. In many cases, your health care provider needs to consider your medical history along with your current health risks and health to decide if symptoms warrant a visit. Much of this can be done over the phone, saving you the time and expense of an office visit.

Remember—these self-care guidelines are not intended as a substitute for your doctor's advice. If you are not sure if these guidelines apply to you or if your symptoms do not seem better with self-care methods, call your doctor's office. You also need to consider your own medical history and health to decide if self-care is a good idea given your symptoms.

EQUIPPING YOUR HOME FOR SELF-CARE

Also refer to p. 4, for information on preparing a first-aid kit.

Stocking your home with some special tools and equipment is the first step in handling health problems successfully. Some of these tools prepare you for treating minor health problems at home. Others give you the information you'll need to decide whether a trip to the doctor is necessary. Here are some basic home medical supplies to keep on hand.

- Medical and self-care reference books

- Thermometer

- A heating pad for treating sore or tense muscles

- An assortment of adhesive bandages, including butterfly-shaped bandages for closing cuts

- Sterile gauze pads for cleaning cuts and scrapes and covering larger wounds

- Paper tape—which pulls off painlessly—for holding gauze pads in place

- An elastic bandage for wrapping sprained ankles or wrists or for supporting and putting pressure on injured, swollen, or sore knees

- A cold-water vaporizer for relieving congestion of colds and coughs (clean vaporizers daily when in use to avoid spreading germs)

- A penlight for examining sore throats

- Two pairs of tweezers: A blunt-tipped pair for such things as removing an object from a child's nose, and a pair with pointed ends for removing splinters

- An ice pack, either the type that holds ice cubes or the newer "cold/hot" packs that can be kept in the freezer

DIGESTIVE, URINARY, AND STOMACH PROBLEMS

Humans eat and digest thousands of pounds of food every year—including a huge variety of meats, produce, grains, and drinks. Your body does an impressive job of processing these foods every hour of the day. This section describes common problems related to your vital digestive and urinary organs and suggests how to take care of nonurgent health problems at home. *This information cannot replace care by your health care providers.*

Your primary care doctor (pediatrician, family practitioner, or internal medicine specialist) can offer advice and treatment for most digestive and urinary problems. If your condition is especially difficult to handle, your primary care doctor may bring in other medical providers who specialize in the diagnosis and treatment of these problems, such as gastroenterologists or urologists.

Use the Decision Guides to see if your symptoms call for medical attention or if they can be handled with self-care. However, you need to consider your own medical history and your current health when deciding whether self-care is right for you. If you have any conditions that do not seem to be healing normally or if self-care steps are not helpful, you should call your health care provider.

ABDOMINAL PAIN

We all know the kind of abdominal pain caused by an occasional attack of vomiting and diarrhea or "stomach flu." Abdominal pain can also point to many other conditions including indigestion, gallbladder disease, appendicitis, ulcers, inflammatory bowel disease, irritable bowel syndrome, and even bowel (or colorectal) cancer.

I thought my pain was indigestion because it often came on after eating. When it got worse, I saw my doctor and discovered I had gallbladder disease.

Barbara

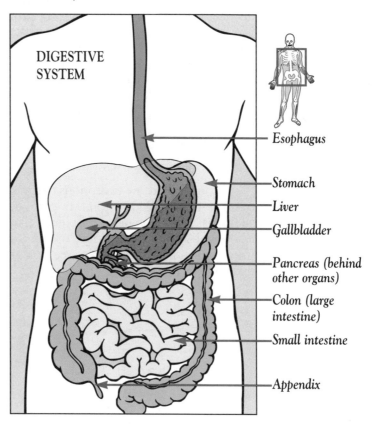

DIGESTIVE SYSTEM

- Esophagus
- Stomach
- Liver
- Gallbladder
- Pancreas (behind other organs)
- Colon (large intestine)
- Small intestine
- Appendix

My stomach often hurt if I went too long without eating. Turns out I have an ulcer.

Jose

The type and location of pain often gives a clue to its cause. Pain that starts at the navel and moves to the lower right side of the abdomen can mean appendicitis. **Symptoms of appendicitis can include:**

• Nausea, vomiting, or loss of appetite

• Tenderness in the lower right side of abdomen

• Not able to walk upright

• Fever ranging from 100° to 102° F

Sharp pain (like heartburn) in the upper middle part of your stomach could be an ulcer. Sharp pain under the right rib cage that's worse after eating points to gallbladder disease. Diverticulitis, a disorder of the intestine, often causes pain in the lower left-hand side of the abdomen. Pain from bleeding or infection is often felt throughout the abdomen. Pain that occurs each month, just before a woman's period, suggests endometriosis. For women of childbearing age, symptoms of an ectopic pregnancy could include sudden sharp, stabbing abdominal pain along with:

• Pain radiating to the shoulder

• Vaginal bleeding

• History of missed or light periods

Of course, there are exceptions to these rules of thumb. Most stomach pain in adults is from common problems like emotional distress, overeating, or the flu (for stomach pain in children, see box at right).

SELF-CARE STEPS FOR MILD ABDOMINAL PAIN

• Eat bland, not spicy, foods.

• Use acetaminophen (Tylenol or Tempra) for pain relief. Children and teenagers should not be given aspirin.

• Avoid irritants such as alcohol, nicotine, caffeine, aspirin, and ibuprofen.

• Take warm baths, or apply a warm water bottle to the abdominal area for comfort.

SPECIAL CONCERNS FOR CHILDREN

Abdominal pain in children can have almost as many different causes as it does in adults. Most stomach upsets in children are caused by overeating or constipation. Often children will complain of a stomachache right before getting a cold, a sore throat, or the flu. Because the digestive tract is sensitive to emotions, children may get "tummy aches" when they are feeling stress or anxiety. Talk to your child about the worries he or she might be feeling. Putting a child's mind at ease may ease the stomach pains. Always consider diet, too, when a child's stomach hurts. Some studies say too much fruit or fruit juice can cause abdominal cramps and diarrhea. Intolerance to dairy products, wheat, eggs, or other foods may also be the culprit.

DECISION GUIDE FOR ABDOMINAL PAIN

SYMPTOMS/SIGNS	ACTION
Mild pain that comes and goes for less than 4 weeks	
Pain that comes and goes for more than 4 weeks	
Sudden abdominal pain, constipation, loss of appetite, or loss of energy	
Sudden, severe pain that worsens over a few hours	
Abdominal pain and fever; jaundice; pale, pasty stools; or dark urine	
Very bad, constant abdominal pain after an injury or sudden black, tarry stools (p. 43)	
Symptoms of appendicitis (p. 42)	
Symptoms of ectopic pregnancy (p. 42)	
Abdominal pain and sudden bright red rectal bleeding or vomiting of blood or a substance that looks like coffee grounds	

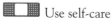 Use self-care

 Call doctor's office for advice

 See doctor

 Seek help now

For more about the symbols, see p. 2.

BLACK OR BLOODY STOOLS

Stools that look tarry, black, or bloody can be caused by drugs, hemorrhoids, bleeding ulcers, colon cancer, or other significant bowel disorders. It's important to recognize when these symptoms are signs of serious illness and when they are a bothersome, but benign condition.

Black or tarry stools may mean bleeding in the upper gastrointestinal tract. Pepto-Bismol, iron pills, or iron-rich foods such as spinach can also cause stools to temporarily turn black.

Hemorrhoids—swollen blood vessels in the anal canal and lower rectum—are a common cause of pain, itching, and rectal bleeding, especially during bowel movements. People with hemorrhoids may notice bright red blood on the toilet tissue or on the stool itself. Hemorrhoids can usually be treated with home care.

Frequent, mucus-covered, bloody diarrhea accompanied by fever and weight loss can be caused by a serious, intestinal disorder called **ulcerative colitis**.

Blood in the stool can be a symptom of **colorectal cancer**. This form of cancer may also cause changes in bowel movements; lower abdominal pain; and thin, pencillike stools. When diagnosed and treated early, colorectal cancer is often curable.

I was relieved to find out that my black stools were caused by the iron pills I'd started taking, and not by a serious illness.

Shirifa

Ever since the births of my children, I've had bouts of hemorrhoids. They're uncomfortable and aggravating, and, quite frankly, embarrassing. I'm still trying to lose weight but I don't have the best diet, which might be making the problem worse.

Lois

SELF-CARE STEPS FOR BLACK AND BLOODY STOOLS

 • Avoid nonsteroidal anti-inflammatory pain relievers, including over-the-counter ibuprofen (Motrin), naproxen (Naprosyn), and aspirin. They may cause intestinal irritation and bleeding.

To avoid constipation that can irritate hemorrhoids:

• Use a stool softener such as Colace, Metamucil, Fibercon, or Citracil.

• Take Metamucil or Citracil with 8 ounces of water for best results.

• Drink at least six to eight glasses of water each day.

• Eat plenty of fresh fruits, vegetables, and fiber.

To relieve hemorrhoid symptoms:

• Use an over-the-counter rectal ointment such as Anusol HC, Nupercainol, (do not use if allergic to novocaine) or Preparation H.

• Soak in a tub of warm water for 10 to 15 minutes three times a day to help relieve pain and to clean and heal the area.

• Apply Tucks pads to the rectal area twice a day and after bowel movements.

• Take acetaminophen (Tylenol, Tempra, or a generic) for pain relief. Do not take aspirin, which may make bleeding worse.

DECISION GUIDE FOR BLACK AND BLOODY STOOLS

SYMPTOMS/SIGNS	ACTION
Symptoms of hemorrhoids (p. 43)	
Symptoms last more than 24 hours	
Hemorrhoids are suspected but have not been diagnosed	
Black, tarry stools unrelated to food or medicine	
Bright red rectal bleeding and abdominal pain (p. 41), fever, changes in bowel habits, recent weight loss, bleeding problems or gastrointestinal bleeding, history of colon problems such as Crohn's disease, irritable bowel syndrome, or colitis	
Red blood in the stool of a person taking a blood thinner	
Person has a bleeding ulcer, had a prior ulcer, or is on aspirin or NSAIDs	
Sudden onset of heavy, continuous, bright red rectal bleeding or black, tarry stools and dizziness; lightheadedness; rapid pulse; cool, clammy skin	

 Use self-care   Seek help now

 Call doctor's office for advice

 See doctor

Emergency, call 911

For more about the symbols, see p. 2.

CONSTIPATION

If you believe what you see on television, constipation is the scourge of modern life, to be banished at first suspicion by laxatives and fiber supplements. In reality, constipation is the passage of hard, dry, or infrequent stools and is usually easy to cure naturally.

Emptying one's bowels ought to be fairly easy. After all, the bowels send a signal when they're ready to pass a stool. Most frequently, the cause of constipation is ignoring this signal. The large intestine draws water from stools, so the longer stools are available, the more water the large intestine will absorb, making the stools harder and more difficult to pass.

The myth that one should have a bowel movement every day is just that: a myth. Each person has his or her own natural schedule. Some people may move their bowels two or three times a day, while others may have a bowel movement once every three to five days. How often doesn't matter (unless the frequency has changed a lot); it is the consistency of the stool or the discomfort that tells you if you're constipated.

Constant worry about constipation may be a sign of depression, anxiety, or obsessive/compulsive disorder. Discuss any concerns with your health care provider.

Children sometimes become constipated, although their parents usually are more worried about it than the children. Stress triggered by toilet training can lead to constipation. Seniors, who may become less active as they age, sometimes complain of constipation. With both age groups, a change in diet can get the bowels back on course. Fresh fruits and vegetables have a natural laxative action and also provide fiber. Foods such as bran, celery, and whole-wheat breads also add fiber, which draws water to the stool. Extra fluids also are a good idea, particularly plain water and fruit juices. Replace soda pop and coffee with plain water. Seniors also may want to exercise more. Walking is an excellent choice.

Sometimes, constipation signals an underlying, more serious problem. Alternating diarrhea and constipation may stem from an irritable colon, a common health problem. **Diverticulitis**, an inflammation of small pockets in the colon wall, causes alternating diarrhea and constipation, fever, and pain in the lower left abdomen.

SELF-CARE STEPS FOR CONSTIPATION

• If you have no other symptoms, relax and wait it out. It's not unusual for bowel movement frequencies and consistencies to vary from time to time.

• Learn to heed the call. Your body will signal you when it's ready for a movement. When you discover the natural time during the day for you to have a bowel movement, try to set aside that time each day. Relax while sitting on the toilet.

• Change your diet. Increase your liquid intake; plain water and fruit juices are best.

Prune juice is especially good for relieving constipation. Add fresh fruits and vegetables and whole-grain breads to your diet.

• Exercise more. Exercise not only helps your bowels move more freely, it helps reduce the stress that may make you temporarily constipated.

• Use a stool softener, mild laxative, or nondietary fiber product to relieve temporary symptoms. Once your bowel movements have returned to normal, use diet modification, exercise, and stress reduction techniques to stay regular.

When I was having a very stressful time at work, I began to notice I was having a really hard time having a bowel movement. I didn't have the time, and that was probably the biggest problem. My solution was to bring a lot of fresh fruit and vegetables to work and put them right on my desk. I'd eat those as I worked and it really helped.

Dena

Mild laxatives, such as milk of magnesia, or enemas, such as Fleets, can relieve temporary symptoms of constipation, but should not be used often as an aid to regular bowel movements. Diet, particularly adding natural fiber, will work as well. Fiber supplements, such as Metamucil (3 tablespoons per day mixed with liquid) can also be used.

DECISION GUIDE FOR CONSTIPATION

SYMPTOMS/SIGNS	ACTION
Constipation without other symptoms	
Constipation and abdominal pain (p. 41), cramps or gas, vomiting (p. 58), fever, or loss of appetite	
Pencil-thin stools, which may suggest a bowel tumor	
Suspicion that a drug is causing the constipation (antacids, antidepressants, antihistamines, antihypertensives, diuretics, and narcotics all can cause constipation)	
Self-care steps do not help after a week, or discomfort increases	
Bowel movement becomes impacted in the rectum; only mucus and fluids will pass	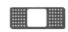

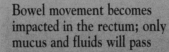 Use self-care

 Call doctor's office for advice

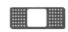 See doctor

For more about the symbols, see p. 2.

DIARRHEA

Diarrhea is perhaps the world's least favorite traveling companion and most unwelcome houseguest. Yet, it seems everyone is occasionally visited by it.

Diarrhea is frequent, loose or watery stools often with abdominal cramps, vomiting, or fever. Stools move so quickly through the intestines that the body is unable to absorb the water in them. Because of this loss of fluid, diarrhea can lead to dehydration.

Diarrhea can be caused by bacteria, viruses, emotional upset, stress, certain drugs, and some chronic bowel diseases. With bacterial infections of the colon, however, diarrhea is usually more severe, lasting longer than usual. Prolonged diarrhea may also be a symptom of conditions such as giardiasis (if you have been traveling), amebic dysentery, Crohn's disease, ulcerative colitis, or food intolerances.

Most diarrhea goes away on its own or with home care within 2 days. When a diet of clear liquids doesn't help, the doctor may prescribe a prescription drug, such as Lomotil, that will slow down activity of the bowel. These drugs aren't recommended for children.

Diarrhea is always unpleasant, but it's usually not a major health concern for healthy adults. It can seriously weaken young children and older people, however, and may even require hospitalization.

SELF-CARE STEPS FOR DIARRHEA IN ADULTS

- Drink room-temperature liquids.

- Avoid alcohol, smoking, caffeine, milk, and fruit juice.

- Don't eat if your stomach feels very upset or crampy.

- Drink only clear liquids such as water, flat nondiet soda (ginger ale, 7 Up, Sprite), clear chicken or beef broth, or noncarbonated Gatorade. Sip a few ounces a bit at a time throughout the day.

- Suck ice chips if other liquids can't be kept down.

- When your appetite returns, but diarrhea continues, choose the following foods: ripe bananas, rice, applesauce, white toast, cooked cereal, potatoes, chicken, turkey, cooked carrots.

- Avoid until diarrhea is gone: fresh fruits, green vegetables, alcohol, greasy or fatty foods (cheeseburgers, bacon), highly seasoned or spicy foods.

- Take over-the-counter drugs such as Pepto-Bismol, Kaopectate, or Immodium, following the product instructions. Note that Pepto-Bismol may temporarily darken the stools or tongue.

- Call your doctor if you believe the diarrhea could be caused by a drug. Diarrhea is a common side effect of the following drugs: nonsteroidal anti-inflammatory drugs, antibiotics, gold compounds, antidepressants (Prozac, Zolof, Paxil).

I had a mild case of diarrhea when I was on a business trip. I took Pepto-Bismol and felt better. The next morning when I went to brush my teeth, I noticed the black coating on my tongue. It really shocked me. I thought I had come down with some strange and horrible disease. I can't tell you how relieved I was to find out it was just a normal part of taking Pepto-Bismol.

Larry

PREVENTIVE STEPS

- Washing your hands after using the toilet or diapering a baby and before eating or preparing food is an important way to prevent the spread of organisms that can cause diarrhea.

- Unpasteurized dairy products and undercooked fish, poultry, eggs, and meat—especially hamburger—can also have bacteria that can cause diarrhea and other gastrointestinal problems. Always cook foods thoroughly and wash cutting boards, utensils, and hands that have touched uncooked meat products in warm, soapy water. Eat only pasteurized dairy products. Be sure to keep hot foods hot and cold foods cold. Harmful bacteria can grow in foods left at room temperature for too long.

- If you have diarrhea, don't prepare food for others unless you wash your hands thoroughly. Do not work as a waiter, waitress, or cook or in any food-handling position until your diarrhea and upset stomach are completely gone and you know you are not contagious.

- Foreign travelers often get diarrhea. About half of North Americans and Northern Europeans who travel to less well-developed areas of the world will get some type of diarrhea during or just after their trip. (Ever wonder why they call them "globe trotters"?)

- Travelers to foreign countries should avoid drinking or cooking with unpurified water. Water can be purified by boiling it for 15 to 20 minutes or by adding iodine or chlorine drops or tablets. It's very important to follow product directions exactly when using water-purifying products. Travelers should also avoid fresh fruits and vegetables unless the foods have been thoroughly washed in purified water or can be peeled. Be wary of foods such as melons, which are often injected with water (most likely contaminated) to increase their weight.

DECISION GUIDE FOR DIARRHEA IN ADULTS

SYMPTOMS/SIGNS	ACTION
Lasts less than 48 hours with mild cramping that's relieved by bowel movements	
Is associated with recent international travel; ingestion of water from lakes, streams, or wells; or blood streaking on toilet paper and no history of hemorrhoids	
Lasts more than 1 week	
Person is elderly or has a chronic illness, such as diabetes	
Persistent mucus or blood in stool	
Intermittent abdominal pain or cramping that lasts 24 hours or more	
Temperature over 101° F	
Black and sticky or dark red stools (p. 43), brief loss of consciousness, dizziness, sweatiness, fast heart rate	
Is associated with severe, constant abdominal pain (p. 41) for longer than 2 hours	
Is associated with signs of dehydration (p. 48)	
Is associated with breathing difficulty	

Use self-care

Call doctor's office for advice

See doctor

Seek help now

For more about the symbols, see p. 2.

In Children

Diarrhea is common in infants and young children because their digestive systems are still developing. Diarrhea in children most often goes away on its own. The parents' job is to closely watch the child with diarrhea and to see that the child gets enough liquids, the right diet, and lots of tender loving care.

Just as in adults, the major concern for children with diarrhea is dehydration. Because of their smaller body size, children can become dehydrated more rapidly than adults. **Be alert to the following signs of dehydration:**

- No urination (more than 8 hours without urinating for children under 1 year old; more than 12 hours without urinating for children 1 year and older)
- Dry mouth
- Absence of tears
- Dizziness or disorientation
- Dry skin that doesn't spring back after being touched
- Dark circles around eyes
- Fever

SELF-CARE STEPS FOR DIARRHEA IN CHILDREN

• Make sure children get lots of fluids. Avoid fruit juices and highly colored drinks (food dyes may make the problem worse). Infants may have breast milk or soy formula. Also offer water and electrolyte solutions such as Pedialyte, Ricelyte, or noncarbonated Gatorade. Older children can have light-colored Kool-aid or flat, clear soda pop. Give small amounts of fluids often—every half hour or so.

• If the child doesn't have an appetite, don't encourage solid foods. When appetite returns, offer small amounts of starchy, easily digested foods such as: white rice, bread, and crackers; potatoes; ripe bananas; cooked carrots, squash, and sweet potatoes; noodles; bland soups such as chicken rice or chicken noodle; turkey or chicken, cooked without the skin.

• Don't give Pepto-Bismol to children or teenagers. It contains aspirin, which has been linked to a serious condition in children called Reye's syndrome.

• Diarrhea can be very hard on the tender skin of young children, especially those still in diapers. To protect the skin, change diapers quickly after each stool. Wash the bottom with plain water or sit the child in a tub with a few inches of warm water (a sitz bath). (You don't need to use soap, but if you do, use mild soap in small amounts and rinse it off well.) For cleanup, use a soft washcloth and plain water or a commercial diaper wipe that has been rinsed out well with water. Dry the area completely by patting with a soft cloth or towel or using a blow dryer on the low/cool setting. A generous layer of petroleum jelly or other ointment will help protect the skin. Since cloth diapers are more gentle on the skin than disposables, consider switching to cloth diapers or lining disposable diapers with cloth ones during prolonged bouts with diarrhea.

DECISION GUIDE FOR DIARRHEA IN CHILDREN

SYMPTOMS/SIGNS	ACTION
Three or more stools per day lasting for over 1 week with no other symptoms	
Temperature over 100.4° F for over 48 hours	
Eight or more stools per day over 48 hours with no improvement after dietary changes	
Intermittent abdominal pain and cramps for more than 24 hours	
Signs of dehydration (p. 48)	
Diarrhea and breathing difficulty, severe and constant abdominal pain or cramps, blood in stools, more than one stool per hour, child acting very sick	

 Call doctor's office for advice

See doctor

 Seek help now

For more about the symbols, see p. 2.

Home care is highly effective in relieving rectal pain and itching. Patients with frequent hemorrhoids and bleeding should see a physician for an examination of the anus and rectum. The hemorrhoids may be removed through one of several outpatient treatments. Major hemorrhoid surgery is reserved for the most persistent problems.

Internist

RECTAL PAIN

Rectal pain may be linked with intense itching, fever, and rectal bleeding with bowel movements. Obesity, pregnancy, chronic diarrhea or constipation, and some infections—especially of the bowel—may contribute to the problem.

Hemorrhoids or "piles" (very swollen veins in the rectal area) or *fissures* (cracks in the skin around the rectum) are the most common causes of rectal pain.

Rectal itching is usually not a medical emergency and, in many cases, can be prevented. Wearing cotton, breathable underwear and loose clothing will help. Also have plenty of water, fresh fruit, and high-fiber foods to soften stools and avoid constipation. Try avoiding certain foods that may contribute to irritation, such as highly spiced or acidic foods, coffee, alcohol, or chocolate.

SELF-CARE STEPS FOR RECTAL PAIN

- Avoid straining during bowel movements.

- Cleanse rectal area well after each bowel movement. Try Tucks instead of, or after, toilet paper. Or use a soothing lotion like Balneol on the toilet paper.

- Use a soft, white, unscented toilet tissue to reduce irritation.

- Try dusting the area with cornstarch or talcum powder.

- Use zinc oxide ointment to decrease chafing and absorb excess moisture.

- Avoid prolonged sitting.

- Raise legs when sitting, especially if obese or pregnant.

- Apply cold compresses (ice packs, Tucks pads, or witch hazel) four times a day for pain.

- Follow cold compress with a warm bath or sitz bath to soothe and cleanse.

- If needed, take aspirin or use medicated suppositories to relieve discomfort.

Note: Anal ointments with a local anesthetic may cause an allergic reaction. These medicines will have the suffix "caine" in the name or ingredients.

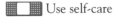 Use self-care

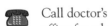 Call doctor's office for advice

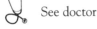 See doctor

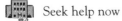 Seek help now

For more about the symbols, see p. 2.

DECISION GUIDE FOR RECTAL PAIN

SYMPTOMS/SIGNS	ACTION
Pain lasts less than 1 week	
Pain lasts for more than 2 weeks with self-care, or itching occurs with bleeding or pain	
Pain is severe or lasts longer than 1 week	
Bleeding is heavy or dark in color	
Heavy bleeding with signs of impending shock (p. 36)	

SPECIAL CONCERNS FOR CHILDREN

Sometimes a child will suddenly awake with rectal pain and itching. This often means pinworms. Seldom seen—but quite common and harmless—these small worms are contagious and may be picked up from contaminated food. Call your health care provider's office for a prescription, and wash hands thoroughly after using the bathroom and before preparing food.

URINARY INCONTINENCE

It's one of those embarrassing problems people don't like to talk about—even with their doctors. But there is help for incontinence. In most cases, the problem is treatable. It can usually be improved if not completely cured.

The first step is understanding the problem. Urinary incontinence is not being able to control leakage of urine. It affects more than 10 million Americans. Incontinence is more common in older people. Childbirth, being overweight, and aging can all weaken the muscles of the pelvic floor, causing incontinence in women. As men age, the prostate gland often enlarges and blocks the flow of urine, which can build up in the bladder until it overflows.

Families who care for elderly relatives sometimes worry that they will be unable to handle the problems of incontinence. But these problems are often reversible, and families can learn about treatment options together.

Symptoms of incontinence are:

- Urine leaks when coughing, sneezing, laughing, lifting, or getting up from a chair
- Urinate often to avoid accidents
- Get up several times at night to use bathroom
- Urinate in a dribbling, weak stream with no force
- Urine leaks during the day, unrelated to lifting or other stresses
- Sometimes can't urinate despite the urge to do so
- Don't feel empty after urinating
- Urinate only in small amounts
- Wet bed during the night
- Feel urgent need to urinate, and sometimes can't get to toilet in time
- Strong need to urinate at least every 2 hours
- Urge to urinate shortly after drinking
- Urine leaks a minute or so after urinating, especially in men

I have suffered with incontinence for more than 20 years. It's gotten worse recently. I use disposable underwear and try to avoid drinking large amounts of liquid or stressing myself. Sometimes I wish I could talk with my physician about this, but I just can't imagine discussing it with anyone.

Joe

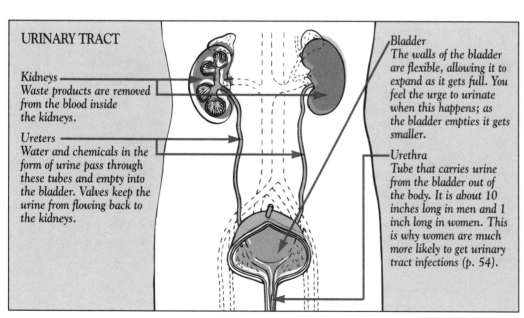

URINARY TRACT

Kidneys
Waste products are removed from the blood inside the kidneys.

Ureters
Water and chemicals in the form of urine pass through these tubes and empty into the bladder. Valves keep the urine from flowing back to the kidneys.

Bladder
The walls of the bladder are flexible, allowing it to expand as it gets full. You feel the urge to urinate when this happens; as the bladder empties it gets smaller.

Urethra
Tube that carries urine from the bladder out of the body. It is about 10 inches long in men and 1 inch long in women. This is why women are much more likely to get urinary tract infections (p. 54).

For several years, I could control my incontinence by doing pelvic floor exercises. Then, after my third child, it seemed the exercises didn't help much anymore. I've got three youngsters to keep up with, and I can't let a problem like this slow me down. I had surgery to correct the problem and would recommend it to anyone in a similar situation.

Beth

Stress incontinence is caused when activities place pressure on the bladder and the muscles that are designed to prevent leaks are weak. People who suffer from stress incontinence leak small amounts of urine when they cough, sneeze, laugh, lift heavy objects, exercise, or even get up from a chair.

Urgency incontinence affects people who suddenly feel the need to urinate so badly that they can't hold back. A bladder infection may be the cause, especially if symptoms of pain and burning accompany urination.

Overflow incontinence occurs when the bladder never completely empties. People with overflow incontinence tend to leak small amounts of urine throughout the day. They often feel the need to go to the bathroom—especially at night—but can only produce small amounts of urine. They don't feel completely "empty" after urinating.

Treatments for incontinence may include exercises, drug therapy, or surgery. Exercises can tone and strengthen sphincter muscles. "Bladder training" techniques help patients empty their bladders as completely as possible and help lengthen the time between trips to the bathroom. Various drugs can help correct some types of incontinence. In postmenopausal women, for example, estrogen may help reduce stress incontinence.

Surgery can help some types of incontinence. One operation for women moves the bladder, allowing the bladder neck (where the bladder opens into the urethra) to return to its normal, closed position. In men, an operation to remove the part of the prostate gland that blocks urination can relieve symptoms of overflow incontinence.

The Self-Care Steps on the following page have special exercises and techniques that may help control incontinence.

FEMALE URINARY TRACT   MALE URINARY TRACT

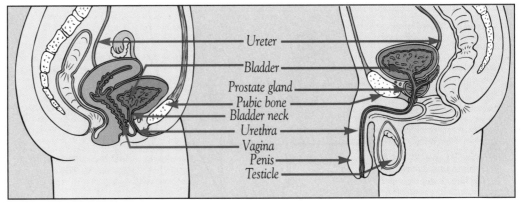

Ureter
Bladder
Prostate gland
Pubic bone
Bladder neck
Urethra
Vagina
Penis
Testicle

Sometimes surgery helps incontinence. One operation for women moves the bladder, allowing the bladder neck to return to its normal, closed position. For men, surgery can be performed to remove the part of the prostate gland that blocks urination.

SELF-CARE STEPS FOR URINARY INCONTINENCE

- Practice starting and stopping the flow of urine several times.

- Tighten the muscles around the anus and urinary sphincter, hold for a few seconds, then relax the muscles. Repeat 20 times. Perform exercises during a daily routine activity—while brushing your teeth, doing dishes, or reading the paper. Doing a set of 20 exercises several times during the day should improve symptoms of incontinence within a few months.

- Set a specific schedule for going to the bathroom—every 3 hours, for example—even if there's no urge to go. Use an alarm or timer to help stay on schedule.

- After urinating, wait a minute, then try to empty the bladder again. People often find they are able to release additional urine this way.

- Try to resist the urge to urinate more often. If this isn't possible without risking an accident, reduce the timing to every 2 hours, and then try to increase to every 4 hours.

- The time between bathroom trips can be extended this way. When you feel the urge to go to the bathroom, contract the muscles of the pelvic floor until the urge goes away. Try to hold off going to the bathroom a little longer each time. Keep track of how long you can wait between urinating. Within 2 to 3 weeks, you should see an improvement.

- If your problem occurs mainly at night, avoid drinking after the evening meal.

- Avoid stimulants such as coffee, especially after dinner.

- Don't stop drinking water—especially when it's hot or when you are working or playing in a hot climate. It is important to drink fluids regardless of the weather.

- If getting to the toilet in time is a problem, keep a portable urinal nearby (you can buy one at a drugstore or medical supply store). Drugstores also carry a variety of absorbent undergarments.

- Keep a record of the symptoms. A record can help your doctor understand the specific problem and recommend the right treatment. For several days, keep a record of each time you drink fluids, each time you urinate, and each time you leak urine—even during the night. Use "D" for drink, "U" for urinate, and "L" for leak. Note the time next to each letter. For every "L," also note the circumstances, for example, "while coughing," or "couldn't get to bathroom in time."

See your doctor if incontinence interferes with your lifestyle. Some people prefer to try self-care techniques before consulting a doctor. Whatever approach you choose, know that incontinence often isn't something you just have to live with. Together, you and your doctor can do something about it.

My incontinence was related to an enlarged prostate. I'd heard most men face that problem sooner or later, so I didn't give it much thought. I assumed it was just part of the natural process of aging. My doctor told me that even though it's very common, prostate problems shouldn't be ignored. My doctor and I have chosen "watchful waiting" as the best approach for me at this time.

Clarence

DECISION GUIDE FOR URINARY INCONTINENCE

SYMPTOMS/SIGNS	ACTION
Symptoms are occasional, manageable	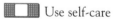
Self-care doesn't improve the problem	
Symptoms are frequent and troublesome and interfere with your lifestyle	

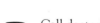 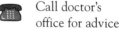 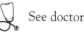

Use self-care

Call doctor's office for advice

See doctor

For more about the symbols, see p. 2.

I've always been prone to urinary tract infections. Since my doctor explained some preventive steps I can take at home, my infections have happened less often. I quit using the diaphragm and switched to a different type of birth control. I also drink a lot of water, which has made a real difference. But when I get an infection, I call my doctor's office right away for advice. I know my infections don't go away on their own, but it's nice to know I may not need an appointment every time.

Clare

URINARY TRACT INFECTIONS

They're bothersome, embarrassing, and painful. Occasionally, they're a sign of a serious health problem. Luckily, most cases of frequent urination can be cleared up quickly—often with just a couple days of treatment.

Some urinary tract infections have few symptoms—not even pain and fever. Recognizing urinary tract infections during pregnancy is especially important. **Symptoms of urinary tract infections are:**

- Frequent and/or urgent urination, especially at night

- A burning feeling during urination

- Blood in the urine

- Pressure in the lower abdomen

- Urine that looks cloudy and/or smells very bad

When a urinary tract infection involves the bladder, the sac where urine is stored before it leaves the body, it's called cystitis. It's often caused by *E. coli* bacteria. This bacteria is common in the bowel and can cause a urinary tract infection if it gets into the urine or bladder and comes into contact with the urethra, the tube through which urine passes. Urinary tract infections are more common in

women because the urethra is shorter and the anus and urethra are closer together than in men. Bacteria may also enter the urinary tract during sexual intercourse or when you use a diaphragm. Perfumed soaps, powders, and bubble bath products also may cause irritation that can lead to infection.

Urinary tract infections can be a problem for men, too, especially those over 50. An enlarged prostate gland, common in older men, can restrict the flow of urine and lead to bacterial growth and infection.

If the infection reaches the kidneys, it's called *pyelonephritis* and can sometimes cause permanent kidney damage.

SPECIAL CONCERNS FOR CHILDREN

Children can suffer urinary tract infections. Their symptoms are the same as those of an adult. Urinary tract infections in children may be more serious and should be checked by a doctor.

Children may urinate often for other reasons, too. Some children have small bladders and need to go to the bathroom quite frequently. If this is the case for your child, tactfully explain the situation to teachers or other caregivers. Stress at school or at home can also cause a child to urinate more often.

PREVENTIVE STEPS

- Drink lots of water. Medical guidelines recommend this.

- Women should urinate often, especially before and after sexual intercourse.

- Wear clean cotton underwear.

- Women should wipe from front to back after using the toilet, to avoid spreading bacteria from the rectal area.

- Avoid bubble bath, perfumed soaps, douches, and deodorant tampons.

- Switch from the diaphragm to another type of birth control if urinary tract infections are a problem.

- Avoid caffeine and alcohol, which can irritate the bladder.

SELF-CARE STEPS FOR URINARY TRACT INFECTIONS

- Avoid caffeine, alcohol, and spicy foods, all of which can make the symptoms worse.
- Drink eight glasses of fluid per day. Water is the best.
- Take tepid or cool sitz baths to relieve the discomfort.
- Call your health care provider. You may be told to have your urine tested, be treated with antibiotics right away, or be scheduled for an appointment. You may be sent to an urgent care center or emergency room if your symptoms include fever and chills.

A urine specimen may be requested to diagnose a urinary tract infection. Check with your doctor to see if this is needed—given your symptoms and history of infections. Some medical guidelines suggest that if you have an uncomplicated urinary tract infection, a short (3-day) course of antibiotics will work. If a urine specimen is needed, you will be asked to first release some urine into the toilet, then collect a midstream "clean catch" in a special sterile container provided at the doctor's office. Results of the urinalysis can often be obtained within an hour, but it may take 24 to 48 hours. If your doctor prescribes antibiotics for the infection, you may be asked for another urine specimen after you have finished the pills. A follow-up urine culture can show if the infection is completely gone. This follow-up test may not be necessary if you have a history of uncomplicated infections.

In some cases, a nurse may ask questions about your symptoms and past problems, and antibiotics will be prescribed without a urine test. More complicated cases may require an appointment with your health care provider.

DECISION GUIDE FOR URINARY TRACT INFECTIONS

SYMPTOMS/SIGNS	ACTION
Suspect urinary tract infection	Use self-care
Symptoms last more than 48 hours	Call doctor's office
Blood in urine	Call doctor's office
Men: Frequent, burning, urgent urination regardless of fever	Call doctor's office
Women: Frequent, burning, urgent urination with temperature above 101° F	See doctor
Nausea and vomiting	See doctor
Shaking chills	See doctor
Four or more urinary tract infections in the past 12 months	See doctor
Person also has diabetes or symptoms of diabetes (p. 214)	See doctor
Pregnant women	See doctor
Person also has compromised immune system (HIV positive or taking radiation or chemotherapy treatments)	See doctor
Person also has kidney disease or kidney stones	See doctor

Women who have frequent urinary infections and who have been evaluated by their health care provider often keep antibiotics at home and begin taking them at the first sign of a bladder infection.

Frequent urination can also be caused by drinking more fluids or taking diuretics (fluid pills). See your doctor if you are thirstier than usual, have blurred vision, feel tired, and have lost weight (also see Diabetes, p. 214).

Antibiotics will clear up a urinary tract infection quickly. It's important to take all of the medicine and drink more fluids. Symptoms will usually disappear within 48 hours after starting the drugs. Recent studies show that most bladder infections will clear up with only a few days of pills. However, complicated urinary tract infections require longer therapy. Also, be sure to tell your doctor if you are pregnant, breastfeeding, or allergic to certain types of medication.

Internal Medicine Specialist

Use self-care

Call doctor's office for advice

See doctor

For more about the symbols, see p. 2.

VIRAL HEPATITIS

Hepatitis, or inflammation of the liver, is most often caused by one of several viruses. Viral hepatitis often begins with flu-like symptoms: fatigue, headache, loss of appetite, nausea, or vomiting, and a low-grade fever (below 101° F). As symptoms get worse, jaundice (a yellow color to the skin and the whites of the eyes), brown urine and pale stools, and pain or pressure on the right side below the ribs may be present. In some cases, however, people with hepatitis have no symptoms at all.

There's no specific treatment for acute viral hepatitis, but you can do several things to get well and avoid spreading the disease to others.

The **hepatitis A** virus is spread through food, water, eating utensils, toys, and other objects that have been contaminated by feces, usually from dirty hands. Prevention of hepatitis A is the main reason restaurant employees and child care workers are required to wash their hands after using the washroom or changing babies' diapers.

After exposure to the virus, symptoms usually do not appear for 2 to 6 weeks. During this time, the exposed person is contagious. Most symptoms usually end within several days or a few weeks, but tiredness can continue for a few months as the liver continues to heal. Complete recovery usually takes a few months. Hepatitis A usually does not permanently damage the liver. However, serious and sometimes fatal complications can occur.

All close family members or close contacts of someone with hepatitis A should get a shot of gamma globulin to prevent or reduce the symptoms of hepatitis A. Your doctor also may prescribe a gamma globulin shot if you are going abroad. A vaccine to protect against hepatitis A is now used in some parts of Europe and is expected to be approved soon in the United States.

Hepatitis B is a more serious form of viral hepatitis. About 10 percent of people with hepatitis B will develop chronic

SELF-CARE STEPS FOR VIRAL HEPATITIS

- Get plenty of rest.

- Eat well. Hepatitis interferes with the liver's ability to help break down food. Therefore, it is very important to eat enough easily digestible food to get enough calories. Fatty food is often poorly tolerated. Try eating mostly carbohydrates (such as grains and fruits).

- Check in with your doctor regularly. He or she may run blood tests for several months to check for recovery or continuing inflammation of the liver.

- Avoid alcohol and drugs that irritate the liver. While you are ill and recovering, alcohol, birth control pills, tranquilizers, some antibiotics, antidepressants, and even aceta-

minophen (such as Tylenol) can also irritate the liver. Until you are fully recovered, check with your doctor or pharmacist before taking any drugs.

- Wash your hands after using the bathroom and before handling food.

- Talk with your doctor about having a hepatitis B vaccination. Many doctors feel everyone should have a vaccination for hepatitis B. Current recommendations say all children should have this vaccine routinely. Risk factors for hepatitis B include being sexually active and not in a mutually monogamous relationship, having HIV, being an IV drug user, being a sexually active gay male, needing dialysis, or being a health care or dental professional.

hepatitis, a long-term inflammation of the liver that in some cases causes worsening liver damage and even cirrhosis.

Hepatitis B spreads mainly through blood and body fluids, sexual contact, and contaminated needles used with intravenous (IV) drugs. It can also be spread if needles used for tattooing, acupuncture, or ear piercing are contaminated. In years past, blood transfusions were also at fault. Since 1972, screening of donated blood has almost wiped out the risk of getting hepatitis B from transfusions and blood products.

Symptoms of hepatitis B are basically the same as those of other forms of hepatitis, but they appear later, may last longer, and may be worse. Symptoms can take up to 2 to 3 months to develop. During this time, hepatitis B is most contagious. A hepatitis B vaccination series before exposure can prevent the illness. Hepatitis B immune globulin, a special type of gamma globulin, given shortly after exposure may prevent or reduce symptoms of hepatitis B.

Hepatitis C, a third form of viral hepatitis, spreads mainly through blood transfusions and through contaminated needles used for IV drugs. It can also be spread by sexual relations and tattooing. Symptoms usually appear 1 to 10 weeks after exposure. Often symptoms are less severe than they are for hepatitis A and B, and jaundice may not develop. Like hepatitis B, hepatitis C can lead to chronic hepatitis.

Until recently, about 2 percent of those who received blood transfusions got hepatitis C. A screening test, however, is now available for detecting hepatitis C in donated blood.

Drinking too much alcohol may predispose one to, or worsen, any form of hepatitis.

DECISION GUIDE FOR VIRAL HEPATITIS

SYMPTOMS/SIGNS	ACTION
Headache, low-grade fever, loss of appetite, nausea or vomiting, fatigue for more than 3 to 5 days	&
Suspected exposure to viral hepatitis	phone
Symptoms persist despite rest and self-care	doctor
Jaundice (p. 56)	doctor
Dark urine and light stools	doctor
Severe symptoms, especially if the person is unable to eat or drink*	doctor

*A brief hospitalization of a few days may be needed if the person is unable to get adequate nutrition or hydration because of nausea and vomiting, but usually a person with viral hepatitis can be cared for at home.

 Use self-care   See doctor

 Call doctor's office for advice

For more about the symbols, see p. 2.

When I found out my girlfriend was sick with hepatitis B, I was angry and scared. Of course, she didn't know she had it until she actually got sick. But that's when she was most contagious. I spoke with my doctor, who gave me some injections to prevent hepatitis. I never developed any symptoms.

Britt

Many parents worry about dehydration when their children have an upset stomach. Be patient. Give fluids in very small amounts at first, and solid foods only after eight hours without vomiting.

Pediatric Nurse

There is no magic choice of foods that will settle an upset stomach. While it is commonly believed that milk can coat the stomach and have a calming effect, the opposite is just as likely. Be careful of caffeinated drinks—such as colas, coffee, and tea— which can irritate the stomach.

Dietitian

VOMITING

Vomiting is usually the result of an infection located anywhere from the stomach to the colon.

More rarely, it is caused by a bacterial infection that would benefit from medical treatment. But in most cases, an upset stomach is a simple virus that will disappear by itself in a few days.

Vomiting can also be the body's reaction to eating spoiled food—for example, food left at room temperature for too long before being refrigerated. Or it can be the side effect of a drug or drinking too much alcohol. Nervousness, emotional stress, or tension can also cause an upset stomach. And, particularly in children, these upsets can be brought on by motion sickness, too much excitement, or too much sun.

It's very important to prevent dehydration while recovering from vomiting. Fortunately, there are sensible and safe home remedies that can satisfy your body's need for fluids and provide relief— over-the-counter drugs are rarely necessary. Although they may make you more comfortable, they won't speed your recovery, and you will get well without them.

SELF-CARE STEPS FOR VOMITING

• Let your stomach rest. Adults should eat nothing for several hours and gradually add liquids as the nausea stops.

• Stay on clear liquids for the first full day. Try water, cracked ice, bouillon, gelatin, chicken soup, or flat nondiet soda, sipping a little at a time during the day.

• Add bland foods on the second day. Choose foods like bananas, rice, applesauce, unbuttered toast, soup, dry crackers, or dry cereals without milk. Eat these foods in small amounts as comfortably tolerated.

• Avoid milk and dairy products. They may prolong the illness. Cigarettes, caffeine, and alcohol should be avoided also.

• Get plenty of rest.

DECISION GUIDE FOR VOMITING

SYMPTOMS/SIGNS	ACTION
Possible motion sickness	▨▨□▨
After eating too much	▨▨□▨
After drinking too much alcohol	▨▨□▨
Possibly stress or tension related	▨▨□▨
Oral temperature over 101° F for more than 48 hours	☎
Possibly pregnant	☎
Listless, less-than-normal activity level	☎
Early signs of dehydration (see box)	☎
Severe, constant pain	☎
Yellowish look to the skin or the whites of the eyes (see Viral Hepatitis, p. 56) and vomiting or diarrhea, dark brown urine, and light stools	☎
Person has diabetes	☎
Signs of dehydration (p. 48)	🩺
Vomiting blood or a substance that looks like coffee grounds	🏥

SPECIAL CONCERNS FOR CHILDREN AND SENIORS

Because dehydration is especially serious for young children and seniors, limit fluids for the first 2 hours only. Then, begin offering fluids by the teaspoon, gradually increasing the amount. For some children, fruit juices can make diarrhea worse—limit juices if symptoms persist.

When a child younger than 2 years of age keeps vomiting for more than 8 hours or has diarrhea (more than five runny stools a day) for more than 2 days, seek medical advice.

For the young and old, medical attention is also important for these **early signs of dehydration:**

• Dark circles around the eyes. Less than normal urination (for infants, less than five *soaked* diapers per day).

• Dry skin that does not spring back normally when picked up between thumb and index finger.

▨▨□▨ Use self-care

☎ Call doctor's office for advice

🩺 See doctor

🏥 Seek help now

For more about the symbols, see p. 2.

Dehydration (loss of fluids), fever, or loss of appetite can lead to serious problems, so it is important to keep enough fluids in the body. Frequent, small sips of clear liquids will ensure that you are getting adequate fluids.

Family Practitioner

EYE, EAR, NOSE, AND THROAT PROBLEMS

This section describes common problems related to your eyes, ears, nose, and throat and suggests ways to take care of nonurgent conditions at home. *This information cannot replace care by your health care providers.*

Your primary care doctor (pediatrician, family practitioner, or internal medicine specialist) can offer advice and treatment for most eye, ear, nose, and throat problems. If the condition is very hard to handle, your primary care doctor may involve other medical providers, such as eye, ear, nose, and throat (ENT) specialists.

Use the Decision Guides to see if your symptoms warrant medical attention or if they can be handled with self-care. However, you need to consider your own medical history and your current health when deciding if self-care is right for you. If you have any conditions that do not seem to be healing normally or if self-care steps do not seem helpful, you should call your health care provider.

BAD BREATH

It's one of nature's cruelest tricks. People who suffer from bad breath often aren't aware of it, and few people are willing to tell them that their breath has, well, quite an impact.

Although there are dozens of possible causes of bad breath (often referred to as "halitosis"), often it is caused by poor dental hygiene. Without proper brushing and flossing, food particles and plaque build up on the teeth, gums, and tongue. Bacteria begin to grow and produce bad mouth odors.

Smoking is another leading cause of foul-smelling breath. Tar and nicotine residues coat the teeth, tongue, inside of the mouth, and lungs, making breath especially smelly.

Bad breath can also be caused by tonsillitis, pneumonia, mouth sores, sore throats, sinus infections, and even the common cold. Stomach problems such as heartburn can produce bad breath, and so can certain drugs.

Breathing through the mouth, talking for long periods, or sleeping with the mouth open can dry out the mouth and turn breath sour. And, of course, eating garlic, onions, cabbage, or hot and spicy foods can leave breath smelling ripe for a day or so after the meal. Foods high in milk and butterfat are also culprits.

As a salesperson, it's important that my breath not offend people. Before calling on a customer, I always check my breath. I cup my hands over my mouth, exhale, and then sniff. If my breath could use some improvement, I'll brush my teeth or use a breath spray. I want customers to remember me and my products, not my breath.

Kristine

SELF-CARE STEPS FOR BAD BREATH

• The best way to fix a bad breath problem is to brush up on your dental hygiene. Brush your teeth after every meal and floss at least twice a day. See your dentist for an exam and cleaning twice a year.

• If your gums bleed when you floss or brush, you probably have gum disease (gingivitis), which can cause bad breath. If the condition doesn't improve after 3 weeks of careful dental hygiene, see your dentist.

• Brush the back of your tongue with a soft toothbrush. The tongue, especially far in the back as it goes down your throat, can have bacteria that cause bad breath. Studies have shown that people who brush the top and back surface of the tongue as well as the teeth have better breath than people who brush only the teeth.

• If you smoke, stop now. You'll need to brush your teeth and tongue twice a day for 2 weeks after you stop smoking before the smelly effects of tobacco are out of your system.

• Drink plenty of fluids to avoid dry mouth. Eat apples, citrus fruits, lettuce, and other raw vegetables that cleanse the teeth. Avoid strong-smelling foods such as onions, garlic, cabbage, and hot and spicy foods.

• Parsley is a natural breath freshener. Mouthwashes, breath mints, and sprays may mask the odor of bad breath temporarily, but they don't get at the source of the problem. Avoid sugary breath mints. They can make bad breath worse. (Bacteria thrive on sugar.)

Do you have bad breath? Do a breath check (cup your hands over your mouth, exhale, and then sniff) to find out. Or, floss your back molars and then sniff the used section of the dental floss. If it smells bad, you've got a problem.

 Use self-care

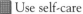 Call doctor's office for advice

For more about the symbols, see p. 2.

DECISION GUIDE FOR BAD BREATH

SYMPTOMS/SIGNS	ACTION
Most cases of bad breath	
Constant or recurring bad breath that doesn't respond to home care	
Bad breath from decayed teeth or gum disease	See dentist

BURNING EYES

Lots of different things can make your eyes burn. Smoke, pollen, or a viral infection such as a cold or the flu can cause eyes to itch, burn, water, and redden. In these cases, the burning and itching usually go away when the irritant is removed. However, age and disease can cause chronic dry eyes, which sometimes leads to burning eyes. Over-the-counter lubricating drops (artificial tears) can relieve this type of burning. Itchy, burning eyelids can also result from infection. Over-the-counter lid scrubs are available to treat this problem at home.

Caustic substances such as paint thinner, dish washing detergent, lye, toilet cleaner, drain cleaner, or gasoline can chemically burn the eyes. Chemical burns are painful medical emergencies that can result in decreased vision and sensitivity to light. Always wear protective eyeglasses or goggles when working with caustic chemicals.

Unprotected eyes can also be burned by the ultraviolet (UV) rays from the sun, tanning lamps, or arc welding equipment. Like sunburns to the skin, the pain isn't felt until hours later. Then the eyes and the area surrounding them swell up. UV rays can damage the retina. The risk of sunburning the eyes is very high when sunlight is reflected off water, sand, or snow. Wear sunglasses with UV protection when in the sun.

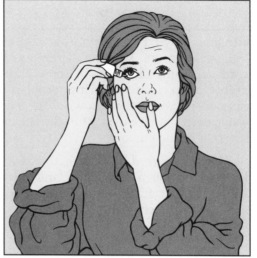

To put eyedrops into the eye, pull down lower lid and look up.

SELF-CARE STEPS FOR BURNING EYES

• If your eyes burn and water, try to trace the source of irritation and then avoid it. Smoke, cosmetics, chemical fumes, and pollen are some possibilities.

• For chemical burns to the eye, see Chemical Burns, p. 9, in the Emergencies and Urgent Care section.

• Apply a cool compress to sunburned eyes. Stay out of the sun until swelling is gone.

SPECIAL CONCERNS FOR CHILDREN

Make sure children wear sunglasses with UV protection. Be sure to shade your baby's eyes from the sun, too. Face infants away from the sun when outside. Store cleaning products and other caustic substances out of children's reach.

DECISION GUIDE FOR BURNING EYES

SYMPTOMS/SIGNS	ACTION
Irritated eyes	🩹
Sunburned eyes	☎ & 🩹
Irritated eyes don't respond to self-care	☎
Pain and swelling from sunburned eyes lasts longer than 24 hours	☎
Any chemically burned eyes (p. 9)	🩺
Impaired vision	🩺
Colored parts of eyes appear whitish or cloudy	🩺
Discharge from the eye (p. 68)	🩺

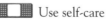 Use self-care

 Call doctor's office for advice

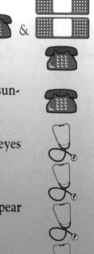 See doctor

For more about the symbols, see p. 2.

Our 18-month-old son awoke suddenly at night with a loud, hacking cough and labored breathing. He had a mild cold with congestion, but no fever. After an hour of pacing and a bottle of diluted juice, the coughing stopped and he dozed off. We called the nursing care line for reassurance.

Karen and Bill

CROUP

Croup is a viral infection that causes inflammation and swelling of the vocal cords in young children. In some children, croup is a recurring problem. Episodes of croup are outgrown as the airway passages grow larger. After the age of seven, it is uncommon.

Croup is marked by a distinctive seal-like barking cough, hoarseness, and difficult breathing. Croup lasts 3 to 5 days and may be accompanied by a cold or fever.

Croup without fever (spasmodic), the most common and mildest type of croup, comes on suddenly during the night. The child may have seemed perfectly healthy during the day or have the mildest cold but suddenly wakes up with a violent fit of croupy coughing.

Croup with fever (laryngotracheo-bronchitis) is a more serious form of croup, which inflames the area around the vocal cords down to the large bronchi (airways). It is usually accompanied by a chest cold. The temperature is usually lower than 102° F. The croupy cough and tight breathing may start slowly or suddenly at any time of the day or night. If your child does not respond promptly to simple home measures, call your doctor.

Epiglottitis is a bacterial infection of the respiratory tract (breathing tube) that sometimes seems like severe croup with a fever. The temperature is usually higher than 102° F. The child will drool and gasp for air, will not respond to the simple measures that bring relief of croup, and must receive immediate medical attention. Epiglottitis usually starts very quickly.

Most children with croup can be cared for at home. Three key elements in treatment are moist air, keeping the child sitting up or propped up, and encouraging plenty of fluids.

SELF-CARE STEPS FOR CROUP

• Put moisture into the air to make it easier to breathe. The simplest method is to take the child into the bathroom, close the door, turn on the hot water faucet of the shower, and sit with the child upright on your lap on the bathroom floor for 15 to 20 minutes, inhaling steam. Other options are a brief walk outdoors or a cold-mist humidifier in the child's bedroom.

• Give plenty of clear fluids, such as water or diluted juice, to help loosen the cough.

• Use a nonaspirin pain reliever to reduce fever and discomfort.

• Elevate the head of your child's bed.

• Remember, a child with croup is often frightened and crying, so try to reassure your child with a hug or distract him or her with a book or favorite game.

Note: Cough medicines and antibiotics are not effective in treating croup.

DECISION GUIDE FOR CROUP

SYMPTOMS/SIGNS	ACTION
Child wakes with a croupy cough but no fever, perhaps makes high-pitched noises when inhaling	▭
Child cannot relax enough to sleep after 20 minutes of steam inhalation	☎
Child has had croup symptoms for more than 3 nights	☎
Child is coughing and breathing with increasing difficulty	☎
Child drools and has great difficulty swallowing	🏥
Child cannot bend his or her neck forward	🏥
Child has blue or dusky lips or skin	🏥
Symptoms of epiglottitis (p. 64)	🏥

▭ Use self-care

☎ Call doctor's office for advice

🏥 Seek help now

For more about the symbols, see p. 2.

EARACHES

There are many possible causes for earaches—the most frequent is an infection of the middle ear. Although uncommon in adults, middle ear infections are an increasing problem for young children. For parents, it's important to be well informed about the care and treatment of children's ears, particularly if their child often has ear pain.

Middle Ear Infections

Middle ear infections result from a buildup of fluid in the middle ear that gets infected. Fluid buildup is caused by congestion that blocks the natural channel (eustachian tube) that allows air and fluid to go in and out of your middle ear. Once the fluid is infected with bacteria, a middle ear infection develops. This condition requires medical attention and treatment with an antibiotic.

Colds or allergies are almost always to blame for the congestion and fluid accumulation. That's why ear infections often occur on the second or third day of a cold. When children tug at their ears, act very irritable, or have a fever after a cold, suspect an ear infection and seek medical attention.

For children with chronic ear infections, regular treatment with low doses of antibiotics is sometimes recommended. Ear tubes may also be considered for recurring problems. With ear tubes, drainage from the ears may be cause for concern.

Swimmer's Ear/Earwax Buildup

An infection of the outer part of the ear canal, known as "swimmer's ear," usually results from water in the ear that gets infected. The symptoms are an itchy feeling, redness of the outer ear, and pain from simply wiggling the ear. Ear pain may also result from a buildup of earwax in the ear canal. Although earwax is normally protective, it can sometimes become impacted and hard to remove.

Many parents become concerned about a middle ear infection when their young children wake at night. Remember that an ear infection usually follows or comes with a cold. If your child has no cold symptoms, consider other causes for wakefulness.

Infectious Disease Physician

Follow-up exams for ear infections are very important, especially for little people who can't tell us if their ears still hurt or if their hearing is back to normal.

Pediatric Nurse

THE EAR

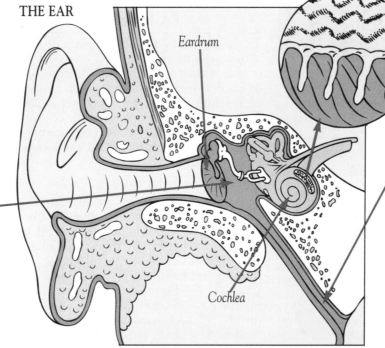

Eardrum

Middle ear

Cochlea

Hair cells in the inner ear can be damaged by long exposure to noise above 86db or one exposure above 140db.

Eustachian tube— *Plugging of eustachian tube leads to fluid buildup in middle ear. Fluid can build up in this tube from congestion caused by colds or allergies. This fluid can become infected with bacteria, resulting in a middle ear infection. Middle ear infections require medical attention.*

SELF-CARE STEPS FOR MIDDLE EAR INFECTIONS

• If your doctor has prescribed an antibiotic, *take as directed* to reduce the risk of recurring problems. That means not skipping doses, measuring doses carefully, and taking all the prescribed amount *even if the symptoms have gone away.* Store the antibiotic as directed—some require refrigeration.

• Follow your doctor's recommendations for follow-up exams or other measures to prevent future ear problems.

• For relief from pain or help with sleep, *use acetaminophen* (Tylenol, Tempra, or a generic) instead of aspirin. Ear drops may also provide temporary relief.

• Since colds are a common cause of ear infections, *teach your children to prevent colds* by avoiding contact with people with a cold. Teach children to wash their hands after contact with someone with a cold.

SELF-CARE STEPS FOR SWIMMER'S EAR/EARWAX BUILDUP

• To prevent swimmer's ear, dry your ears after a swim with a clean towel or hair dryer. You may also want to use drying ear drops if your doctor recommends them.

• If earwax has built up, *do not probe in the ear with swabs like Q-tips—they often jam earwax farther into your ear, causing even more problems.* Instead, direct a warm (never hot) shower at

your ear to loosen the wax and then wipe it out with a clean towel. Sometimes gently squeezing warm water into the ear using a soft rubber-nose syringe helps. Don't try to wash your ear if you think you have ruptured your eardrum or if you have ear drainage.

• A heating pad or a warm cloth on the ear may also provide relief.

Stuffiness/Airplane Ears

The pilot says, "We will now begin our descent," but your ears already have told you there's something going on. Sound is muffled and there's a painful, uncomfortable feeling in your ears. You have *barotitis*, commonly called "airplane ears." As the plane descends, the air pressure inside your ears is lower than the air pressure outside your ears. This creates a vacuum inside your ears, pushing your eardrums inward and making your ears feel full or stuffed up.

If you have allergies or a cold when traveling by plane, descent can cause real pain. Some doctors advise postponing a trip by air when you or your child have an upper respiratory or ear infection.

Other than momentary discomfort, "airplane ears" shouldn't cause any lasting harm. Sometimes there is bleeding into your middle ear. This acts like an infection, may be quite painful, and takes several days to heal.

🩹	Use self-care
🩺	See doctor

For more about the symbols, see p. 2.

DECISION GUIDE FOR EARACHES

SYMPTOMS/SIGNS	ACTION
Swimmer's ear (p. 65)	🩹
Ear stuffiness (p. 67)	🩹
Mild wax buildup (p. 65)	🩹
Discharge of fluids from the ear or any type of severe, constant ear pain	🩺
Symptoms of a middle ear infection (p. 65)	🩺
Ear stuffiness or blocked ear passages that do not respond to self-care steps within 3 days	🩺
Temperature over 101° F	🩺
Child with ear pain	🩺
Painful, itchy outer ear	🩺
Earwax can't easily be dislodged (p. 66)	🩺
Hearing loss	🩺

It never fails. I have to take a business trip, I get a cold. I used to be in agony during landings until I talked to my doctor. She suggested I take a decongestant or use nose spray. Now I'm not afraid to fly no matter how I feel.

Rhiannon

Avoid smoking at all, but especially near children. Cigarette smoke is irritating to breathing passages and can increase the chance of congestion—and ear infections—in your children.

Family Practice Physician

SELF-CARE STEPS FOR EAR STUFFINESS/AIRPLANE EARS

- Clear your ears by swallowing, yawning, or chewing gum.

- Another ear-clearing technique isn't beautiful, but it's the one pilots use. Squeeze your nostrils shut, take a big gulp of air, and clamp your mouth shut; then try to blow the air out against your closed mouth and nose. If you're successful, you'll feel your ears pop.

- Don't sleep during descent. You don't swallow as often when you're asleep. Ask the flight attendant to wake you.

- Give children too young to chew gum something to drink. That will make them swallow.

- If you must fly when you have an upper respiratory infection, take an oral decongestant like Sudafed about 2 hours before you expect to land. This will give it time to work.

- Use a nasal decongestant spray. Use it an hour before landing and then again 5 to 10 minutes later. (Sprays should not be used for more than 3 days.) Do not use nasal decongestant sprays if you have high blood pressure.

EYE DISCHARGE

Have you ever awakened in the morning with your eyes stuck shut? That memorable experience is most often caused by **conjunctivitis,** also known as pinkeye. This eye infection can produce a sticky discharge that leaves eyelids crusty in the morning.

Conjunctivitis is an infection of the membrane that lines the inside of the eyelids and covers the surface of the eye. Along with discharge, conjunctivitis can cause red, swollen, itchy, watery eyes. Eyes may burn or feel like they have sand in them.

Conjunctivitis can be caused by viruses, bacteria, allergies, pollution, or other irritants. Some forms of pinkeye can be contagious. Conjunctivitis caused by allergies, pollution, or irritants is not contagious, but a viral form of pinkeye can be very contagious. Doctors treat conjunctivitis with antibiotic ointments or eye drops (antibiotics have no effect on viruses), but the infection will often clear up on its own within 5 days. However, if left untreated for long, some forms of conjunctivitis can seriously damage the eyes. The most common form of conjunctivitis is caused by a virus similar to the type that causes a cold.

SELF-CARE STEPS FOR EYE DISCHARGE

• Warm compresses applied to the eyes will help relieve irritation and buildup of the discharge.

• A cold compress will help relieve itching.

• Wipe away the discharge or crust with a washcloth or cotton ball and warm water.

• Don't rub your eyes. It can spread the infection from one eye to the other.

• Keep it to yourself. Don't share towels, washcloths, or anything else that touches the eyes. Wash these items separately in hot water. Wash your hands frequently and thoroughly if you have conjunctivitis, if you are caring for someone who does, or even if you are around someone who has the infection.

SPECIAL CONCERNS FOR CHILDREN

Take your child out of school or day care when you notice symptoms of conjunctivitis, and keep the child away from other people as much as possible. Follow your school or day care policy on when the child can return to class. Be very careful to avoid contact between an infected child and infants, other children, elderly people, and those with chronic illnesses or damaged immune systems.

DECISION GUIDE FOR EYE DISCHARGE

SYMPTOMS/SIGNS	ACTION
Infection is mild and lasts less than 5 days	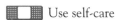
Eyes are sensitive to light	☎
Pinkeye and cold sores	☎
Discharge is thick and yellow or greenish	🩺
History of recent eye injury or foreign object in eye	🩺
Infection is worse rather than better after 3 days	🩺
Unclear vision	🩺
Infection recurs	🩺
True pain, rather than irritation, in the eye	🩺
Pupils are different sizes	🩺

 Use self-care

☎ Call doctor's office for advice

🩺 See doctor

For more about the symbols, see p. 2.

FOREIGN OBJECT IN THE EYE

Pain is the body's way of getting our attention, and nothing grabs attention quite like an object that becomes trapped in the eye. It simply cannot be ignored.

If you feel something in your eye, don't rub it. Rubbing can damage the cornea, the clear tissue covering the eye.

Wash your hands and take a look in the eye. If you find any of the following, put a patch over your eye (without putting pressure on the eyeball), and see the doctor right away: **A piece of glass or metal; an object that has penetrated the eyeball or is stuck on or embedded in the eye; or an object floating or stuck on the colored part of the eye—the iris or pupil.**

If the **object is on the cornea** (the clear layer covering the iris and pupil), you need to be seen by a doctor at once.

If the object is on the white part of the eye, try the Self-Care Steps on the next page.

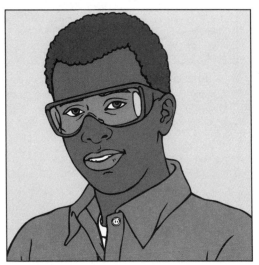

Always wear eye protection when working around flying objects or caustic chemicals.

I was working on a carpentry project in my basement and got some wood shavings in the white part of my eye. I got them out with the corner of a handkerchief and everything was fine. But it was a painful reminder. Now I never forget to wear my safety glasses.

Steve

SELF-CARE STEPS FOR A FOREIGN OBJECT IN THE EYE

• Wash the eye with water dropped from an eyedropper or squeeze bottle. The object may loosen and flow out of the eye with the water.

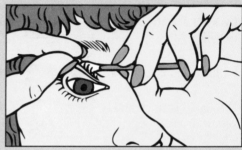

• Fill the sink or other large open container with lukewarm water. Hold your breath and plunge your face into the water with eyes open. Roll your eye and move your head around until the object floats away. (Don't try this with young children who don't know how to hold their breath.)

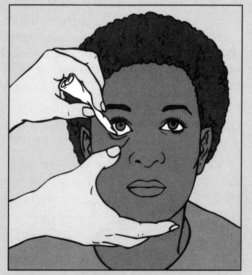

• Roll the corner of a clean handkerchief, tissue, paper towel, or other clean cloth to a point and gently push the object out of the eye with the cloth.

• If the object feels as though it is stuck on the inside of the upper lid, pull the lid out and down over the lower lashes and hold for a few seconds. This may help dislodge the object.

• The following technique works best when someone else helps you. Look up and pull the lower lid down while your helper looks under the lower lid. Then look down at your shoes and pull the upper lid up by the lashes while your helper looks under the upper lid. A Q-tip can help you grasp the upper lid (*see illustration*). **Never insert** a toothpick, matchstick, tweezers, or other hard object into the eye itself to remove an object.

• You can remove something stuck on the under surface of your upper eyelid with a moistened Q-tip if care is taken to avoid brushing the cornea (the clear layer over the colored part of the eye).

SPECIAL CONCERNS FOR CHILDREN

Try to help the child understand that rubbing the eye will make the problem worse. Give the child something to squeeze or hold onto to keep those little hands occupied while you examine the eye. It's also important for the child to stay calm so he or she can follow your directions. Speak soothingly and stay calm yourself.

DECISION GUIDE FOR A FOREIGN OBJECT IN THE EYE

SYMPTOMS/SIGNS	ACTION
Object is on the white part of the eye	🩹
Home care methods fail to remove the object	☎
Pain continues after the object has been removed	☎
Eye becomes red, warm, swollen; is increasingly painful; and discharges a yellow/green pus	🩺
Object is on the colored part of the eye	🩺
Eye is bleeding	🩺
Object is a piece of metal or glass	🏥
Impaired vision	🏥
Object sticks to the eye or is embedded in or penetrates the eyeball	🏥

🩹 Use self-care

☎ Call doctor's office for advice

🩺 See doctor

🏥 Seek help now

For more about the symbols, see p. 2.

HOARSENESS/LARYNGITIS

You never realize how much you need your voice until it's gone. When laryngitis strikes, you can't talk on the phone, read the kids a bedtime story, or even join in a conversation.

Laryngitis is the swelling of the vocal cords. It keeps the vocal cords from vibrating normally, so the sounds they produce are far from normal. The voice may sound hoarse or husky or disappear altogether.

Hoarseness or laryngitis is usually caused either by overuse of the vocal cords or a viral infection. Cheering your team on at a sporting event, shouting, singing, and speaking for long periods can all cause temporary hoarseness or loss of voice. Occasional hoarseness often afflicts teachers, singers, actors, salespeople, politicians, and others who use their voices for long periods. A cold, sore throat, or other upper respiratory infection can also rob you of your voice if the infection spreads to the voice box.

Hoarseness that is caused by overuse or by a cold or other infection will usually go away on its own within 2 weeks. To prevent attacks of hoarseness, avoid straining your voice and stop talking as soon as you begin to feel hoarse.

Smoking, alcohol, and air pollution can dry the vocal cords and cause hoarseness. Constant or repeated hoarseness not linked to overuse or an infection may be something more serious, such as cancer of the larynx. See your doctor if hoarseness doesn't go away within a month.

I always seem to get laryngitis at the end of a cold, when the other symptoms are almost gone. It's annoying, but it doesn't make me feel as ill as the other cold symptoms do. For me, hoarseness is a sign that it's almost over. I start to sound awful just when I'm beginning to feel better.

Rob

SELF-CARE STEPS FOR HOARSENESS/LARYNGITIS

• Give it a rest. Avoid talking and whispering as much as possible. (Whispering strains vocal cords as much as talking.) Use a pencil and paper and lots of hand gestures to communicate.

• Drink plenty of fluids. Water is best to keep your vocal cords well hydrated.

• Don't smoke or drink alcohol. Both can dry out and irritate vocal cords.

• Humidify your home.

• If you have to go out in extremely cold weather, wear a scarf or mask over your mouth.

DECISION GUIDE FOR HOARSENESS/LARYNGITIS

SYMPTOMS/SIGNS	ACTION
Hoarseness or loss of voice caused by overuse or infection associated with cold symptoms	
Repeated bouts of hoarseness not caused by overuse or infection associated with cold symptoms	
Hoarseness that lasts longer than 1 month, particularly if you are over 40 and smoke	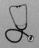

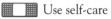	Use self-care		See doctor
	Call doctor's office for advice	*For more about the symbols, see p. 2.*	

MOUTH SORES

Mouth sores can be painful, unsightly, and slow to heal, but most of them go away on their own in a couple of weeks. People don't die of canker sores, but we need to find ways to treat the pain, promote healing, and keep new sores from forming.

Canker sores and cold sores are the two most common types of mouth sores. **Canker sores** are found on the wet surfaces inside the mouth, on the gums or inside the lips or cheeks. They can be red or yellowish white with a red border. No one knows what causes them.

Cold sores usually crop up outside the mouth, on or around the lips. More than half of us have had these before we are out of high school. They are caused by the herpes simplex virus type 1 and can start before or during a cold or the flu. Because cold sores can easily spread from one person to another, kissing someone with a cold sore should be avoided. Often an early warning signal is given—the affected area will itch, tingle, or burn before the sore forms.

Both cold sores and canker sores are more apt to develop when you are under stress. Fatigue, frustration, emotional upset, poor nutrition, and other stress may weaken the body's defenses enough for a mouth sore to form.

SPECIAL CONCERNS FOR CHILDREN

The virus that causes cold sores can be dangerous to newborn babies. Keep newborns away from anyone who has a cold sore or the itching, burning symptoms that precede a cold sore.

SELF-CARE STEPS FOR MOUTH SORES

• Apply over-the-counter products such as Anbesol for canker sores, and try Carmex or Blistex for cold sores. These won't make the sores heal any faster, but they may reduce the pain.

• Avoid eating acidic foods such as citrus fruits or tomatoes. Salty, spicy, or vinegary foods may irritate mouth sores, too. Also avoid foods with sharp edges, like potato chips.

• Cold sores are contagious. If you have one or feel one coming on, avoid skin-to-skin contact with anyone else until the sore has healed.

Hand-foot-and-mouth disease is a summertime disease that mostly afflicts children. Symptoms include sores on the mouth, hands, and feet. These sores are caused by a virus. Mouth sores that don't heal within 3 to 4 weeks may be a more serious problem—like mouth cancer. See your doctor if you have mouth sores that won't heal.

There isn't much you can do to prevent mouth sores. Good general health practices are the best precaution. Eat a nutritious diet with lots of vitamin-rich fruits and vegetables. Get enough rest and exercise. Try to avoid getting colds and the flu. Wash your hands often with warm, soapy water. Don't share glasses or utensils with someone who has a cold.

DECISION GUIDE FOR MOUTH SORES

SYMPTOMS/SIGNS	ACTION
For canker sores: One or more red, craterlike sores inside the mouth, on gums, or inside of lips or cheeks	
For cold sores: One or more blisters on the outside of the mouth area	
Recurring mouth sores	
Mouth sores caused by poorly fitting dentures or rough or broken teeth	See dentist
Mouth sores that don't heal within 3 weeks	
Small whitish, lacy sores (oral lichen or leukoplakia)	
Creamy yellow patches on inside of mouth that may be sore or painful	
Large, bleeding, and painful ulcers on gums (trench mouth)	

Use self-care

Call doctor's office for advice

See doctor

For more about the symbols, see p. 2.

SORE THROATS

Sore throats can be annoying, but they usually can be improved with a few simple self-care steps. Low humidity in your home, failing to drink enough fluids, winter dryness, or smoke can be the culprits, but often, sore throats are a sign of infection.

During an infection, your throat fights back by increasing the blood flow to your neck. This is what causes the swelling, soreness, and cough that often accompany a sore throat.

Two types of infections cause sore throats: the more common viral infection; and the less common—but more serious—bacterial infection, known as strep throat. Here are the usual differences between the two:

Viral Sore Throat

- Caused by a virus
- Usually causes a dry cough and a lighter colored mucus
- Less likely to be accompanied by a fever
- Often associated with cold or flu

Strep Throat

- Caused by bacteria
- Throat appears very red with white patches or pus and swollen tonsils and neck glands
- Often produces a temperature of over 101° F
- Requires treatment with antibiotics

Viral sore throats will go away in a few days, but up to 7 to 10 days is not uncommon. These do not need to be treated with antibiotics. With strep throat, however, you need to be careful. Strep throat may lead to more serious problems, although it happens rarely. It is best to call your health care provider when you have symptoms of strep throat.

NOTES FOR CHILDREN

- Fluids are very important for children. Be sure to give them plenty of soups, juice, or water.

- Fever doesn't necessarily mean serious illness in children. Be more concerned with changes in eating or sleeping habits or an unhealthy appearance. Acetaminophen (Tylenol, Tempra, or a generic) can be used for fever.

- If a child doesn't feel too tired, staying active is fine.

- Teach your children to prevent sore throats and other infections by washing their hands often and keeping their hands away from the face. If your children have been with friends who are infected, these preventive steps may keep the illness from spreading to themselves and others.

SELF-CARE STEPS FOR SORE THROATS

- Drink fluids. Drinking at least eight glasses of fluid a day will soothe your throat and loosen mucus for a more productive cough.

- Gargle with warm salt water. Add about a half teaspoon of salt to 8 ounces of water. Mouthwashes don't prevent or relieve a sore throat and are no more effective than salt water.

- Suck on hard candies or cough drops and take aspirin for fever or discomfort if you need to. For children or teenagers, use acetaminophen (Tylenol, Tempra, or a generic) instead of aspirin.

- Increase the humidity with vaporizers or hot showers. However, since vaporizers can transmit infection, it is important to keep them very clean.

DECISION GUIDE FOR SORE THROATS

SYMPTOMS/SIGNS	ACTION
Temperature below 101° F	
Cough that comes and goes	
Dry, sore, itchy throat	
Seems like a cold	
Cough that gets worse	☎ & ▭
Swollen glands	☎
Throat very red with white patches or pus and swollen glands	☎
Temperature over 101° F that lasts longer than 48 hours	☎
Sore throat develops into chest symptoms with cough getting worse	☎
Difficulty breathing	🏥
Unable to swallow saliva	🏥

Note: To determine if you have strep, your doctor may recommend that you have a throat culture. Be sure to tell your doctor if you have recently been exposed to someone with strep or if you are allergic to any antibiotics.

 Use self-care   🏥 Seek help now

☎ Call doctor's office for advice   *For more about the symbols, see p. 2.*

STIES

A sty is a red, tender bump on the eyelid. It can make the lid swell and feel itchy. Sties are normally smaller than a pebble, but the discomfort and swelling tend to make them feel huge.

A sty appears when an oil gland at the base of an eyelash becomes clogged. Over a few days, a sty usually comes to a head —like a pimple—and drains on its own.

Sometimes a sty will persist for weeks without coming to a head. In these cases, a doctor may choose to open and drain the sty. Good hygiene can help hair follicles from becoming clogged and forming sties.

Growths on the eyelid that are not red and painful are usually cysts, rather than sties. Although any unusual lump or growth should be checked by a doctor, most eyelid cysts are harmless and do not need to be removed.

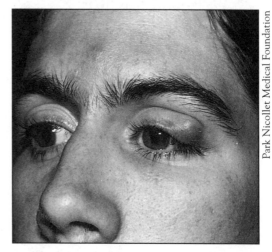

A sty on the upper eyelid.

Park Nicollet Medical Foundation

SELF-CARE STEPS FOR STIES

• Hot compresses will help a sty come to a head and drain. Place a clean washcloth in water as hot as you can stand it without burning yourself. Wring out the cloth and place it on your eye for 5 to 10 minutes. Repeat three or four times a day.

• If pus discharges on its own or during the self-care process, carefully clean the entire area.

SPECIAL CONCERNS FOR CHILDREN

A child's skin is much more sensitive to heat than is an adult's. Use lukewarm compresses instead of hot ones to treat a child's sty. Allow the child to test the temperature of the compress before you apply it.

DECISION GUIDE FOR STIES

SYMPTOMS/SIGNS	ACTION
Red, swollen, itchy lump on eyelid	
Lump on eyelid that isn't painful	
Sty persists and remains painful for a week or more	
Sty returns	

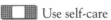 Use self-care   See doctor

 Call doctor's office for advice   *For more about the symbols, see p. 2.*

SWOLLEN GLANDS IN CHILDREN

Swollen glands are a good news/bad news story. The good news is that your child's glands probably are swollen because they're busy fighting an infection in your child's body. The bad news is that, because they get larger quickly, they may be painful.

Lymph glands ordinarily are about the size of a pea, and they produce the antibodies your child uses to fight viruses and infections.

The location of the swollen gland can tell you where the virus or infection is. An infection in the feet, legs, or genital area—and it can be as simple as athlete's foot or an ingrown toenail—will cause glands in the groin to swell. A swollen gland in the armpit might be from an infected cut on the arm or finger.

Most people connect the term "swollen glands" with the glands between the ear and the angle of the jaw, that often swell during sore throats and ear infections. Swollen glands down the sides and/or back of the neck might be from an infection in the scalp, German measles, or mononucleosis.

When lymph glands enlarge quickly, it may cause some tenderness. If the gland feels fairly soft and somewhat mobile, as well as tender, the infection probably is minor. The soreness will get better in a few days, although the gland may remain somewhat swollen for several weeks. It simply takes longer for it to return to its natural size than it does for it to grow.

Swollen glands usually need no treatment. But sometimes a bacterial infection will lodge in the glands themselves, making them red, hot, very tender, and very sore. Infected glands may require antibiotics. Most often, swollen glands are caused by viral infections and the only treatment is acetaminophen to relieve pain.

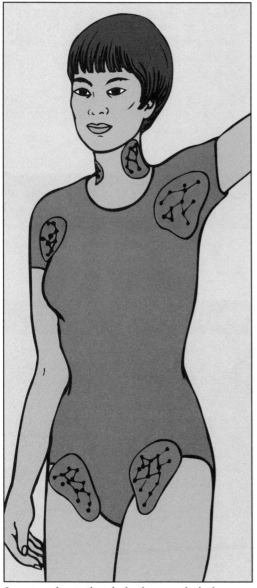

Location of major lymph gland sites in the body

DECISION GUIDE FOR SWOLLEN GLANDS IN CHILDREN

SYMPTOMS/SIGNS	ACTION
Swollen glands without more serious symptoms, such as redness and extreme tenderness	
Swollen glands with a sore throat and/or temperature higher than 100° F	
Swollen glands are very tender and red	
Swelling lasts for more than 2 weeks	
Difficulty opening the mouth, or moving the neck	
Difficulty breathing and swallowing	

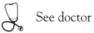 Use self-care   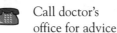 Seek help now

 Call doctor's office for advice   Emergency, call 911

See doctor   *For more about the symbols, see p. 2.*

My toddler woke up from his nap crying, which was very unusual. When I went in to get him, he was hot and the glands under his jawline were large and tender. I called his pediatrician, who said to start him on Tylenol. The Tylenol took away the fever and eventually the glands went down in size. It was kind of weird how fast it came on, but it went away pretty quickly.

Roberta

It seemed like, when I was a kid, my glands were never the normal size. I had chronic tonsillitis. I never knew what I really looked like until my tonsils finally came out. Then I finally discovered I had a normal jawline and neck after all.

Tim

I had a throbbing toothache. Unbelievable. And even the short time that passed before I could get in for a root canal was too much. It was a good motivator. I floss daily now and brush after every meal. I never want to go through that again.

Pablo

TOOTHACHE

At the painful peak of a toothache, you may be moved to vow that you'll never go a day without flossing again. *Ever.*

Whether or not you ever feel that much pain, you should promise to floss daily (see p. 79 for proper flossing technique) because tooth decay is at the root of most toothaches. Good dental hygiene, together with regular cleanings and checkups at the dentist's office, works like nothing else to prevent decay and the toothaches caused by it.

Toothaches can also be caused by cracked teeth, hypersensitive teeth, food stuck between the teeth, or old and crumbling dental work. Sometimes pain in the upper teeth may be caused by sinusitis. So once again, don't put off your regular checkups.

Emergency Steps for a Lost Permanent Tooth

If you should happen to have a tooth knocked free from its normal place in your mouth, the following actions are very important.

- **Act quickly.** The longer a tooth is out of its socket, the harder it is to successfully reimplant.

- If the tooth is dirty, gently rinse under water. Do not scrub, and remember to plug the sink.

- Replace the tooth, even though it won't be securely anchored, by gently teasing it back into its socket. Hold the tooth in place while you get to the dentist.

- If you can't replace the tooth in its socket, put it in a glass of milk or salt water solution.

SPECIAL CONCERNS FOR CHILDREN

Ask your dentist if dental sealants are a good preventive treatment for your child.

SELF-CARE STEPS FOR TOOTHACHE

- First figure out if your tooth pain is caused by an object or food particle wedged between your teeth. Try to remove it by flossing carefully. If this doesn't work, call your dentist. Don't try to remove a tightly wedged particle on your own. You could do even more damage.

- If your pain lingers, call your dentist as soon as possible. Swelling should always be seen by your dentist immediately.

- For temporary relief of pain, you may try the following techniques:

- Take acetaminophen (Tylenol, Tempra, or a generic) or ibuprofen (Advil, Nuprin, or a generic) to relieve the pain. Children and teenagers should not take aspirin due to the pos-sibility of Reye's syndrome. Be sure to swallow the pill. Do not rub it on the sore area. That home remedy can cause acid burns to an already sore mouth.

- Apply small amounts of oil of cloves to the tooth. Also called eugenol, oil of cloves is a nonprescription remedy available at drug stores. Over-the-counter anesthetic gels with benzocaine can also be used to numb tooth pain.

- If your gums become swollen, an infection may be present. Apply a cold pack on the outside of the cheek to reduce the swelling and pain. Ice cubes wrapped in a towel will work. If nothing else is available, hold a cold can of soda to your cheek. Swelling can mean a serious problem, so be sure to call your dentist.

- If milk or salt water solution is not available, place the tooth in a plastic wrap, wet towel, or glass of water.

- **Do not allow the tooth to air dry.**

- If the tooth is a baby tooth, have the child seen by a dentist. The tooth will *not* be reimplanted.

Chipped Tooth

A chipped tooth, though inconvenient, is seldom a serious medical problem. There are a variety of ways to fix this physical and cosmetic problem. Have your mouth and tooth seen by your dentist as soon as possible. Be very aware of how your "bite" may have been affected, since a blow hard enough to chip may also cause some position problems.

Wisdom Teeth

For temporary relief of pain, rinse your mouth with warm salt water and take an anti-inflammatory medication such as acetaminophen (Tylenol, Tempra, or a generic) or ibuprofen (Advil, Nuprin, or a generic) to relieve the pain. If there is any swelling, call your dentist right away.

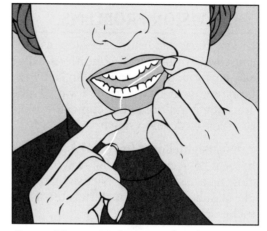

Correct Flossing Technique—*Insert floss and curve in a "C" shape against tooth; from base of tooth, shimmy floss back and forth while pulling away from gum. (The action is similar to drying the back with a towel.) Do this on either side of each tooth.*

DECISION GUIDE FOR TOOTHACHE

SYMPTOMS/SIGNS	ACTION
Dental appointment has been scheduled	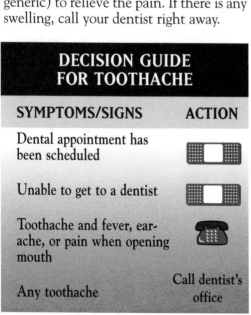
Unable to get to a dentist	
Toothache and fever, earache, or pain when opening mouth	
Any toothache	Call dentist's office

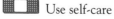 Use self-care

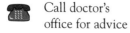 Call doctor's office for advice

For more about the symbols, see p. 2.

VISION PROBLEMS

Blurry, fuzzy, or distorted vision can be caused by a number of conditions. Most can be corrected. If your vision suddenly blurs, see your doctor right away. These are some conditions that can cause blurry vision to develop slowly.

Nearsightedness (myopia) is difficulty in seeing objects that are far away. Objects close up are seen clearly. Nearsighted people may hold reading material just a few inches from their noses.

Farsightedness (hyperopia) causes nearby objects to appear fuzzy. Objects at a distance are seen clearly. Farsighted people often hold their reading material at arms length.

Astigmatism can cause areas of blurry vision because the lens in your eye is not smooth. People with astigmatism may find it hard to see vertical, horizontal, or diagonal lines clearly.

Presbyopia is a problem of aging. As we get older, the eye lens hardens and loses its flexibility, making it hard to focus on near objects. Eyeglasses with bifocal lenses can correct most cases of presbyopia.

Cataracts cloud the lens of the eye, impairing vision. They usually start very slowly over several years. Most cataracts are a result of aging but they can also be caused by injuries, birth defects, too much heat or ultraviolet (UV) light, drugs, and diabetes. Lenses affected by cataracts can be replaced by surgery if necessary.

Glaucoma, a major cause of blindness, is increased pressure within the eyeball. This pressure can damage the optic nerve, which controls sight. Symptoms of glaucoma include loss of vision to each side (peripheral vision), halos around lights, pain in the eye, blurred vision, and then blindness. Glaucoma destroys peripheral vision first, so it often is not caught until a good deal of vision is lost. Early diagnosis through routine glaucoma checks after age 40 is the key to treating this problem.

Macular degeneration is the leading cause of blindness in the United States. It causes increasingly blurred central vision and most often strikes elderly people. If diagnosed early, laser treatment can sometimes keep it from getting worse.

SPECIAL CONCERNS FOR CHILDREN

Children should have their first eye exam at 3 or 4 years of age unless you suspect a vision problem earlier. If a school-age child starts having headaches or is having trouble at school, he or she may have a vision problem.

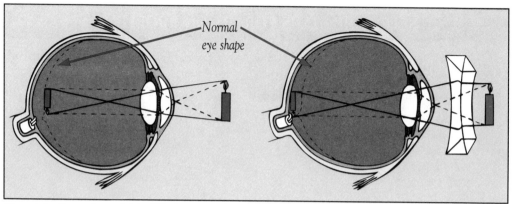

Nearsightedness (myopia) is difficulty seeing objects that are far away. It happens when the eyeball is longer than normal. The focal point falls short of the retina, causing objects at a distance to appear blurry. Eyeglasses with lenses that curve in (concave) bend the light rays so that they fall on the retina.

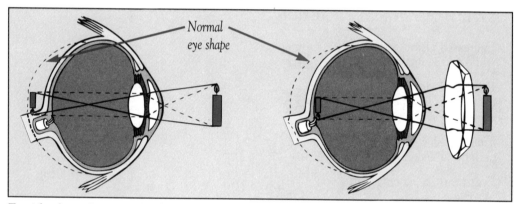

Farsightedness (hyperopia) is difficulty seeing objects up close. It happens when the eyeball is shorter than normal. The focal point falls beyond the retina, causing objects up close to appear blurry. Eyeglasses with lenses that curve out (convex) bend the light rays so that they fall on the retina.

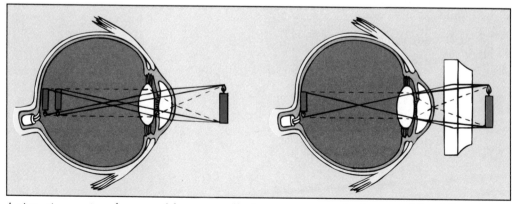

Astigmatism, an irregular curve of the cornea and/or lens, can cause two focal points to fall in different locations. This makes objects up close and at a distance look blurry. A person can have astigmatism combined with nearsightedness or farsightedness. Cylindrical lenses make up for the structural defects in the eye.

SELF-CARE STEPS FOR VISION PROBLEMS

• Have regular eye exams—every 3 to 5 years if you don't have vision problems, every 2 years if you wear glasses, contact lenses, or have other vision problems. More frequent exams may be recommended by your doctor or eye specialist.

• Wear safety glasses or goggles whenever you use power tools.

• Wear sunglasses with UV protection when you are out in bright sunlight. Be especially careful when sunlight is reflected by water or snow. Too much UV light has been linked to cataracts.

DECISION GUIDE FOR VISION PROBLEMS

SYMPTOMS/SIGNS	ACTION
Decreased vision began while taking medication	
Decreased vision in person over age 50 (suspect cataracts)	
Tunnel vision or loss of peripheral vision	
Eyes protrude or bulge out of sockets	
Sudden loss or blurring of vision	
Loss of vision associated with injury to head or eyes	
Seeing flashing lights or black spots	

 Call doctor's office for advice

 Seek help now

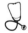 See doctor

For more about the symbols, see p. 2.

HEART AND LUNG PROBLEMS

Your heart and lungs are the organs that offer the most dramatic evidence of your body's well-being. This section describes common problems of these vital organs and suggests how to take care of nonurgent conditions at home. *This information cannot replace care by your health care providers.*

Your primary care doctor (pediatrician, family practitioner, or internal medicine specialist) can offer advice and treatment for most heart and lung problems. If your condition is very hard to handle, your primary care doctor may involve other medical providers who specialize in these problems, such as cardiologists, pulmonologists, or surgeons.

Use the Decision Guides to see if your symptoms warrant medical attention or if they can be handled with self-care. However, you need to consider your own medical history and your current health when deciding if self-care is right for you. If you have any conditions that do not seem to be healing normally or if self-care steps do not seem helpful, call your health care provider.

ACUTE BRONCHITIS

A cold or flu usually lasts about a week, but after all the other symptoms are gone, you may find yourself with a cough that lingers a while longer. The cough may be "productive," meaning you cough up mucus (usually yellow or gray instead of clear), or dry and hacking. Such a cough is often a sign of acute bronchitis.

Bronchitis occurs when the lining of the tubes leading to the lungs gets inflamed and begins making too much mucus. When this happens, your body must cough to clear out the extra mucus.

Acute bronchitis in an otherwise healthy person may be caused by viruses or bacteria. These organisms can also cause pneumonia. Airborne irritants—such as smoke, dust, chemical fumes—or even cold weather may cause bronchitis. People with asthma may also develop bronchitis more easily when they have a respiratory infection.

Because bronchitis is so closely related to pneumonia, it is important to see your doctor to rule out pneumonia if symptoms get worse instead of better or if they last longer than a week. Often a chest exam is all that is needed, but your doctor may also order chest X-rays or a mucus culture. If your doctor prescribes an antibiotic, take it until it is gone, even if you feel better.

I'd been fighting the flu for a week. My nose finally stopped running, and all the aches and pains went away, but I still had a cough. By the end of my first day back at work, I felt miserable. I was coughing hard, my chest felt tight, and it hurt to cough. I also was running a low fever.

When I called the doctor's office, the nurse said I probably had bronchitis. She recommended acetaminophen for the fever, drinking lots of fluids, and suggested a cough suppressant with an expectorant. She said that if I wasn't feeling better in a week or if I started to feel worse, I should see the doctor. I followed her advice and slowly my cough cleared up. In a week, I felt a whole lot better.

Maria

SELF-CARE STEPS FOR ACUTE BRONCHITIS

The best treatment for bronchitis is to drink plenty of fluids. By drinking six to eight glasses of clear liquids (not milk) a day, you will help keep the mucus from "gumming" up your bronchial tubes. When the mucus is thin and fluid, it is easier to clear away by coughing. And when the bronchial passages are clear and the inflammation has gone away, so too will the cough.

Here are some other things you can do on your own to treat bronchitis:

• Watch for signs of pneumonia. This includes: coughing; shaking and chills; temperature (sometimes as high as 104° or 105° F); white, yellow, green, blood-streaked, or rust-colored mucus; shortness of breath; chest pain; and fatigue. Because pneumonia left untreated can be life threatening, it is important to see your doctor if your bronchitis becomes worse or you start to have the above symptoms. Severe cases of pneumonia require hospitalization.

• Get plenty of rest. Listen to your body. You may be able to continue your daily routine while you have bronchitis, but don't overdo it. If you feel tired, rest.

• Avoid alcohol and caffeine. Either can make you lose body fluid, which you need to keep the mucus thin.

• If you feel you need medicine, choose a cough suppressant or an expectorant. Some cough medicines contain antihistamines or other preparations you probably don't need or want when you have bronchitis. Look for a cough preparation that has only the cough suppressant dextromethorphan. If you are coughing up mucus you might also try one with the expectorant guaifenesin.

Acute bronchitis usually lasts 1 to 2 weeks. But even after the inflammation in the bronchial tubes is gone, a dry cough, sometimes with wheezing, remains for as long as 4 to 6 weeks. During this time, exposure to cold, dry air, smoke, or dust can irritate the bronchial tubes and bring on coughing. Over-the-counter cough suppressants and decongestants may help relieve this nagging cough, or your doctor may prescribe other drugs. A cough that lasts longer than 4 to 6 weeks should be checked by a doctor.

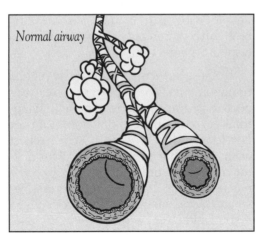

Normal airway

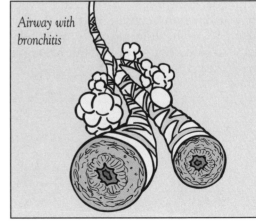

Airway with bronchitis

DECISION GUIDE FOR ACUTE BRONCHITIS

SYMPTOMS/SIGNS	ACTION
Productive or dry cough after a cold or flu, no fever, and tiredness	(self-care)
Cough worsens or lasts longer than 1 week	(self-care) & (phone)
Temperature 101° F or higher or any fever lasting longer than 3 days	(phone)
Blood in phlegm	(see doctor)
Cough lasts longer than 4 to 6 weeks	(see doctor)
Shortness of breath and heavy coughing	(see doctor)
Person has asthma (p. 207) and gets symptoms of bronchitis	(see doctor)
Person has chronic obstructive pulmonary disease (p. 212) and gets symptoms of bronchitis	(see doctor)

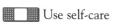 Use self-care

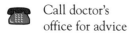 Call doctor's office for advice

 See doctor

For more about the symbols, see p. 2.

CHEST PAIN

Feelings of pain or pressure in the chest area could signal a problem as simple as indigestion or as serious as a heart attack. Pay attention to those signals, and call your doctor's office if you are unsure of what the symptoms mean.

Heart Pains

A **heart attack** can cause chest discomfort, such as a feeling of heaviness, burning, crushing, squeezing; chest pain; or pressure in the middle of the chest area. Sometimes pain spreads to the jaw, arms, neck, or back. A heart attack is often accompanied by sweating, shortness of breath, anxiety, dizziness, nausea and/or vomiting, and an irregular or rapid heartbeat.

Angina is a similar type of pressure or pain in the heart, but it comes and goes. Angina is a warning signal that the heart isn't getting the oxygen it needs. Resting or taking prescribed drugs usually relieves this type of pain.

Pain from a heart attack, on the other hand, doesn't go away so quickly. It usually lasts longer and is much worse. Rest and drugs don't completely relieve the pain. Sometimes the pain will ease, but then come back later. The risk factors for a heart attack include a family history of early coronary artery disease, diabetes, or hypertension.

Other Chest Pains

Sudden chest pains that last half an hour or less in people under 35 years of age are often panic disorder. **Panic disorder** can include chest pain symptoms such as heart palpitations (a fast, strong or uneven heartbeat) and shortness of breath. Other symptoms of panic disorder are anxiety and fear of suffocation or dying.

At first, it wasn't very painful at all—just like a little angina. But, I hadn't been exerting myself; it came out of the blue. When a nitroglycerin pill didn't stop the pain, I knew this was a heart attack. I felt a little silly calling 911 for an ambulance because I felt perfectly capable of driving myself to the hospital. By the time the paramedics arrived, though, the pain was much worse. The doctor said she wished all her heart attack patients could get to the hospital as quickly as I did.

Domingo

I found him sitting in the kitchen at 2 a.m. drinking Alka-Seltzer. He kept saying, "I'm fine, I'm fine. It's just a little heartburn." I knew something was very wrong. His face was gray and he was all sweaty. We got to the hospital just in time. He was having a heart attack.

Ruth

I get bronchitis every winter. Last year, I'd been coughing hard for weeks. One night my chest hurt so much, I was afraid I was giving myself a heart attack from coughing. I called the hospital and talked to a nurse. She asked me about my symptoms and said it wasn't a heart attack, but I should see my doctor at the clinic the next day. It turns out I had developed pneumonia with pleurisy.

Tran

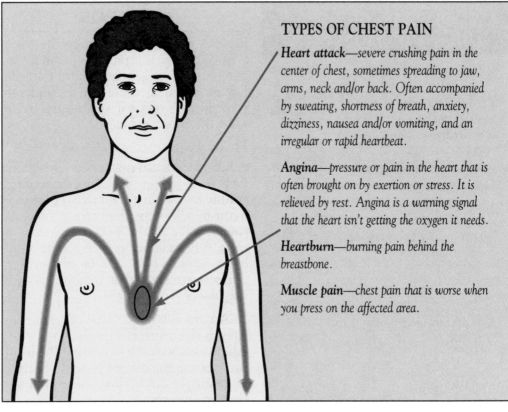

TYPES OF CHEST PAIN

Heart attack—severe crushing pain in the center of chest, sometimes spreading to jaw, arms, neck and/or back. Often accompanied by sweating, shortness of breath, anxiety, dizziness, nausea and/or vomiting, and an irregular or rapid heartbeat.

Angina—pressure or pain in the heart that is often brought on by exertion or stress. It is relieved by rest. Angina is a warning signal that the heart isn't getting the oxygen it needs.

Heartburn—burning pain behind the breastbone.

Muscle pain—chest pain that is worse when you press on the affected area.

The muscles, ligaments, cartilage, and other tissues in the chest wall can become quite painful from strains caused by exercise, by a fall, or even from coughing. Called **chest wall pain**, this type of chest pain usually feels worse when you press on the sore area.

Indigestion or heartburn, which often occurs after eating a heavy or spicy meal, can cause chest pains that seem similar to those of a heart attack.

A brief, sharp pain that lasts only a few seconds or a pain at the end of a deep breath is fairly common. Although they are unexplained, these pains are usually harmless.

Ulcers and gallbladder problems may also cause spreading pains in the chest. **Ulcer pains** are worse if the stomach is empty. **Gallbladder pains** are usually worse after a meal high in fat and often occur in the upper right side of the body.

Pulmonary embolism is a clot blocking one of the leading arteries from the heart to the lungs. A pulmonary embolism is unusual and mainly occurs in bedridden patients. Symptoms include sudden shortness of breath, sudden chest pains that are worse when breathing deeply, and sometimes a bloody cough and sweating.

Know the Signs of a Heart Attack

- A crushing, squeezing, burning pain in the chest
- Feeling of pressure in the chest
- Pain that spreads to the jaw, arms, neck and/or back
- Rest or prescribed drug doesn't relieve pain
- Pain lasts longer than 15 minutes
- Nausea, vomiting, shortness of breath, sweating

- Pain occurs at rest or awakens you from sleep

If you think you could be having a heart attack, **call 911** or your local emergency response team and get to the hospital as quickly as possible. **Do not drive yourself!**

Know the Signs of a Pulmonary Embolism (a blood clot in your lung)

- Sudden onset of shortness of breath that is often associated with chest pains that are worse when you breathe deeply

- A bloody cough

- Pain and swelling of the calf

- Anxiety, sweating, and rapid heartbeat (see Hyperventilation, p. 27)

Call 911 or your local emergency response team and get to a hospital immediately if you think you are having a pulmonary embolism.

Risk factors for pulmonary embolism are surgery within the past 6 weeks, a cast, or some other immobilization.

Keep Your Heart Healthy

Heart-related chest pains are caused by clogged arteries in your heart. Good health habits can help prevent or correct the problem. Exercise regularly, eat a low-fat diet, don't smoke, lose weight if you are overweight, learn to relieve stress, and get your blood pressure and cholesterol levels checked. Lifestyle changes can't prevent all cases of heart disease, but they can greatly reduce your risk of heart attack.

Be Prepared

If someone in your family suffers from heart disease, learn CPR (cardiopulmonary resuscitation, p. 12) and be prepared to use it in an emergency. It could save a life.

SELF-CARE STEPS FOR CHEST PAIN

Chest Wall Pain
- If your chest pain appears to be related to muscle strain from exercise, a fall, or other accident, and the pain is worse when you press on the affected area, take an anti-inflammatory such as ibuprofen (Advil or a generic) or acetaminophen (Tylenol or a generic). Heat and rest are also helpful.

Indigestion and Heartburn
See Heartburn, p. 92.

COLDS (VIRAL UPPER RESPIRATORY INFECTIONS)

Coming down with another cold is hardly a surprise. Neither is having a runny nose, congestion, fever or cough, or feeling just plain miserable. Although myths abound about this common annoyance, the fact is you can't catch a cold by walking in the rain, failing to bundle up in the cold, or sitting by a draft. Simply put, a cold is a *viral* infection.

The easiest way to catch these viruses is from other people: by shaking their hands, being near their sneezes, or touching things they have touched. That's why it is more common to catch a cold in the winter. The best way to prevent the spread of the common cold is to avoid people with colds. *Wash your hands if you have physical contact with someone with a cold.*

Fortunately, a cold will rarely require medical attention. Remember the following facts about colds:

- Because the common cold is a viral infection, there are no medicines that will cure it or shorten its length.

SELF-CARE FOR COMMON PROBLEMS

Frankly, when it comes to colds, my advice as a doctor is not much better than what your mother tells you. You can spend a lot of money trying drugstore remedies, but I think you can't do better than chicken soup. Be a good citizen when you have a cold by washing your hands often and not sharing your food with others. If you have a sore throat, gargle with slightly salted, warm water.

Infectious Disease Specialist

Antibiotics are only effective for treating bacterial infections.

- Bacterial infections complicate only a small number of colds.

- "Sinus congestion," colored nasal discharge, and headaches frequently accompany the common cold and do not always mean a serious infection.

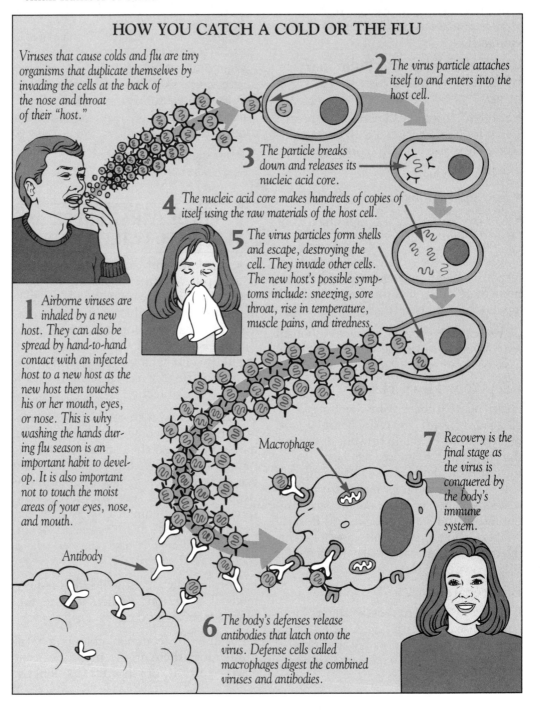

HOW YOU CATCH A COLD OR THE FLU

Viruses that cause colds and flu are tiny organisms that duplicate themselves by invading the cells at the back of the nose and throat of their "host."

2 *The virus particle attaches itself to and enters into the host cell.*

3 *The particle breaks down and releases its nucleic acid core.*

4 *The nucleic acid core makes hundreds of copies of itself using the raw materials of the host cell.*

5 *The virus particles form shells and escape, destroying the cell. They invade other cells. The new host's possible symptoms include: sneezing, sore throat, rise in temperature, muscle pains, and tiredness.*

1 *Airborne viruses are inhaled by a new host. They can also be spread by hand-to-hand contact with an infected host to a new host as the new host then touches his or her mouth, eyes, or nose. This is why washing the hands during flu season is an important habit to develop. It is also important not to touch the moist areas of your eyes, nose, and mouth.*

Macrophage

7 *Recovery is the final stage as the virus is conquered by the body's immune system.*

Antibody

6 *The body's defenses release antibodies that latch onto the virus. Defense cells called macrophages digest the combined viruses and antibodies.*

- Symptoms start quickly. They worsen during the first 3 to 5 days and then slowly improve.

- A cold will usually go away naturally in 7 to 14 days, regardless of what you do.

- Some loss of appetite or difficulty sleeping is normal with colds, especially for children.

A cold is uncomfortable, but it is usually just an inconvenience. Commonly used cold remedies do not cure or shorten the length of a cold, but the Self-Care Steps below list a variety of measures you can take to help relieve your symptoms while you wait for a cold to pass.

Many parents are surprised to learn that a fever with colds is not necessarily harmful. It helps the body's immune system fight off the cold virus. If a child with a cold has fever and otherwise seems well, there is no medical reason to treat the fever. However, if a child is uncomfortable, a parent may want to use a medicine such as acetaminophen (Tylenol, Tempra, or a generic) to bring the fever down.

Pediatrician

SELF-CARE STEPS FOR A COLD

- Raise the humidity at home. You can sit in the bathroom with a hot shower running or use a humidifier/vaporizer (a cool mist is preferred). If using a humidifier, empty and clean it daily following the manufacturer's instructions.

- Drink extra fluids. Warm fluids are especially soothing for irritated throats.

- Sleep with your head raised on pillows to relieve nasal congestion.

- Gargle with salt water or suck hard candy. Homemade salt water ($1/4$ teaspoon salt dissolved in 8 ounces warm water) or a store version will help relieve a sore throat. Hard candy is as effective for sore throats as cough drops.

- Try saline nose drops or sprays (e.g., Ocean or Salinex).

- Remain up and about. You will benefit from extra rest, but generally, you'll feel better by staying moderately active.

- Over-the-counter nasal sprays or decongestants may provide temporary relief. Because of potential side effects, be sure to follow the recommended dosage and precautions. If you have high blood pressure, diabetes, thyroid disease, or asthma, check with your health care provider before using decongestants.

- Temperatures during a cold are usually lower than 101° F and last less than 3 days. Use medicine for discomfort as recommended by your doctor or nurse.

SPECIAL CONCERNS FOR CHILDREN

- Children have colds more frequently than adults—five to eight colds each year is not unusual.

- Over-the-counter medicine is not recommended for children without a doctor's advice.

- Encourage children to drink a lot of fluids and stay active if they do not feel too tired.

- It is important to assess fever in the context of other cold symptoms. A fever is defined for children as a rectal temperature over 100.4° F (38° C) or an oral temperature over 99.5° F (37.5° C).

- For infants younger than 3 months of age, call your health care provider when rectal temperature is over 100.4° F, if infant is feeding poorly, can't be comforted, can't stay awake, or has a weak cry.

DECISION GUIDE FOR COLDS

SYMPTOMS/SIGNS	ACTION
Sore throat (p. 74), cough	Use self-care
Congestion, general achiness	Use self-care
Scratchy throat, runny/stuffy nose	Use self-care
Symptoms worsen after 3 to 5 days	Call doctor
Symptoms don't improve and still bother you after 7 days	Call doctor
Symptoms not resolved after 14 days	Call doctor
Children: Bothersome cold symptoms and a fever (p. 90) lasting longer than 72 hours or associated with symptoms of ear infection	Call doctor
Difficulty breathing, wheezing, or difficulty swallowing	Seek help now
Infants/young children: Less responsive, poor eye contact	Seek help now

Use self-care   Seek help now

Call doctor's office for advice   *For more about the symbols, see p. 2.*

FEVERS

From shivers and shakes to sweating and aches, your body's temperature is an important barometer of how well you are dealing with germs, stress, exertion, or extreme changes in weather. For good health, the body works best at a temperature of about 97° to 99° F.

Although body temperature rises slightly during the day, this change is not important unless your temperature is over 100.4° F. In fact, many people have a temperature that is always a little above or below the 98.6° F considered "normal."

By itself, a high temperature is not necessarily cause for concern—it can actually be a perfectly normal way for your body to defend itself against infection. Your body shivers to help produce the heat it needs to fight germs and sweats to regulate the rise in temperature.

A fever is a special cause for concern in infants under 3 months of age, the elderly, and those with a history of heart and lung disease. But for most people, there is no medical reason to try to reduce a fever unless it is accompanied by *other symptoms* of illness.

SELF-CARE STEPS FOR FEVERS

• With no other symptoms, drugs are not necessary. But if the fever makes you uncomfortable, take aspirin or acetaminophen (Tylenol, Tempra, or a generic). For children, use acetaminophen (Tylenol, Tempra, or a generic), not aspirin.

• Drink eight glasses of fluid a day. When you have a fever, you lose bodily fluids, so it's important to prevent dehydration.

SPECIAL CONCERNS FOR CHILDREN

- Fever is not necessarily harmful, nor does it mean serious illness. Be more concerned with changes in eating or sleeping habits, coughing, pain, or other marked changes in a child's behavior.

- Fluids are very important for children so be sure to give plenty of soups, juice, or water.

- Because a dangerous condition called Reye's syndrome can occur when children or teenagers take aspirin, use acetaminophen (Tylenol, Tempra, or a generic).

- In children between 6 months and 5 years of age, seizures or "fits" sometimes result from fever. These seizures are seldom harmful. During a seizure, try to protect your children from hurting themselves. Keep them away from nearby objects, and make sure they are breathing freely.

- When a child under 3 months of age has a rectal temperature over 100.4° F, call your health care provider.

How to Take a Child's Temperature

Since most children under 2 years of age cannot keep their mouths closed or remain still for an oral temperature, it is best to take their temperature rectally. Apply petroleum jelly to the thermometer for comfort, insert it about an inch into the rectum (until you can no longer see the silver end) for about 3 minutes. Be certain you hold onto the thermometer while it is in the child's rectum so that the child doesn't roll over or move and puncture his or her colon. If you seek medical advice, let your doctor or nurse know what the temperature was and if it is an oral or rectal temperature. A rectal temperature is normally 1 degree higher than an oral temperature.

DECISION GUIDE FOR FEVERS

SYMPTOMS/SIGNS	ACTION
Fever for less than 3 days without other symptoms	
Oral temperature less than or equal to 100.4° F	
Fever with sore throat, earache, or frequent cough	
Fever lasts 3 days or more	
Fever with vomiting	
Shaking, teeth-chattering chills	
Back pain or painful urination and fever	
Oral temperature over 100.4°F	
Older people with fever who are suddenly confused	
Fever with stiff neck	
Lower abdominal pain and fever for more than 2 hours	

 Use self-care   See doctor

 Call doctor's office for advice   Seek help now

For more about the symbols, see p. 2.

Through endless trips to the doctor with my kids, I've learned that fever without other symptoms is probably a viral infection that will go away within a few days. The best method of dealing with infection is rest. Put a cool cloth on the forehead, use common sense, and make sure your children save some energy to heal themselves.

Mother of eleven

Fever is only one of the many signs of childhood illness and is probably less important than the associated symptoms. Very high temperatures may be frightening to parents but are not necessarily dangerous to the child. Acetaminophen may be used for the child's complaints or symptoms, but is rarely needed for fever alone.

Pediatrician

Fever in the very young or very old is of concern and often needs medical attention. For the rest of us, plenty of fluids and a little time may be all that is needed.

Family Practitioner

I never even knew what heartburn was until I was pregnant. My daughter was breech, with her hard little head pushing up against my stomach and esophagus. In my ninth month, everything gave me heartburn, even water.

Roberta

HEARTBURN

That hamburger topped with tomatoes and raw onion with a big basket of fries sure tasted good, but 2 hours later, you feel like it's ripping a hole in your chest. Is it your stomach taking revenge? Nope—it's heartburn. And it has nothing to do with your heart.

When you eat, the muscle (sphincter) at the lower end of your esophagus relaxes and opens to admit food to your stomach. The sphincter then closes to prevent stomach acid from washing back up the esophagus. Heartburn occurs when the sphincter at the end of the esophagus doesn't close completely. Acid and bile from the stomach then come back up the esophagus, causing a burning sensation.

Nearly everyone has heartburn once in a while. Although heartburn can be treated easily with changes in diet and over-the-counter drugs, it also can be a symptom of more serious problems. Heartburn that just won't go away needs medical attention, because it may be a sign of ulcers or other gastrointestinal problems.

There are many things you can do that will reduce or relieve the symptoms of heartburn. Using the Self-Care Steps below will help cut down acid levels in your stomach, reduce pressure on your stomach or esophagus, and neutralize the effects of acid.

SELF-CARE STEPS FOR HEARTBURN

- Don't smoke.
- Don't overeat. Try eating smaller meals, more often. And don't eat within a few hours of going to bed.
- Make mealtimes relaxed. Eat slowly and chew thoroughly.
- Lose weight if you're overweight. That will reduce the pressure on the esophagus.
- Loosen or remove tight-fitting clothing when you eat.
- Don't lie down immediately after eating.
- Sleep with the head of your bed elevated.
- Avoid alcohol, caffeine, decaffeinated coffee, and any other drinks or foods that regularly cause heartburn for you.
- Avoid aspirin, ibuprofen (such as Advil), naproxen (Naprosyn), and other arthritis medications except acetaminophen.
- If needed, use over-the-counter antacids to relieve heartburn symptoms.

DECISION GUIDE FOR HEARTBURN

SYMPTOMS/SIGNS	ACTION
No relief after 2 weeks of self-care	
A drug may be causing your heartburn	
Heartburn with symptoms of heart attack, p. 86. (If you are under 35 years of age with a low risk of having a heart attack, call your doctor first. You could be having a panic attack.)	

 Call doctor's office for advice   Emergency, call 911

For more about the symbols, see p. 2.

PALPITATIONS

How many love songs speak of hearts skipping a beat? What sounds romantic can feel frightening, however.

Heart palpitations, the feeling that the heart has skipped a beat, usually are not dangerous and, in fact, everyone has them from time to time. However, a rapid heart rate or persistent palpitations should be discussed with your doctor. If you have palpitations that may be caused by panic disorder—a common cause of chest pain in people under 35 years of age—tell your doctor.

When the heart beats normally, the two smaller chambers contract together and then the two larger chambers contract together. This produces the familiar two-thump heartbeat sound. Heart palpitations, known in medical terms as arrhythmias, occur when the beating heart gets out of step. **Arrhythmias** vary from the feeling that the heart has skipped a beat to feeling that the heart is racing or fluttering.

Many arrhythmias are caused by common culprits: caffeine, nicotine, alcohol, stress, and worry. Relieving or ridding yourself of any or all of these can correct your heartbeat.

Keep in mind that serious heart conditions usually are marked by other symptoms too.

SELF-CARE STEPS FOR PALPITATIONS

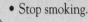

- Stop smoking.
- Avoid caffeine and alcohol.
- Exercise relieves heart palpitations for many people. When you exercise, be sure to warm up gradually, and allow yourself a cool-down period. This helps your heart return to its normal rate gradually.
- Practice stress- or anxiety-reducing techniques such as meditation, biofeedback, or yoga.

DECISION GUIDE FOR PALPITATIONS

SYMPTOMS/SIGNS	ACTION
Persistent heart palpitations or a rapid heart rate; write down exactly what happened before you call	
Palpitations and dizziness, shortness of breath, or sweating	
Palpitations and chest pain (p. 169)	

 Call doctor's office for advice   Emergency, call 911

For more about the symbols, see p. 2.

I can't tell you how many doctors I saw when I started having palpitations. I went from one to another, convinced there was something exotic wrong with me that no one could spot. It was exotic, all right—it was anxiety about my heart palpitations that was causing me to have heart palpitations. Once I learned to control my anxiety, I stopped having palpitations.

Newt

I have always prided myself on not drinking alcohol, but I drank about 20 cups of coffee and smoked two packs of cigarettes a day. One day I was sitting at work and my heart started to pound and then skip a beat. I thought I was having a heart attack. When I got to the emergency room, they did an EKG, which was normal. Then the doctor asked about coffee and cigarettes, and said those were probably the cause. I stopped smoking immediately and cut way back on drinking coffee and I've never had another "heart attack" again.

Greg

WHEEZING

If you hear a whistling sound that feels as if it's coming from your chest when you breathe out, you are wheezing.

Wheezing is caused by narrowing airways in the lungs. It's a sign that there is difficulty breathing. A common symptom of asthma (p. 207), wheezing can also be caused by bronchitis, smoking, allergies, pneumonia, sensitivities to chemicals or pollution, emphysema, lung cancer, heart failure, or even an object trapped in the airways.

The conditions that cause most cases of wheezing require medical attention. If you are under a doctor's care for asthma, for example—and have developed an action plan with your doctor—you don't have to run to the doctor's office when you start to wheeze. Just follow the physician's recommendations. If you do not have asthma and develop wheezing, call your doctor.

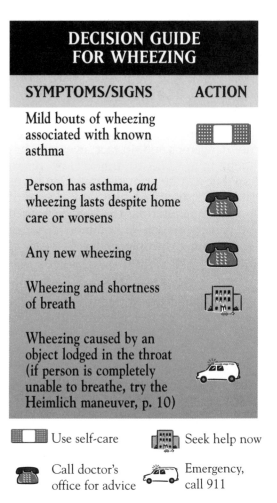

DECISION GUIDE FOR WHEEZING

SYMPTOMS/SIGNS	ACTION
Mild bouts of wheezing associated with known asthma	🔲
Person has asthma, *and* wheezing lasts despite home care or worsens	☎
Any new wheezing	☎
Wheezing and shortness of breath	🏥
Wheezing caused by an object lodged in the throat (if person is completely unable to breathe, try the Heimlich maneuver, p. 10)	🚑

🔲 Use self-care   🏥 Seek help now

☎ Call doctor's office for advice   🚑 Emergency, call 911

For more about the symbols, see p. 2.

MUSCLE AND JOINT PROBLEMS

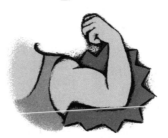

Your muscular and skeletal systems have remarkable jobs. From everyday tasks like typing to dramatic athletic feats like windsurfing and gymnastics, your muscles and bones perform day after day and year after year. Although you may complain about the aches and pains that come with aging, you are lucky to have a musculoskeletal system that signals when you have pushed too hard. This section describes common problems of your muscles and joints and suggests ways to take care of nonurgent conditions at home. *This information cannot replace care by your health care providers.*

Your primary care doctor (pediatrician, family practitioner, or internal medicine specialist) can offer advice and treatment for most muscle and joint problems. If your condition is very hard to handle, your primary care doctor may involve other medical providers who specialize in those problems, such as physiatrists, physical therapists, orthopedists, or sports medicine specialists.

Use the Decision Guides to see if your symptoms warrant medical attention or if they can be handled with self-care. However, you need to consider your own medical history and your current health when deciding if self-care is right for you. If you have any conditions that do not seem to be healing normally or if self-care steps do not seem helpful, you should call your health care provider.

ACHES AND PAINS IN MUSCLES AND JOINTS

Whether it's your shoulder, ankle, or some joint in between, pain in or around joints has similar causes and treatments throughout the body. Of course, a broken bone will cause pain and limit movement, but more often joint pain and limited mobility are caused by an injury to muscles, ligaments, or connective tissue. Knowing what happened before the pain started gives you an important clue to the problem. The following are common causes of muscle and joint pain.

Accidents

A fall, bump, blow, or sudden twist can cause bruising of soft tissues; bone fractures; joint dislocations; or torn muscles, tendons, or ligaments.

Repetitive Motions or Prolonged Overuse

All good things require moderation—including work and play. Too much of any activity—such as pitching too many games of softball, or working long hours typing at a computer—can cause inflammation and pain to the joint and surrounding tissues.

Overdoing It

If you've been indoors and inactive for months, a 25-mile bike ride or a day digging in the garden is apt to cause some muscle soreness. Injuries from overdoing it occur most often when people do

I cross-country and downhill ski in the winter and do a lot of bicycling in the summer. Some of the guys at work give me a hard time because at least once a year I'll show up at work wrapped in an elastic bandage or on crutches. My response is this: If you're serious about fitness, you're probably going to have some minor injuries once in a while. If you just watch TV all the time, you are less likely to get injured, but a lot more likely to die of a heart attack. I'll take the sprains and strains any day.

Richard

strenuous activities without slowly building the strength and endurance needed. In addition, older people may be likely to injure themselves due to aging tissues.

Muscle Imbalance

When muscles on one side of the body are much stronger than those on the other side (for example, biceps that are stronger than triceps), they put added stress on weaker muscles, often causing injury. For example, a weight lifter who overdevelops the chest and arm muscles, but neglects the muscles that support the upper back and shoulder blades, may wind up with a back or neck injury. The reason: the chest muscles overpower the back, causing constant tightness and muscle or joint pain.

Referred Pain

Sometimes pain felt in one area of the body originates in a different area. For example, pain in the left shoulder or arm may be a sign of a heart attack. Likewise, knee pain may be caused by a hip or foot problem. Whenever pain appears suddenly without an apparent cause, such as accident or injury, call your doctor. If you feel sudden left-arm pain, chest tightness, shortness of breath, or pain in the jaw with no apparent cause, **call 911** immediately.

SPECIAL CONCERNS FOR CHILDREN

Muscle and joint pains in children are treated much the same as they are in adults. Children and teenagers, however, should be given acetaminophen (Tylenol) to relieve pain. *Do not give aspirin, ibuprofen (Advil), or naproxen (Aleve) because these drugs can cause Reye's syndrome.* If the child can't move the joint, or pain increases with movement, call a doctor. Inability to bend a joint can be a sign of a fractured bone or infection in the joint—both are serious conditions.

Until a child reaches maturity, the long bones in the body (arms and legs) have growth plates, called *epiphyses*. The epiphysis allows the bone to grow or lengthen. A fracture or dislocation can damage the epiphysis. This may slow or stop a bone's growth or make the bone grow crooked. Although it is common sense that any suspected broken bone should be seen by a doctor, this is very important if the child complains of pain around a joint. A fracture to the epiphysis can occur without trauma, often through overuse (pitching too many fast balls or lifting heavy weights).

Broken bones and other injuries aside, it is common for children having growth spurts to have vague aches and pains for no apparent reason (see Lower-Leg Pain, Special Concerns for Children, p. 128).

SELF-CARE STEPS FOR ACHES AND PAINS IN MUSCLES AND JOINTS

With a few exceptions, the **RICE** (Rest, Ice, Compress, Elevate) method explained below will reduce pain and help speed recovery of joint and muscle injuries.

Rest. For most injuries, rest the area until the pain stops. For simple sore muscles, however, gentle stretching will reduce stiffness more quickly. Hold the stretch for 30 to 60 seconds, then rest and repeat 5 to 10 times. Do this several times a day.

Ice. Ice is the most effective treatment for reducing inflammation, pain, and swelling of injured muscles, joints, and connective tissues—such as tendons, ligaments, and bursas. The cold helps keep blood and fluid from building up in the injured area, reducing pain and swelling. Apply ice as soon as possible after injury, even if you are going straight to the doctor. To speed recovery and ease pain, raise the injured area and apply ice for 20 minutes (10 to 15 minutes in children) every 2 to 3 hours while awake. For best results, use crushed ice in a moist towel as an ice pack. Use an elastic bandage to hold the pack in place. During the first 48 to 72 hours, or as long as there is any swelling, *do not apply heat* to an injury. Heat increases blood flow to the affected area, which makes swelling and pain worse.

Compress. Between icings, wrap the injured area with an elastic (Ace type) bandage to help control swelling and provide support. Begin wrapping at the farthest point away from the body and wrap toward the heart. For example, to wrap an ankle you would begin at the toes and wrap to the mid-calf. Don't sleep with the wrap on, unless told to do so by a doctor. And **don't wrap too tightly!** If the wrap begins to cause pain or numbness, or if toes are cool or white, remove the elastic bandage and wrap it more loosely.

Elevate. Raising the injured area above your heart will allow gravity to help reduce swelling by draining excess fluid. At night, place a pillow under the area to support and raise it.

In addition to RICE, there are several other things you can do to promote healing and relieve pain of most muscle and joint injuries. These are the basics to remember, but check the section on the next pages that addresses the joint where you are having pain.

If you need to, take NSAIDs (nonsteroidal anti-inflammatory drugs). Acetaminophen, aspirin, and NSAIDs often effectively treat muscle and joint injuries. Sometimes NSAIDs and aspirin work best because they reduce inflammation. Acetaminophen doesn't reduce inflammation. Aspirin and other NSAIDs are often more irritating to the stomach and bowel so that acetaminophen is better for patients with ulcers or other gastrointestinal problems or for those who try NSAIDs and suffer gastric problems. When using aspirin, choose buffered aspirin or enteric-coated aspirin. All aspirin and NSAIDs should be taken with food. If NSAIDs cause minor gastrointestinal upset after 7 to 10 days of use, stop medication, take antacids, and call your doctor. Children and teenagers with muscle or joint injuries should be given *acetaminophen only*, unless your doctor says otherwise. Because of the risk of Reye's syndrome, they should not be given aspirin, ibuprofen, or naproxen.

Slowly strengthen the injured area. Slow strengthening of the injured area after it has healed is advisable for keeping most injuries from occurring again. Your doctor or a physical therapist can recommend specific exercises, including range-of-motion exercises, muscle stretches, and specific weight training.

Heat before, ice after. Once the swelling has subsided—often it takes weeks—and you are working to strengthen the recovering area, you may apply heat before exercise to prepare the muscles, joint, and connective tissues for the workout. Apply ice soon after your workout to prevent inflammation and swelling.

I sprained my knee skiing last winter and had to use crutches. I was the most popular kid at school the day I showed up with those crutches. Everyone wanted to try them out. While my friends took turns on the crutches, I limped around on my sore knee. That night it started to swell up again pretty bad. I had to go back to the doctor and have the water drained from the knee. That really hurt. So, I'd tell other kids with sprained knees not to let anyone else use your crutches. It's important not to put weight on a sprained knee.

Anna, age 9

I've fallen and hurt myself a number of times recently. I'm 76 and, at my age, I don't heal up as fast as I once did. After I sprained my wrist last spring, the doctor suggested I start exercising to build up my strength. Now I go for a walk every morning. At night while I'm watching TV, I use a resistance band—it's like a big rubber band—on my arms and legs. I really think it's helped. I don't feel quite so fragile anymore.

Latisha

DEFINITIONS OF COMMON MUSCLE AND JOINT PROBLEMS

Arthritis Inflammation, pain, swelling, stiffness and redness, or damage in joints. Arthritis may involve one joint or many joints, and has a number of causes.

Bruise Bleeding and damage to tissue underneath the skin, from a blow or fall. *Treatment:* apply ice right after injury.

Bursitis Swelling and inflammation of a bursa, causing pain and, occasionally, loss of motion. Bursas are fluid-filled sacs that lubricate and cushion joints. Bursitis can be caused by pressure (leaning on elbow), friction from overuse, or an injury. *Treatment:* RICE method (p. 97); see a doctor if symptoms persist more than 7 days.

Dislocation Separation of a joint, usually with tearing of the ligaments and capsule that support it. Dislocations can often accompany fractures. Deformity is usually visible, and movement is restricted. *Treatment:* leave the joint alone—*do not try to put it back!* However, try to support the limb in a comfortable position if possible. Apply ice and **call 911**, or if the patient can walk, take him or her to an emergency room.

Fracture A break in a bone, most often caused by a blow or fall. This may range in seriousness from a hairline fracture to a compound fracture (bones protrude through skin). Symptoms may include point tenderness over a bone, shooting pain, visible deformity, increased pain with movement, and, in severe cases, bone protruding through the skin. *Treatment:* if fracture is suspected, see a physician. If a spinal injury is suspected or the patient cannot walk, **call 911**.

Do not move the person. Until help arrives, apply ice to the area. If there is bleeding, apply pressure to stop the bleeding.

Ganglion A soft, fluid-filled cyst on the sheath of a tendon that may range from marble to golf-ball size. It is commonly found in the wrist, fingers, and foot; however, it may occur anywhere. Treatment is needed only if a ganglion is painful. Ganglions often disappear on their own.

Gout A disease that causes pain, swelling, redness, and extreme tenderness of a joint. An acute attack usually affects a single joint, most commonly in the big toe. Other joints commonly affected include those of the foot, ankle, knee, or wrist. Pain worsens within the first 24 to 36 hours and may be so severe that the touch of a bedsheet is too much. Gout can be treated with prescription drugs. Call your doctor as soon as possible.

Muscle cramp/spasm An involuntary shortening of a muscle, creating a painful spasm. Cramps can be caused by overuse, too much sweating, lactic acid buildup during or after exercise, or poor circulation (nighttime leg cramps). *Treatment:* stretch the muscle very slowly, apply ice, and drink plenty of fluids.

Muscle soreness/stiffness Usually results from overuse and is caused by microscopic muscle damage or lactic acid building up in the muscles. *Treatment:* drink plenty of water and move as much as is comfortable (such as walking or stretching). Stretch before and after exercise. Heat and massage can also be helpful.

DEFINITIONS OF COMMON MUSCLE AND JOINT PROBLEMS

Repetitive motion injuries These injuries can affect any tendon or muscle in the body. (Severe, long episodes may cause joint damage.) They are usually caused by too much of a particular motion—throwing, squeezing, lifting, pushing, or pulling. The injury may be a combination of tendinitis, bursitis, or trauma to specific tissues. *Treatment:* limit or stop the motion, alternately apply cold and heat, take anti-inflammatory medications, engage in physical therapy and exercise. Sit, stand, or move in ways that avoid stress on affected joints and tendons.

Rotator cuff injuries The term "rotator cuff injuries" is often used as a catch-all to describe more than one problem, including tiny tears of the tendons supporting the shoulder (the rotator cuff) and impingement syndrome (compressing the tendons between bones, resulting in painful inflammation). The cause, result, and treatment, however, are similar. Repetitive overhead motions, such as throwing a softball, painting a ceiling, or swimming, often cause rotator cuff injuries. Symptoms include shoulder pain at night and pain when raising or lowering the arm between waist and shoulder height. If impingement occurs, pain may be worst when the arm is raised with the palm turned down—as when emptying a soda pop can. Tingling or numbness in the arm or fingers may also be felt.

Sprain Stretching or tearing a ligament beyond the normal range of motion. Ligaments connect bone to bone. Sprains may occur at any joint, but are most common in ankles, knees, wrists, and fingers. Symptoms include swelling, pain, and bruising. *Treatment:* RICE method (p. 97) for at least 72 hours, or until swelling begins to decrease.

Strain Stretching or tearing a muscle or tendon past its normal range of motion. Strains most often occur in the middle of the muscle. Symptoms include pain, swelling, muscle spasm, and limited movement. *Treatment:* ice, massage, and gently stretch the muscle three to five times a day.

Tendinitis Painful inflammation of the tendon. It is usually caused by overuse or an injury. Symptoms may include pain, tenderness, minor swelling, and sometimes limited motion. *Treatment:* RICE method (p. 97) and anti-inflammatory drugs.

ACUTE ARTHRITIS

The word *arthritis* means "inflammation of the joint." It is used to describe more than 100 different conditions, each of which has symptoms and an individual treatment plan based on your doctor's diagnosis.

When people feel joint pain, most think the symptoms are arthritis. Not all joint pain is due to arthritis, however. Often, joint or muscle pain is caused by problems with the structures around the joint, such as tendons, bursas, ligaments, or muscle.

Common Symptoms

In deciding what kind of self-care may be right for joint pain, it is helpful to learn the difference between pain that is likely to be caused by arthritis and pain that is probably a result of other problems.

Joint pain that is *not* due to arthritis (often caused by tendinitis, bursitis, or muscle strains) usually has the following features:

- Usually no swelling or joint damage

- Joint can usually be moved without a lot of difficulty

- Often follows a recent bout of activity

The kind of **joint pain that *is* due to arthritis** usually has one or the other of the following features:

- Fluid buildup and swelling about the joint

- Change in the physical appearance of the joint

Joint pain due to arthritis may last for many weeks, months, or longer.

NORMAL JOINT   ARTHRITIC JOINT

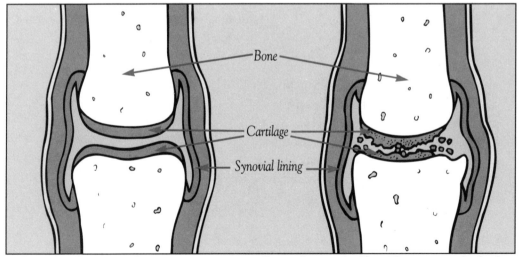

Arthritis, the inflammation of a joint, can cause pain, swelling, stiffness, and redness. There are many kinds of arthritis. The illustration on the right is typical of osteoarthritis, where the protective cartilage cushion on the bone breaks down and the bones of the joint rub against one another.

Types of Arthritis

There are two main types of arthritis: inflammatory and noninflammatory. Each has features that set it apart from other types of joint pain.

Inflammatory Arthritis

There are three main types of inflammatory arthritis: *rheumatoid arthritis, gout,* and *arthritis caused by infections*. Signs of inflammatory arthritis include:

• Swelling

• Redness, warmth, tenderness

• Loss of motion or function of the joint

• Often causes joint damage

The start of inflammatory arthritis varies from person to person. For some people, this type of arthritis pain can be sudden and intense. For others, the pain is gradual.

Noninflammatory Arthritis

The most common type of noninflammatory arthritis is osteoarthritis. Signs of osteoarthritis include:

• Minor to nonexistent swelling

• Changes in the joint cartilage, which can lead to joint damage, pain, loss of function

Osteoarthritis starts slowly, usually over many months to years.

SELF-CARE STEPS FOR ACUTE ARTHRITIS

For a detailed discussion, see Self-Care Steps for Chronic Arthritis, p. 204.

DECISION GUIDE FOR ACUTE ARTHRITIS

SYMPTOMS/SIGNS	ACTION
Pain without swelling or fever	
Pain lasts and obviously affects your normal activities	
Sudden, intense joint pain that lasts for more than 1 hour	
Sudden and/or a lot of swelling	
Temperature of 100.4° F or higher, combined with sudden, intense joint pain lasting for more than 1 hour and/or sudden or significant swelling	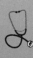

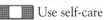 Use self-care   See doctor

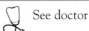 Call doctor's office for advice *For more about the symbols, see p. 2.*

I twisted my ankle walking down a flight of stairs. I don't know how I did it, but it really hurt. After a few minutes, the pain wasn't as bad and I could walk with a limp. I thought I was OK, but a friend said I should put ice on it right away to decrease any swelling. She was right. After a while my ankle began to swell and bruise. I kept my foot raised, iced it four to five times a day, and kept it wrapped between icings. The swelling stopped and I was able to walk. About 3 days after I sprained it, I started doing gentle ankle stretches each day. The stiffness went away and the strength in my ankle returned.

Tony

ANKLE PAIN

The ankle is one of the most commonly injured joints of the body. Strains and sprains reign in ankle injuries, but tendinitis, bursitis, and fractures also happen.

The ankle is the juncture of three bones: the tibia and fibula of the lower leg and the talus of the foot (the ankle bone). Held together by ligaments and tendons, the ankle allows the foot a wide range of motion. Because of the ankle's crucial role in walking and standing, ankle injuries should be taken seriously and treated properly.

Strains, Sprains, and Fractures

Twisting your ankle may cause stretching or tearing of the ligaments and tendons (for definitions of strains, sprains, and fractures, see p. 98). This most often occurs on the outside of the ankle. Mild strains or sprains may cause mild to moderate pain and little or no swelling. The ankle can support weight, but usually a limp is apparent. Moderate sprains hurt more when you move, and swelling and tenderness increase. Walking is hard and often crutches are needed for a few days.

A sprain is generally severe when the ligament and tendons are stretched or

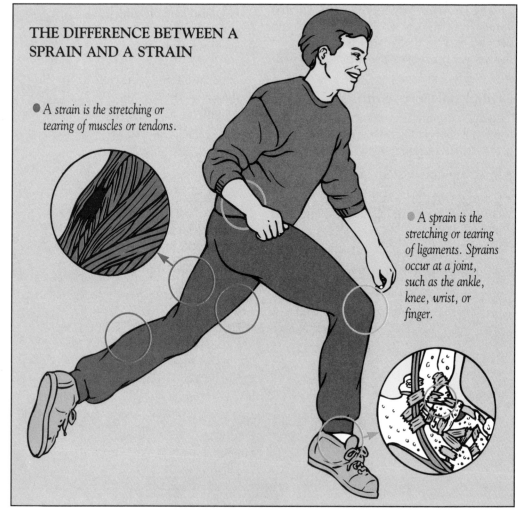

THE DIFFERENCE BETWEEN A SPRAIN AND A STRAIN

● *A strain is the stretching or tearing of muscles or tendons.*

● *A sprain is the stretching or tearing of ligaments. Sprains occur at a joint, such as the ankle, knee, wrist, or finger.*

completely torn (ruptured). Severe sprains are accompanied by severe pain, swelling and tenderness, limited motion, bruising, and inability to walk or bear weight on the ankle. Moderate and severe sprains also may cause bruising in the foot and toes, and up the side of the leg.

With a strain, sprain, or fracture, you may hear or feel a snap, pop, or crack at the time of injury. The RICE method (p. 97) is the right first step for both. A fracture is very difficult to diagnose without an X-ray. A severe injury should be seen by a doctor. Unless the ankle is obviously deformed, very painful, or unable to bear any weight, a sprained ankle can be treated safely at home for the first 24 hours using the RICE method and avoiding weight on the sprain. With a mild or moderate sprain, swelling should stop within 24 hours and the ankle should begin to improve (although not be healed) within 48 hours. If it doesn't, see a doctor.

Because of the strength of the ligament on the inner ankle, often bone will give way before the ligament does. Pain on the inner ankle can often be a fracture and should be X-rayed in most cases.

Achilles Tendinitis and Bursitis

Tendinitis and bursitis at the back of the ankle are very much alike. The treatment, causes, and symptoms of the two are similar. The Achilles tendon is a large strong band that attaches the calf muscle to the heel. Underneath the Achilles tendon are bursas that may also become inflamed.

Symptoms of **Achilles tendinitis** include pain in the calf and ankle, which is worse when you wake up in the morning and generally gets better as the ankle is "warmed-up" with use. Occasionally, with an improper warm-up or sudden movement, the Achilles tendon can tear or even rupture. Any deformity in the calf should be seen by a doctor right away. **Bursitis** usually causes a soft, fluid-filled lump at the back of the ankle, along with pain similar to that of tendinitis.

Common causes of tendinitis and bursitis in the ankle include tight calf muscles, overuse, sudden stress from a quick movement, and repeated motion, such as running. But you don't have to be athletic to have either problem. Shoes are often the culprit. Switching from high heels or cowboy boots to flat shoes or wearing shoes that fit poorly or provide

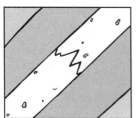

Simple Fracture
Bone breaks but does not puncture the skin.

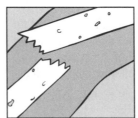

Compound Fracture
Bone breaks and punctures the flesh and skin.

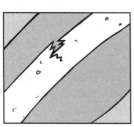

Greenstick Fracture
One side of a bent bone breaks; usually occurs in children.

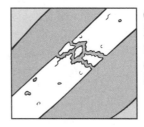

Comminuted Fracture
Bone shatters into more than two pieces; most often caused by a heavy blow.

inadequate support and cushioning can also inflame tendons and bursas in the ankle.

Gout

Sudden pain, swelling, redness, and extreme tenderness in a joint are usually the signs of an acute attack of gout. Most often gout begins in the big toe, but may move up the leg to other joints, including the ankle and knee. If you have these symptoms of gout (see definition, p. 98), call your doctor. Gout can be treated effectively with prescription drugs.

Swelling without Injury

Sitting or standing for long periods without moving may cause the ankles and feet to swell. This type of swelling usually goes away overnight or lasts only a few days. But swollen ankles can also be a sign of something more serious, such as phlebitis (p. 126) or congestive heart failure (p. 126). If your ankles remain swollen for more than 3 days or if just one leg is affected, call your doctor.

SELF-CARE STEPS FOR ANKLE PAIN

As with other joint injuries, the first step in treatment for most ankle injuries—including sprains, strains, and Achilles tendinitis and bursitis—is the RICE method and anti-inflammatory drugs (p. 97). But there are some other things you can do to treat sprains and other injuries:

Sprains
• Stay off the ankle as much as possible until the swelling stops, usually about 24 to 48 hours.

• Use the RICE method (p. 97).

• Use crutches if bearing weight is painful.

• If swelling lasts longer than 3 days, alternately soak the ankle in cold water (45° to 60° F) for 1 minute and then in warm water (100° to 105° F) for 2 or 3 minutes. Do this for 15 to 20 minutes total, and stop if swelling

increases. Print the alphabet in the air with your big toe to help increase range of motion.

• As the swelling and pain decrease, begin gentle stretching and strengthening exercises to regain range of motion.

Other injuries
Strains Follow the RICE method (p. 97) and avoid bearing weight on the ankle for 24 to 48 hours. If pain and swelling are worse after 24 hours, call your health care provider. If you still can't bear weight on the ankle after 48 hours, see your health care provider. As the swelling and pain decrease, begin gentle stretching and strengthening exercises to regain range of motion (see illustration on this page).

Tendinitis Decrease activity for 1 to 2 weeks or until fairly pain free. Apply heat to the area before stretching, and ice when you have finished. If there is no improvement in 10 to 14 days, call your doctor.

Gout Raise your legs and apply ice, if you can stand it. Call your doctor for prescription drugs.

Swelling If your ankles swell after you've been sitting or standing for a long time, raise your legs. Increase activity and movement to prevent swelling. If swelling continues longer than 3 days or if there is pain without injury, see your health care provider immediately.

RANGE OF MOTION EXERCISE

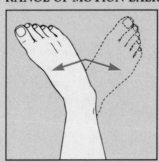

Keeping your leg still, bend your ankle back and forth from left to right ten times. Repeat this exercise several times a day.

DECISION GUIDE FOR ANKLE PAIN

SYMPTOMS/SIGNS	ACTION
Swelling, pain, and possible bruising from sudden twist or force	
Pain at back of ankle—begins slowly and may be worse when you wake up (Achilles tendinitis)	
No improvement of tendinitis symptoms after 10 to 14 days	
Unable to bear any weight after hearing or feeling a pop/snap/crack	
Pain and swelling increasing 24 hours after injury	
Red/warm/swollen ankles; fever; feeling ill or having recently been ill with a sore throat or skin infection	
Chronic swelling in ankles, feet or lower legs; difficulty breathing (see congestive heart failure, p. 126)	
Swelling in only one ankle or leg with pain, no injury (see phlebitis, p. 126)	
Pain on inner side of ankle; ankle twisted inward when injury occurred (see fracture, p. 102)	

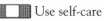 Use self-care

 See doctor

 Call doctor's office for advice

For more about the symbols, see p. 2.

BACK PAIN

Backaches are one of the most common reasons for a visit to a doctor. Studies show that four out of every five people in the U.S. will suffer a serious bout of back pain at some time in their lives. Back pain is rarely the result of one incident. Rather, most back problems result from a lifetime of stress or strain to the back a little at a time.

Poor posture, improper lifting habits, prolonged standing, a stressful job, or declining physical fitness can all add up to a bad back. One episode of disabling back pain may simply be a cue that you have put more stress on your back than it can handle.

Weakened or strained muscles, over time, are responsible for most back pain. Only about 10 percent of back complaints are linked to pressure on the nerves in your back—this type of pain tends to spread more into your buttocks or legs.

Patience is your greatest healer when your back has been strained. You may be surprised that often your doctor cannot find the exact muscles or ligaments injured. The doctor can find out if the problem is not in the muscle/skeletal system. However, we do know that most patients do well with a week or two of self-care.

Family Practitioner

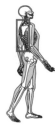

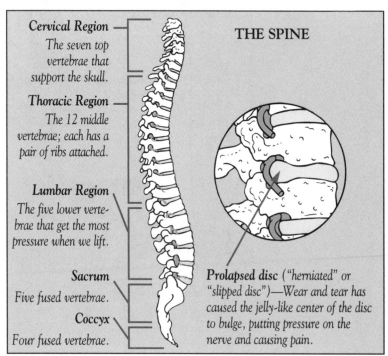

THE SPINE

Cervical Region
The seven top vertebrae that support the skull.

Thoracic Region
The 12 middle vertebrae; each has a pair of ribs attached.

Lumbar Region
The five lower vertebrae that get the most pressure when we lift.

Sacrum
Five fused vertebrae.

Coccyx
Four fused vertebrae.

Prolapsed disc ("herniated" or "slipped disc")—Wear and tear has caused the jelly-like center of the disc to bulge, putting pressure on the nerve and causing pain.

I have found that for many cases of frequent backache a good swimming or water aerobics routine three times a week can help. Remember to start slowly and don't expect too much too soon. It can take 4 to 6 weeks to improve conditioning and reduce back pain.

Rehabilitation Specialist

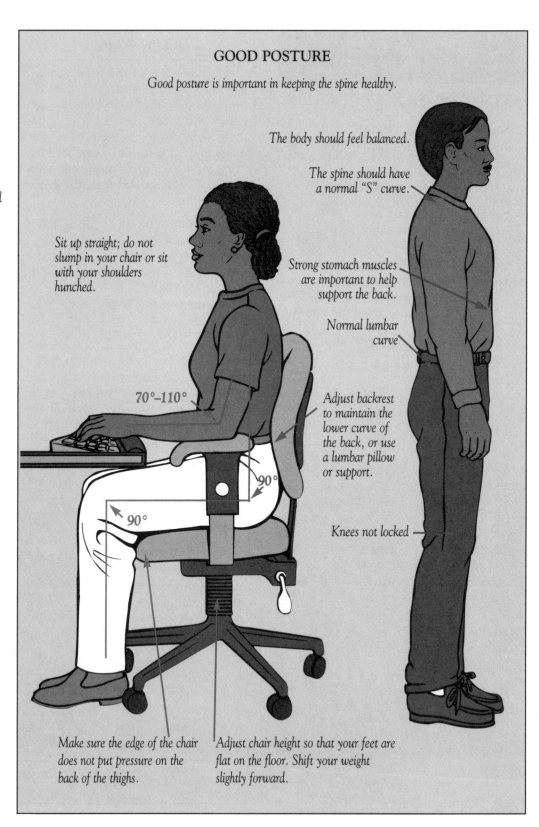

GOOD POSTURE

Good posture is important in keeping the spine healthy.

The body should feel balanced.

The spine should have a normal "S" curve.

Sit up straight; do not slump in your chair or sit with your shoulders hunched.

Strong stomach muscles are important to help support the back.

Normal lumbar curve

70°–110°

Adjust backrest to maintain the lower curve of the back, or use a lumbar pillow or support.

90°

90°

Knees not locked

Make sure the edge of the chair does not put pressure on the back of the thighs.

Adjust chair height so that your feet are flat on the floor. Shift your weight slightly forward.

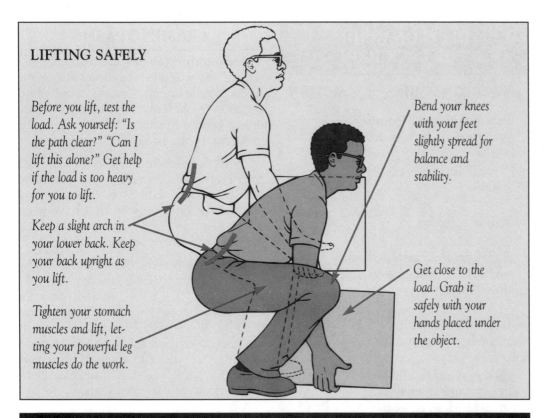

LIFTING SAFELY

Before you lift, test the load. Ask yourself: "Is the path clear?" "Can I lift this alone?" Get help if the load is too heavy for you to lift.

Keep a slight arch in your lower back. Keep your back upright as you lift.

Tighten your stomach muscles and lift, letting your powerful leg muscles do the work.

Bend your knees with your feet slightly spread for balance and stability.

Get close to the load. Grab it safely with your hands placed under the object.

Getting back to work or your usual daily activity within a few days is an important part of healing. You can start with either "light" duties or limited activities. It probably will be a little uncomfortable, but limited activity prevents your back from becoming weak and stiff.

Rob, back pain patient

SELF-CARE STEPS FOR BACK PAIN

• The most important health care treatment is *the care that you give to yourself.* If you fail to take an active role in treating your back, a bad cycle can develop. To protect yourself from pain, you may tend to become less active. But if you are inactive, your muscles become weaker and more susceptible to strains or sprains. So it's just as important to practice exercises and postures that protect your muscles for the *future* as it is to rest your back when you need to.

• Take aspirin. Although no drug can speed up the healing process, aspirin should relieve occasional pain. For children and teenagers, use acetaminophen (Tylenol, Tempra, or a generic) instead of aspirin.

• Take it easy for the first few days. Ice packs on the sore area will keep the inflammation down, and bed rest may help. If lying down is uncomfortable, try keeping your knees raised.

• Use warm packs to increase circulation and healing after the first few days. Light massages or warm baths may help to provide relief.

• Carefully add activities back into your day as you begin to recover from the worst of your back pain. Gradual stretches and regular walking are good ways to get back into action.

• Learn safe back exercises like modified sit-ups and low back stretches, and do them regularly.

• Take time to relax. Tension will only make your back feel worse.

I always scoffed at my inactive brother who complained about his back. I was a runner and general exercise junkie, and I was treating my body right, by golly. Imagine my surprise when I became nearly incapacitated with back and leg muscle spasms after running a marathon. The pain was terrible. My trainer suggested changes in diet and more liquids, and that helped.

Ron

DECISION GUIDE FOR BACK PAIN

SYMPTOMS/SIGNS	ACTION
Pain from tension, "posture" pain, soreness from exercise	
"Usual" back or neck soreness	
Pain lasts for days	
Back pain and temperature over 100° F lasting longer than 48 hours	
Back pain and nausea, vomiting, or diarrhea	
Back pain and painful or frequent urination, menstrual bleeding, or stomachache	
Pain traveling down leg or arm; paralysis or numbness of a lower limb	
Paralysis, confusion, or shock (see Shock, p. 36)	

Note: Worker's Compensation regulations require that any injury occurring at work be reported.

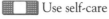 Use self-care   See doctor

 Call doctor's office for advice   Seek help now

For more about the symbols, see p. 2.

CRAMPS/SPASMS

There's nothing to propel you out of bed with a shout in the middle of the night like a muscle cramp. Cramps occur when the muscle suddenly contracts. Why they often happen in the middle of the night, however, is one of life's little mysteries.

Both activity and inactivity can lead to cramps and spasms. Muscles that have been overused, such as in exercise, may cramp. Similarly, muscles that have been underused, such as by sitting in the same position too long, also may cramp.

There are several theories about why muscles cramp. One theory is that cramps are the result of dehydration. Another theory is that cramps result from low levels of calcium and/or potassium. Because these are just theories, and evidence of the effectiveness of treatment may vary, you may find that nothing works to relieve your cramps.

Most muscle cramps aren't signs of a serious problem. Still, dealing with them promptly may help provide relief from pain—and there's no ignoring the pain from a muscle cramp.

SELF-CARE STEPS FOR CRAMPS/SPASMS

 • Stretch out the cramped muscle. For a leg cramp, sit with your leg flat on the floor and pull your toes toward you. For a foot cramp, walk on it.

• You can easily locate the muscle that's cramping. Gently but firmly massage the cramp.

• Another pain management technique that works for some people is pinching the upper lip. Tightly squeeze the skin of your upper lip, just below the nose, between your thumb and index finger.

• Take acetaminophen or ibuprofen for pain that continues after the cramp.

• Drink plenty of liquids before, during, and after exercise. Although water is best, any other drinks (except caffeinated ones, which cause dehydration) are fine. Drink an hour before exercising, and then every 12 to 15 minutes during exercise.

• Be sure to warm up and cool down before and after exercising.

• Changes in diet are sometimes recommended for controlling cramps. Try to add more calcium- and potassium-rich foods to your diet. Eat low-fat dairy products to increase calcium; foods such as dried apricots, whole-grain cereal, dried lentils, dried peaches, bananas, citrus fruits, and fresh vegetables are good sources of potassium. Even if these changes do not help your cramps, it won't hurt to get more variety into your diet.

DECISION GUIDE FOR CRAMPS/SPASMS

SYMPTOMS/SIGNS	ACTION
Occasional cramps that come and go	
Prevention steps don't relieve episodes of muscle cramps or spasms after several weeks	
Heaviness and pain deep in the leg or calf muscle (also see Lower-Leg Pain, p. 126) or swelling, redness or unusual warmth	
Neck or back spasm plus numbness, tingling, or weakness	

 Use self-care

 Call doctor's office for advice

For more about the symbols, see p. 2.

ELBOW PAIN

The elbow lets the hand turn from palm up to palm down, position itself to write, turn a screwdriver or doorknob…and the list goes on.

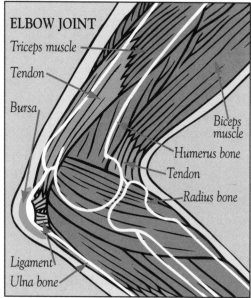

ELBOW JOINT
Triceps muscle
Tendon
Bursa
Biceps muscle
Humerus bone
Tendon
Radius bone
Ligament
Ulna bone

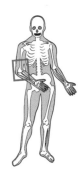

The elbow is the junction of three bones: the humerus in the upper arm and the ulna and radius in the lower arm. Tendons and muscles provide mobility and more support, and bursas within the joint cushion and lubricate the elbow's movement. The bony point at the back of the elbow is the end of the ulna, and two smaller bony points on either side are called *epicondyles*.

Pain in the elbow can occur from overuse, a fall or blow to the joint, or a force that causes the elbow to bend backward. Some common elbow injuries are discussed on the next page.

My husband and I had planned a wonderful rafting trip with friends. I don't normally work out at all, but I didn't think rowing a raft on a fairly fast-running river would be very strenuous. I was wrong. About 2 hours into the expedition, I could feel a "clicking" on the inner side of my right elbow. By the time we pulled out of the water, I could barely row. That night in our tent, a sharp pain began in my elbow. It hurt so bad, I could barely sleep. I iced down the elbow and took some aspirin. In the morning, the pain wasn't so bad, but another day of rowing was out of the question. A friend happened to have an elastic bandage; wrapping the elbow helped. After returning home, I called the doctor's office. They said it was probably tendinitis and recommended some exercises and stretches to help strengthen the area and prevent future injury.

Joanne

Tendinitis

Elbow tendinitis is called by many names—tennis elbow, golfer's elbow, pitcher's elbow—but can be caused by any number of repeated motions. The action isn't as important as the repetition.

Tendinitis pain usually is concentrated at the inside or outside of the elbow and may spread up or down the arm, depending on which tendon is inflamed. Often the pain occurs only with certain movements, such as lifting objects in certain ways, rotating your hand, or

SELF-CARE STEPS FOR ELBOW PAIN

• Tendinitis, bursitis, and hyperextended elbow in adults can usually be treated effectively using the RICE method and anti-inflammatory drugs (p. 97) until the pain and swelling decrease. Rarely is a doctor's care needed for these conditions.

• It is very important to rest from the activity that caused the pain in the first place. But this might not be possible if the injury is from a task that's a normal part of a job (for example, hammering for carpenters). If this is the case, consult your doctor.

• Gentle stretching and strengthening exercises are also an important part of recovery and preventing future injury. Stretches, along with arm curls using light weights or squeezing a rubber ball in the palm of your hand, are examples of exercises you can do to regain strength and range of motion after the pain is better. Ask your doctor to recommend specific exercises for you.

SPECIAL CONCERNS FOR CHILDREN

Elbow injuries aren't common in children, but when they occur they can be serious. If left untreated, a fractured elbow from a fall or blow or elbow overuse injuries—often from baseball pitching and weight training—can interfere with bone growth.

The term "Little League Elbow" refers to a variety of overuse injuries in the elbows of young baseball players—especially pitchers—and sometimes in gymnasts. On the milder end is tendinitis at the inner side of the elbow. Pain and stiffness usually build gradually over several days. Until the pain and tenderness disappear entirely, the child should not throw a ball or exercise the elbow. This may take as long as 6 weeks to 6 months. Continued throwing may cause the growth center in the bone to separate

from the main bone. If the separation becomes too great, the bone may begin to grow crooked or stop growing entirely.

In severe cases, overuse injuries of the elbow can cause fragments of bone and cartilage to break off into the elbow joint, causing pain, stiffness, and even occasional grinding or clicking sounds. Left untreated, this can cause permanent damage to the joint.

Because of its potential seriousness, elbow pain in children and adolescents should always be evaluated by a doctor. To prevent injury, young baseball players should follow league rules limiting the number of practices and games they can pitch.

clenching or squeezing something in your fist. Treatment is the same, no matter which tendon is involved (see Self-Care Steps p. 110).

Bursitis

Inflammation of a bursa causes a soft, fluid-filled lump at the point of the elbow. Bursitis can be quite painful, especially at the tip of the elbow. Acute bursitis, if not adequately treated, can lead to chronic bursitis and small, painful lumps at the point of the elbow can form. With self-care, acute cases will usually heal within 7 to 10 days. See your health care provider if the bursa is red or hot, the elbow looks infected, or pain and swelling do not improve by this time.

Cubital Tunnel Syndrome

A blow to the "funny bone" isn't really funny. In fact, it can be very painful. But more than that, if often repeated (for example, in contact sports), blows to the back of the elbow may cause scar tissue to form over the ulnar nerve, which runs along the "tunnel" or groove between the inner side of the elbow and the point of the elbow (the ulna). Cubital tunnel syndrome causes loss of strength in the hand and numbness and tingling that spread from the elbow down to the ring and little fingers. Because the pressure on the nerve is usually caused by scar tissue, surgery may be needed to free the nerve.

Hyperextended Elbow

This occurs when the elbow is "bent backward" by force, such as from a fall or a backhand tennis swing that goes awry. The result is pain and swelling in the joint capsule and soft tissues at the front of the elbow. A splint or sling to support the elbow may be needed until the pain stops. With self-care (described on p. 110), recovery can be expected within 3 to 6 weeks.

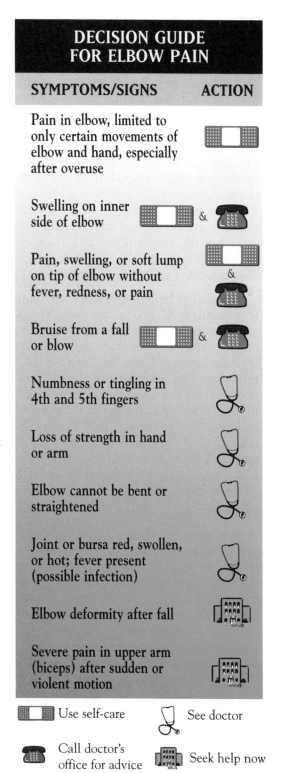

DECISION GUIDE FOR ELBOW PAIN

SYMPTOMS/SIGNS	ACTION
Pain in elbow, limited to only certain movements of elbow and hand, especially after overuse	Use self-care
Swelling on inner side of elbow	Use self-care & Call doctor's office
Pain, swelling, or soft lump on tip of elbow without fever, redness, or pain	Use self-care & Call doctor's office
Bruise from a fall or blow	Use self-care & Call doctor's office
Numbness or tingling in 4th and 5th fingers	See doctor
Loss of strength in hand or arm	See doctor
Elbow cannot be bent or straightened	See doctor
Joint or bursa red, swollen, or hot; fever present (possible infection)	See doctor
Elbow deformity after fall	Seek help now
Severe pain in upper arm (biceps) after sudden or violent motion	Seek help now

Use self-care

See doctor

Call doctor's office for advice

Seek help now

For more about the symbols, see p. 2.

FOOT PAIN

The foot is one of the most complex parts of the body; so complex, in fact, that a medical and surgical specialty—podiatry—is devoted solely to treating and studying foot problems. The main source of most foot pain involves improper foot function or biomechanics. Shoes rarely cause foot deformities, but may irritate them. A properly fitting shoe, with good arch support, cushioning, and a "toe box" that doesn't pinch and squeeze the toes or ball of the foot will prevent irritation to bony joints and the skin over them that can cause problems and pain.

Flat feet or high arches can contribute to painful problems in the feet, knees, and even hips. When the arch is too high or low, other structures in the foot and leg have to work longer and harder than intended. The added stress, weight, and poor motion can cause fatigue, pain, and inflammation. Arch supports (orthotics) and exercises to stretch and strengthen the arch and lower leg help relieve many problems related to weak arches. But for many people, having flat feet or high arches never causes a problem.

Heel Pain

Two closely related conditions—heel spurs and plantar fasciitis—are common sources of pain in the heel and arch of the foot. They involve the heel bone and the *plantar fascia*, a strong band of connective tissue at the bottom of the foot that runs from the heel to the base of the toes. Its job is to help maintain or hold the arch together and serve as a shock absorber during activity.

Overstretching of this band of tissue can result in strain and later inflammation where it's attached to the heel bone. **Plantar fasciitis** is marked by a dull ache in the arch or pain in the heel. The pain is worst when you wake or after resting.

Walking may hurt at first, but once the plantar fascia is "warmed up," the pain may decrease.

Plantar fasciitis most often occurs when activity suddenly increases, or is due to shoes with poor support. Switching from high heels or cowboy boots to flat shoes or athletic shoes can irritate the fascia, causing pain. Gaining 10 to 20 pounds can have the same effect. Working out or standing and walking on hard surfaces, such as concrete, or wearing shoes that do not have good arch support can also lead to the problem.

Overstretching the plantar fascia can cause heel spurs. A **heel spur** is bone growth on the heel bone where it connects to the plantar fascia. As the plantar fascia is pulled and stretched, it pulls the lining of the heel bone away from the main bone, causing a bony growth, or spur, to develop. The pain stems from the irritation of the plantar fascia pulling on the bone. The spur does not necessarily require removal to relieve heel pain.

Heel pain and plantar fasciitis often have similar symptoms and are sometimes considered together as **heel spur syndrome**. In some cases, however, heel spurs may cause a deep tenderness in the bottom of the heel when weight is placed on the foot. Self-care (see p. 115) and rest will sometimes relieve heel spurs and plantar fasciitis. If symptoms continue despite these measures or if pain is severe, see your doctor. Steroid injections may help relieve inflammation. Surgery is a last resort and warranted only in worst and prolonged cases.

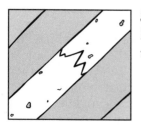

Simple Fracture
Bone breaks but does
not puncture the skin.

Stress Fractures

Sometimes it's not the connective tissues in the foot that give way or get inflamed, but the bones themselves. Stress fractures occur most often in the second metatarsal. The metatarsals are the long bones that connect to the toes.

High-impact activities such as running, basketball, or high-impact aerobics pose particular risk for stress fractures of the foot. Postmenopausal women with lower bone density, women with absent or infrequent periods, or anyone on long-term steroid or hormone therapy may be more likely to have stress fractures.

Stress fractures most often appear several weeks into a new or more intense training schedule or from landing wrong after jumping. At first, pain may be mild enough that it can be ignored. After time, however, the mild pain gives way to sudden, intense pain. Both the top and bottom of the foot may be tender to the touch.

Treating stress fractures in the foot mostly involves time—usually at least 1 month—to allow the bone to heal. With the exception of fractures in the fifth metatarsal, a cast is usually not needed. A wooden shoe or postoperative shoe is usually worn to allow the fracture to heal. A stress fracture in the fifth metatarsal can be serious because it often resists healing. Fractures may need a cast, and crutches may have to be used for 6 weeks to several months. In some cases, surgery may be needed.

Morton's Neuroma

Morton's neuroma is a benign, fibrous enlargement of one of the nerves running between the metatarsal bones (long bones of the foot). The enlargement occurs when the nerve is squeezed between the bones, sometimes from narrow, tight shoes or stress from repeated motions. Most often, neuromas develop between the metatarsal bones leading to the third and fourth toes (called the third intermetatarsal space). Occasionally, they may develop between the second and third metatarsals.

Morton's neuroma causes local swelling and tenderness. A person with this condition may feel as though he or she is walking on a lump, especially when barefoot. Pain may spread to the toes or toward the heel. Pressure makes the pain worse, and if constant, may cause numbness, burning, and tingling in the toes, between the toes, or at the ball of the foot (see Self-Care Steps, p. 115).

Corns

These yellowish calluslike growths develop on tops of the toes in spots where shoes rub. If the rubbing continues, corns can become red, inflamed, and painful. The best way to prevent corns is to wear shoes with a toe box—the area surrounding the toes and ball of the foot—large enough to comfortably fit your foot without rubbing.

I work in a department store, standing all day long on carpet-covered concrete. By the end of the day, my feet are swollen and ache. My back often hurts, too. I usually wear pumps with fairly low heels—about an inch high. But still, my feet are killing me at the end of each day. A friend suggested I find a pair of dress shoes with more cushion in the sole. I have to wear dress shoes, so comfortable athletic shoes are out. I finally found a pair that didn't pinch my toes and had a cushioned sole and only a small heel. The salesperson recommended adding arch-support inserts. With the new shoes and putting my feet up during breaks, I'm finally making it through the day without hurting!

Margaret

Bunions

A bunion is a swelling on the side of the foot that is usually a symptom that the foot isn't working properly, often because of a flat-foot condition. Instability and muscle imbalance cause the big toe to slant in toward the other toes. The joint where the big toe connects to the foot (the end of the first metatarsal) pokes out on the inner side of the foot. This is caused by poor alignment and is not a growth of bone. The bunion may also become inflamed and sore, especially if rubbed by a shoe. A similar problem, called a "tailor's bunion," may develop on the opposite side of the foot, where the little toe meets the fifth metatarsal. For bunions that cause persistent pain despite self-care (see p. 115), steroid injections or surgery may provide relief.

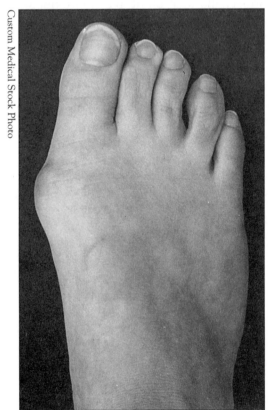

Custom Medical Stock Photo

A bunion on the inner side of the foot.

Hammertoe

Hammertoe is a deformity in which the toe buckles, causing the middle joint of the affected toe to poke above the other toes. The deformity may also cause the toe to become bent at the middle joint so that it turns in toward the toe next to it. Tight shoes can rub and put pressure on the raised portion of the hammertoe, often making a corn form. Hammertoes may cause no problems at all, or they can be a source of pain, especially if the person wears tight or ill-fitting shoes. If self-care (see p. 115) fails to relieve the symptoms, surgery may be needed to straighten the toe or remove the bony protrusion.

Plantar Warts

Plantar warts, like warts in other areas of the body, are caused by a virus. Weight bearing causes plantar warts to grow inward. The result is a painful lump on the bottom of the foot that feels like you are walking on a pebble. Children and teens are more likely than adults to get plantar warts. Plantar warts are often difficult to treat, but a slow approach is best (see Self-Care Steps, p. 115). If plantar warts interfere with walking, you should see your doctor or a podiatrist to have them removed.

SELF-CARE STEPS FOR FOOT PAIN

Good shoes can be important in preventing and relieving foot pain. Shoes should support the arch and cushion the heel, ball, and outside of the foot. They shouldn't pinch the foot or toes or be so loose your feet slide around in them. A good heel height is generally between $1/2$ and $1^1/_2$ inches. For shoes that don't already offer enough arch support or cushioning, commercial arch-support and cushion inserts may be worth buying.

With the exception of plantar warts or trauma to the foot, checking the shoes you've been wearing is the first step in caring for foot pain. Anti-inflammatory drugs (aspirin, ibuprofen, or naproxen) will help relieve pain and inflammation. Other treatments for specific conditions are discussed below.

For heel spurs and plantar fasciitis
• Rest the foot, avoiding high-impact activities for 3 to 6 weeks. Switch to low-impact activities, such as walking, biking, or swimming. Walking is particularly good.

• Apply ice to the heel two to three times daily.

• Support the arches of your feet to protect them from further stretching and tearing. Place arch supports even in your slippers and put them on first thing when getting out of bed.

For stress fractures
• See your doctor if pain continues or worsens after a week or two of nonimpact activity and anti-inflammatory drugs.

• Avoid high-impact activities. Switch to weight-bearing, low-impact or nonimpact activities, such as walking or low-impact aerobics. Weight bearing strengthens bones and prevents bone loss. Resume your regular workout or other activities slowly after pain gets better and the fracture heals.

For Morton's neuroma
• Avoid the original activity that caused the pain, and other high-impact activities, for 3 to 6 weeks. Resume the original activity only after pain is gone.

• Try wearing shoes with a wider toe box to prevent pressure on the nerve.

For corns
• Soak feet in a solution of Epsom salts and water for 15 minutes. Dry carefully and apply a moisturizer. Rub the corn with a clean nail file or pumice stone, using a side-to-side motion. Repeat daily until the corn is gone.

• Use a nonmedicated corn pad to relieve pressure on the area.

For hammertoes
• Wear shoes with a toe box large enough to accommodate the hammertoe.

• Treat accompanying corns as described below.

For bunions
• Choose shoes with a larger toe box (squared or rounded toe).

• Put a piece of foam or cotton between the affected toes to see if it eases the pressure.

• Place padding around the bunion to relieve pressure and rubbing from shoes. Moleskin and bunion pads are available at most drugstores.

• Try using an arch support to stop the jamming of the long bone and the big toe.

• See your doctor if pain lasts, interferes with walking, or is not relieved with self-care.

For plantar warts
• Soak foot for 10 minutes in a solution of 2 tablespoons mild household detergent (such as dish soap) and $1/2$ gallon warm water. Cut a piece of 40 percent salicylic-acid plaster (available at drugstores) the size of the wart and apply it to the wart. Cover with tape or a bandage. Remove the plaster in 2 days. Brush the wart with a toothbrush soaked in soap and water. Repeat this procedure for 2 weeks until the wart is gone.

• If warts remain despite self-care, or if they interfere with walking, see your doctor.

• Do not try to *cut* warts out!

DECISION GUIDE FOR FOOT PAIN

SYMPTOMS/SIGNS	ACTION
Foot pain from overuse or injury; can bear weight	🩹
Unable to move foot or bear weight after a trauma, such as a blow or fall	☎
Pain in heel or arch, especially upon awakening; tender points on bottom of foot between heel and ball (see heel spurs or plantar fasciitis p. 112)	☎
Corns, plantar warts, bunions, or hammertoes	☎
Pain, burning, tingling, or numbness in the toes, between the toes and at the ball of the foot; swelling at the top of the foot; symptoms get worse with pressure (see Morton's neuroma p. 113)	☎
Heel spurs or plantar fasciitis not relieved with self-care within 3 to 6 weeks	🩺
Suspected stress fracture	🩺

🩹 Use self-care   🩺 See doctor

☎ Call doctor's office for advice   *For more about the symbols, see p. 2.*

HIP AND THIGH PAIN

The hip is one of the most stable joints in the body. A "ball-and-socket" joint, the hip is surrounded by large muscles and a deep socket. Because of its stability, few problems occur with the hip joint. Most often, pain in the hip and thigh involves injury to muscles, tendons, or bursas, usually from a fall, a blow, or overuse of some kind. Some common hip injuries are discussed below.

Hip Pointer

A hip pointer is a bruise or tear in the muscle that connects to the top of the ilium, the crest of the pelvis just below the waist. Symptoms include local pain, tenderness, and possibly swelling. Climbing stairs may be difficult, and it may hurt to walk. A hip pointer can be caused by a blow, a fall, or a quick twist or turn of the body. Often the pain increases several hours after the injury. This can be a very debilitating injury that takes a long time to heal.

Groin Pull

This is a pull of the muscles that bring your leg back to the body (adductors). Groin pulls are fairly common among those who play sports such as hockey, tennis, or basketball. A groin pull can cause pain, tenderness, and stiffness deep in the groin, making activity difficult.

Pulled Hamstring

The hamstring is a group of muscles at the back of the thigh that attach at the pelvis and just below the knee. Pulls or tears may occur from a sudden forceful move, such as sprinting to steal a base. Hamstring injuries most often occur in the center of the muscle, but the hamstring can also tear from the pelvic bone, just under the buttocks. Hamstring pulls and tears cause pain and sometimes bruising or a lot of swelling.

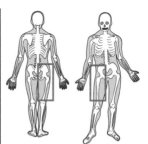

REAR VIEW OF HIP & THIGH   **FRONT VIEW OF HIP & THIGH**

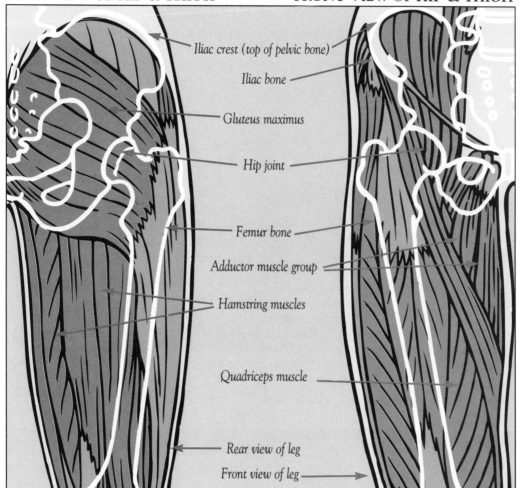

Iliac crest (top of pelvic bone)

Iliac bone

Gluteus maximus

Hip joint

Femur bone

Adductor muscle group

Hamstring muscles

Quadriceps muscle

Rear view of leg

Front view of leg

Avulsion Fractures

Avulsion or "occult" fractures are closely related to hip pointers and groin pulls. Instead of a blow or fall affecting just the muscles, a fragment of bone breaks away from the pelvis or femur (upper leg bone). Symptoms are similar to those of a groin pull or hip pointer. For this reason, any time hip pointer or groin pull symptoms do not improve within 7 to 10 days, you should see a doctor to check for an avulsion fracture. This is especially important for children and teens.

Bursitis

The hip actually contains 13 different bursas. But most often, bursitis in the hip involves the "hip socket." It causes ten-

derness, pain, and swelling on the outer part of the hip where some of the large buttock muscles attach. Bursitis in the hip can cause pain that spreads to the buttocks and down as far as the ankle. It can be caused by activities (such as speed walking, aerobic dance, or carrying a baby on your hip) or conditions (such as one leg being shorter than the other) that alter the normal tilt of the pelvis. To keep it from happening again, you must correct the problem causing the abnormal tilt, for example, by wearing a "shoe lift" insert if one leg is a bit longer than the other.

Charley Horse

A charley horse is a painful muscle cramp caused by bruising of the thigh. In addition to cramping, charley horses are often accompanied by swelling, pain, stiffness, and skin discoloration (from the bruising). Apply the RICE method (p. 97) right after any significant blow to the thigh.

Myositis Ossificans

A serious muscle bruise or repeated bruising in the same area can cause bone growth within the muscle tissue. This condition, called *myositis ossificans* (which means "bone forming in muscle") causes pain, swelling, and limited range of motion of the thigh muscles. This condition needs to be evaluated and treated by a doctor to prevent further bone growth. Aggressive physical therapy is recommended, and the area should be protected from further injury. Once again, apply the RICE method (p. 97) right after any significant blow to the thigh.

Muscle Tightness

Any time you tighten a muscle repeatedly, as when running or hammering, or hold it in one position for a long time, as when squatting or working at a computer, it may become stiff. Often stiffness and pain aren't felt until the next day. The tensor fasciae latae muscle, which runs along the outside of the upper leg and allows the leg to move outward to the side, is a common site for muscle tightness. But other muscles, including those in the buttocks and in the inside, front, and back of the thigh, can also become tight. Usually, muscle tightness lessens with a warm bath, stretching, and drinking plenty of water.

Piriformis Syndrome

The piriformis muscle is one of several smaller muscles lying underneath the larger muscles of the buttocks. Overuse, such as from sitting or standing for long periods, or repeated motions over time can irritate the smaller underlying muscles of the buttocks, causing the piriformis muscle, in particular, to tighten and have spasms. When this happens, pressure may be placed on the sciatic nerve, a large nerve serving the lower body. The irritation, called *piriformis syndrome*, can cause pain, numbness, and tingling from the buttocks, down the back of the leg to the foot.

The symptoms of this are often confused with those of disc disease in the spine. One way to tell if the problem is piriformis syndrome is to lie on your stomach with your knees together and bent, so your feet are in the air. Gently allow your feet to spread apart, toward the floor. If you feel a pain in your buttocks as your feet move apart, your problem is probably piriformis syndrome.

Chronic Hip Pain

Many other conditions can cause hip and thigh pain. Some, like arthritis or chronic bursitis, involve the hip directly. But low back problems, hernias, and inflammation of the urinary tract, reproductive system, or intestine can also cause hip pain—sometimes with little or no symptoms in the area of the body with the real problem. Whenever hip or thigh pain lasts more than 7 to 10 days, call your health care provider.

SPECIAL CONCERNS FOR CHILDREN

Children can have most of the same hip and thigh problems as adults—most of which involve the muscles and connective tissues of the hip, thigh, and buttocks. But several problems unique to children may affect the bones directly. And because children are still growing, these problems require medical attention to prevent long-term problems. Any time a child or teenager has a limp that lasts more than a few days, he or she should see a doctor. For any child or teenager involved in athletics, proper stretching (smooth, slow stretches, not bouncing) and slow strengthening of muscles are important to prevent injuries in the hips and legs, as well as other parts of the body. Conditions of the hip that affect children are described below.

Legg-Calvé-Perthes Disease

Named for the doctors who first described it, Legg-Calvé-Perthes disease is a breakdown of the ball (femoral head) of the femur—the long thigh bone with a "ball" on top that fits in the hip joint. Loss of blood supply to the hip causes part of the femoral head to die and deteriorate, but no one knows exactly what interrupts the blood supply. Symptoms may include limping, pain in the groin area or inner thigh, and knee pain. Rest usually relieves the pain, while activity makes it worse. The hip may also be stiff and the thigh may be weak.

Old bone is absorbed by the body, and new bone grows in its place naturally. But if the femoral head is not held in proper position, the new bone may grow in too large, too flat, or in the wrong shape. The hip "socket" provides a natural mold for the new bone to grow. In some cases, a child with Legg-Calvé-Perthes disease may need to wear a cast or brace, or require rest, traction, or even surgery to make sure the new bone on the femoral head grows properly. But in other cases, especially when only a small area is affected or in children age 4 or younger, monitoring by a doctor is all that's needed.

Unless the hip is inflamed or the doctor recommends traction, a child with Legg-Calvé-Perthes disease may play as usual. The deterioration caused by Legg-Calvé-Perthes disease usually heals completely, and the disease does not recur once healed.

Slipped Capital Femoral Epiphysis

In this condition, the femoral head actually slips out of place, along the growth plate (epiphysis) of the upper leg bone (femur). This condition usually occurs in children at about the time puberty begins (between the ages of 9 and 12). The slip may be slow over several months or occur suddenly following a fall or other significant injury to the hip. Symptoms are similar to those of Legg-Calvé-Perthes disease (see above).

Your child's doctor may recommend bed rest or traction to help reduce inflammation. Surgery is usually needed to stabilize the slip. Treatment for slipped capital femoral epiphysis is usually very effective. Left untreated, however, the condition can lead to arthritis in early adulthood.

Synovitis

Synovitis is an inflammation of any joint. In children, synovitis of the hip occurs most commonly between the ages of 6 and 10. Care by both a pediatrician and an orthopedist or by an orthopedist specializing in children is often required.

I spent most of Saturday pulling weeds from my flower and vegetable gardens. I even dug up a good number of dandelions in the yard. By Sunday night, though, I was paying the price of doing too much in one day. All that squatting on Saturday left the front of my thighs so stiff and sore I could barely walk down the stairs. I tried applying ice to the area and doing gentle stretches to relieve the tightness. Aspirin also seemed to help. By Tuesday, my legs were pretty much back to normal. The next time I pull an all-day stint in the garden, I plan to stretch out well before and afterward, as well as several times throughout the day, and drink plenty of fluids.

Terry

SELF-CARE STEPS FOR HIP AND THIGH PAIN

Simple muscle tightness is probably the most common injury in the hips and thighs. The RICE method (p. 97), anti-inflammatory drugs (p. 97), and gentle stretching of the tight and painful muscles will help speed recovery. Stretching before and after an activity and slowly strengthening muscles before demanding major efforts from them are effective ways to prevent muscle tightness—and most other hip and thigh injuries—in the first place. Below are specific things you can do to speed recovery of other hip and thigh injuries.

Hamstring stretch—*Lie on the floor on your back with your left leg bent. Grab the back of your right knee. Slowly straighten your leg. Feel the stretch on the back of your thigh. Hold for a count of five. Switch to your left leg and repeat.*

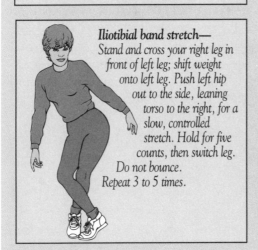

Iliotibial band stretch—Stand and cross your right leg in front of left leg; shift weight onto left leg. Push left hip out to the side, leaning torso to the right, for a slow, controlled stretch. Hold for five counts, then switch leg. Do not bounce. Repeat 3 to 5 times.

For a hip pointer and groin or hamstring pulls or tears
The RICE method and anti-inflammatory drugs (p. 97) usually reduce pain. Depending on the

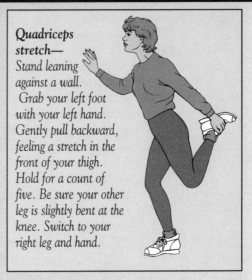

Quadriceps stretch—Stand leaning against a wall. Grab your left foot with your left hand. Gently pull backward, feeling a stretch in the front of your thigh. Hold for a count of five. Be sure your other leg is slightly bent at the knee. Switch to your right leg and hand.

damage to the muscle tissue, you may need crutches for a few days.

For bursitis
Use the RICE method and anti-inflammatory drugs (p. 97). Avoid the activity that started the inflammation.

For a charley horse or myositis ossificans
Apply ice to the entire muscle (or as much of it as you possibly can) right after the injury to slow blood flow and swelling. Rest the area; don't work through the pain. Use the RICE method and anti-inflammatory drugs (p. 97). If not better in 7 to 10 days, see a doctor.

For piriformis syndrome
Stretching and strengthening muscles in the buttocks and leg will help relieve this condition. While lying on your stomach, raise one leg from the floor, toes pointed. Repeat as many times as you can, and then do the same with the other leg. Gradually work on raising your leg higher and increasing the number of repetitions.

For chronic hip pain
Because excess body weight can stress the hip joint, losing weight can often help relieve hip and thigh pain from chronic conditions. Walking is a good way to lose pounds and strengthen hip and thigh muscles. But any time hip or thigh pain lasts more than 7 to 10 days, you should see a doctor.

DECISION GUIDE FOR HIP AND THIGH PAIN

SYMPTOMS/SIGNS	ACTION
Overuse or injury pain that lasts less than 7 days	🩹
Pulled or torn muscle causing tenderness to touch; stiffness; pain; difficulty walking, running, or climbing stairs	☎️
Pain on outside of hip, possibly down to the knee	☎️
Swelling, pain, or stiffness after a blow to the thigh	🩺
Any of the above symptoms do not improve within 7 to 10 days	🩺
Dull pain in hip and groin while walking or climbing stairs	🩺
Severe pain in buttocks with exercise; pain stops when activity stops	🩺
Pain interrupts sleep	🩺
Severe pain after a fall or blow	🏥

🩹 Use self-care   🩺 See doctor

☎️ Call doctor's office for advice   🏥 Seek help now

For more about the symbols, see p. 2.

KNEE PAIN

The knees are a common spot for injuries in athletes and nonathletes, alike. They bear a great deal of the stress from high-impact activities, such as running, aerobic dance, skiing, and other sports. Even everyday activities such as squatting, stooping, kneeling, lifting, and climbing stairs can take their toll. In addition to wear, tear, and sudden twists, the knees are open targets for blows, especially during contact sports.

The knee is composed of four bones: the femur (thigh bone), the tibia and fibula of the lower leg, and the patella (kneecap). The ends of the femur and tibia meet at the knee to form the joint. They are held together with four ligaments. The medial collateral ligament runs along the inner side of the knee and the lateral collateral ligament on the outside. Two cruciate ligaments run diagonally within the knee.

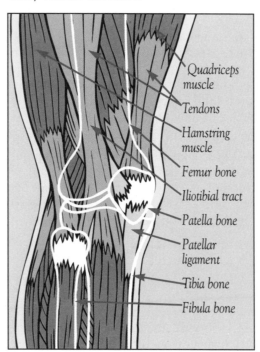

KNEE JOINT

Three-quarter view of front right knee

Quadriceps muscle

Tendons

Hamstring muscle

Femur bone

Iliotibial tract

Patella bone

Patellar ligament

Tibia bone

Fibula bone

Cartilage provides a protective, lubricating "cover" over the bone surfaces of the joint. Two discs of cartilage, called *menisci*, attach to the cartilage of the knee and fit into the joint to form shock-absorbing cushions. The cartilage prevents the tibia and femur from rubbing against one another. The tendons of the hamstring and quadriceps support and help hold the knee in place. The patella is located in the tendon of the quadriceps.

Most knee injuries involve a blow, sudden twist, or a hard landing after a jump. Complex injuries are not unusual. A single strong blow in just the right place may tear cartilage and sprain several ligaments. Except for overuse injuries such as runner's knee and mild sprains, knee injuries should be seen by a doctor to find out how bad the injury is and exactly what structures are affected. Common injuries are described below.

Sprains

A blow or sudden twist of the knee can sprain ligaments on either side of the knee, causing swelling (usually within an hour), pain, and difficulty walking. The sprained side may be tender to the touch. Even mild knee sprains often take 2 to 3 weeks to fully heal.

A strong blow to the inner or outer side of the knee will sprain the ligament on the opposite side as the knee is forced to bend sideways. If pain is felt on the side where the blow occurred, it's probably a bruise and not a sprain.

Anterior Cruciate Ligament (ACL) Injuries

ACL injuries are the second most common sports injury, after ankle sprains. If the force from a blow, twist, or hard landing is strong enough, the anterior cruciate ligament within the knee can be stretched or torn. ACL injuries are common in contact sports, skiing, or basketball or as a result of a trip or fall. You may hear or feel a loud pop when the injury occurs. ACL injuries often bring sudden pain, knee instability, rapid swelling, and limited movement. But in some cases, symptoms may take as long as 6 to 12 hours to appear.

ACL injuries should be seen by a doctor within 24 hours to find out how bad the ligament damage is. If it is bad enough, surgery may be needed to reconstruct the ligament.

Torn Cartilage

The same traumas that can result in sprains can also tear the menisci. Often, cartilage tears occur with sprains. This is especially true of ACL injuries. Repeated squatting or kneeling can also weaken cartilage, increasing the risk of injury. Swelling may be immediate or appear within 24 hours of injury. Continuing pain and a clicking or locking with knee movement are other symptoms of torn cartilage.

Once the cartilage is torn, the knee may buckle or lock without warning, putting surrounding ligaments and tendons at risk of injury. Wearing a brace during activity can help protect the knee from further injury, but surgery may be needed to remove pieces of torn cartilage. Unlike bone, tendons, and ligaments, cartilage does not knit back together once it is torn.

Terrible Triad

The "terrible triad" is a combination of torn cartilage, ACL injury, and a sprained ligament at the inner side of the knee—all from a single blow. Damage this bad usually requires surgery.

Joint Mice

Joint mice are loose bodies—often pieces of torn cartilage or bone chips—floating within the knee. When they get trapped between moving bone, they cause sudden pain and even cause the knee to lock or buckle. A strong blow to the knee may cause a small portion of bone surface to die. Pieces of dead bone then fall away from the main bone to become "joint mice." Often symptoms take as long as a year to appear after a trauma.

Dislocations

With a strong enough blow or twist, either the kneecap or the femur and tibia may dislocate. Dislocations of the knee or kneecap cause very bad pain and visible deformity. Both conditions are serious and require prompt medical attention. But a dislocated knee (the femur and tibia out of alignment) is particularly serious because it can prevent blood from flowing to the lower leg. Immediate surgery is required to realign the bones and ensure that blood vessels are not damaged or pinched.

The kneecap normally rides in a groove at the end of the femur, where it is held in place with tendons attached to the quadriceps muscle in the front of the thigh and lower leg. A blow, quick pivot, or twist can knock the kneecap out of its groove, usually to the outer side of the knee. A dislocated kneecap may pop back into place on its own, but you should still see a doctor to check for fractures. If the kneecap is broken, surgery may be needed to wire the bone together so it can heal.

Runner's Knee (Chondromalacia Patella)

The most frequent cause of knee pain and the most common overuse injury in the knee is runner's knee. This condition can be brought on by any number of activities that place stress on the knee. Wearing shoes that provide inadequate support may contribute to it.

Runner's knee develops because the kneecap fits incorrectly in its groove at the end of the femur. The misalignment is often caused by the foot rolling too far inward. If not properly centered, the kneecap rubs against the femur, causing wear and tear on the cartilage behind the kneecap. Aching and swelling may be present around the kneecap or at the back of the knee, especially during and after activity. Squatting or sitting with the knees bent for a long time can also be painful. Grinding or popping may be felt as the knee bends and straightens.

Jumper's Knee (Patellar Tendinitis)

This condition is an inflammation of the quadriceps tendon at the top of the kneecap or the patellar tendon, attached at the bottom. Jumping is a common cause of inflammation and tearing.

Housemaid's Knee (Prepatellar Bursitis)

This is fairly common in people who work on their knees. Carpet layers, roofers, and people who install flooring are candidates for prepatellar bursitis, which is also called housemaid's knee or milkmaid's knee. Symptoms include a squishy, swollen area in front of the kneecap, pain, and stiffness. In more severe cases, swelling may extend above and to the sides of the kneecap. An inflamed bursa may break internally on its own. If this happens, the body absorbs the excess fluid and the swelling and inflammation usually stop. The best prevention for housemaid's knee is wearing knee pads whenever working on your knees for any length of time.

Iliotibial Band Syndrome

The iliotibial band consists of a muscle that begins at the top rim of the pelvis (the portion of the hip felt just below the

I'd made a resolution this year to run a marathon. I began training, running 45 minutes 4 days a week. By the end of the first month, my right knee was swollen, hurt, and I couldn't run. Even sitting at my desk at work made my knee hurt. When I called the doctor's office, they suggested the RICE method, anti-inflammatory drugs, and 30-degree leg extensions to strengthen my inner thigh muscles. After the inflammation went down, I took a more moderate approach to training. I did the leg extensions regularly and slowly worked my way up toward my mileage goals. I bought shoes that better supported my feet, and I apply ice after each run. I won't make the marathon this year, but next year I expect to be in good shape!

David

waist) and a tendon that fits into the outside of the knee. Exercise can cause the band to tighten, irritating the knee and sometimes the point of the hip. The pain usually begins 10 to 20 minutes into a run or other exercise routine and stops when the activity stops. Iliotibial band syndrome often grows worse, with pain increasing and starting sooner in a workout. Stretching and ice are the keys to relieving the syndrome (see Self-Care Steps, p. 125).

Arthritis
See Acute Arthritis, p. 100.

SPECIAL CONCERNS FOR CHILDREN

Osgood-Schlatter Disease

Osgood-Schlatter disease occurs during adolescence. It is a self-limited syndrome that causes pain for the growing teenager, but generally no long-term problems. It is marked by a dull ache that comes and goes with changes in activity level and by swelling and tenderness on the bony spot just below the knee (tibial tubercle), where the kneecap (patellar) ligament connects.

In normal teenagers, growth spurts cause the tibial tubercle to grow. At the same time, the ligament is growing and trying to attach new tissue to the tubercle. Running, jumping, and other high-impact activities stress the ligament and frustrate its efforts to connect to the growing bone. Muscle imbalance and immature cartilage and bone also contribute to the syndrome. The ligament becomes inflamed, which increases blood flow to the area. This stimulates bone growth at the tibial tubercle, forming an enlarged bump. The on-and-off pain and inflammation of Osgood-Schlatter disease stops by about the age of 16 or 17. But the bony knob just below the knee is permanent.

Because the syndrome causes no permanent harm, a young person with Osgood-Schlatter disease can be as active as he or she likes, using pain as a guide (if it hurts too much, stop). Icing the area after activity will help prevent swelling and pain. Acetaminophen or ibuprofen may also help relieve pain. If the condition flares up, resting for a few days is advised. Exercises to strengthen the leg, such as straight leg lifts, can help prevent inflammation.

Other Knee Injuries

As with adults, knee injuries are common in young athletes. Wearing knee pads and supportive shoes can help prevent such injuries. But when they do occur, the young person should not be allowed to continue playing until the injury is examined by a doctor to rule out a growth plate fracture (see p. 96 for further discussion of epiphyseal fractures).

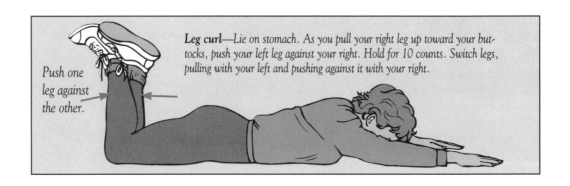

Push one leg against the other.

Leg curl—Lie on stomach. As you pull your right leg up toward your buttocks, push your left leg against your right. Hold for 10 counts. Switch legs, pulling with your left and pushing against it with your right.

SELF-CARE STEPS FOR KNEE PAIN

Overuse injuries, such as runner's knee, tendinitis, and bursitis, can usually be treated safely at home with the RICE method, anti-inflammatory drugs, and exercise to strengthen the area after the pain is gone (see p. 97).

With the exception of mild sprains, knee injuries from trauma should be seen by a doctor to find out how bad the damage is. **Injuries that should be seen immediately include dislocations of the knee or kneecap and "terrible triad" injuries, in which the knee swells severely and cannot be moved.** Most knee injuries, however, do not require a trip to the emergency room. Here is how to treat common knee injuries on your own and when to see a doctor.

For mild sprains

• Follow the RICE method (p. 97). Rest the knee as long as it aches. After the first 72 hours, soak your knee in a warm whirlpool or bath. Use crutches if needed.

• After the pain is better, work to strengthen the muscles around your knee. Leg curls (p. 124), leg extensions (below), and riding a stationary bike are good strengthening exercises. If you choose a stationary bike, set the seat high enough so that your knee doesn't bend much and set the controls so that there is no drag.

• See your doctor if symptoms do not improve within 3 to 4 days.

For severe sprains, ACL injuries, and cartilage tears

• Follow the RICE method (p. 97) and take anti-inflammatory drugs for pain and swelling. Use crutches if needed. See your doctor within 24 hours of injury.

For runner's knee, tendinitis, bursitis, and joint mice

• Follow the RICE method (p. 97) and use anti-inflammatory drugs. Check your shoes to make sure they provide proper support (see p. 115 for information on how to choose footwear). If self-care corrections fail to do the trick, your doctor may prescribe custom-made inserts.

• After the pain is better, exercise to strengthen the area. Recommended exercises are illustrated on p. 124 and below.

• If swelling from bursitis lasts or is very bad, a doctor may drain the fluid with a needle and then inject the bursa with cortisone. After this procedure, watch for signs of infection, such as redness, swelling, and local heat. Surgery may be required if bursitis lasts despite other treatment.

For iliotibial band syndrome

• Stretching is the key to relieving this problem. Stretch the iliotibial band (see illustration p. 120), holding the stretch for 20 to 30 seconds and repeating three to six times. Do this three to five times a day until you no longer feel pain with running. To prevent it from happening again, do this stretch before and after each run.

• If symptoms are not better within 10 to 14 days with the stretching routine, see your doctor.

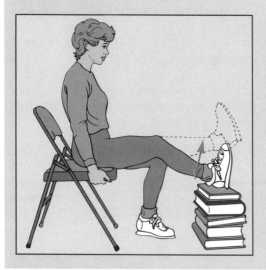

Leg extension—Sit with knees bent at a 60-degree angle; straighten leg; hold for count of five, then slowly bend leg to rest on stool or pile of books. Switch legs. You can add leg weights for added resistance.

DECISION GUIDE FOR KNEE PAIN

SYMPTOMS/SIGNS	ACTION
Pain after sudden twist or blow to side of knee; swelling; can bear weight, but may limp	*(use self-care)*
Tendon below kneecap inflamed; pain going up stairs or jumping	*(call doctor's office)*
Soft, squishy swelling beginning in front of knee; pain; stiffness (see Prepatellar bursitis, p. 123)	*(call doctor's office)*
Pain around or under kneecap; pain increases when you are climbing stairs or sitting for long periods	*(see doctor)*
Bursitis symptoms do not improve within 7 to 10 days; or signs of infection appear (local heat, redness, increased swelling, pain and tenderness)	*(see doctor)*
Pain after sudden twist or blow to side of knee; swelling; cannot bear weight	*(seek help now)*
Pain after sudden twist or blow to side of knee; rapid swelling; limited movement	*(seek help now)*
Severe blow or injury to knee; severe swelling; unable to move knee; visible deformity of knee	*(seek help now)*

Use self-care

Call doctor's office for advice

See doctor

Seek help now

For more about the symbols, see p. 2.

LOWER-LEG PAIN

The lower leg is made up of two bones, the tibia and the fibula. As with other parts of the leg, pain in the lower leg can be caused by overuse, overexertion, or trauma from a fall or blow. In addition to orthopedic problems, the lower leg can also be affected by heart and circulatory diseases, such as congestive heart failure, or blood clots and inflammation in the veins of the legs. The main symptom of such diseases is swelling in the legs and feet from extra fluid (edema).

Swelling (Edema) in the Lower Leg

Occasional swelling in the leg is common. It can occur from sitting or standing for long periods, water retention related to a woman's period or during pregnancy, allergies, varicose veins, or even sitting in the sun too long. In most cases, it goes away on its own overnight. Chronic swelling, however, can be a sign of the following serious conditions that require medical care.

Phlebitis

Phlebitis is an inflammation of a vein, sometimes accompanied by a blood clot. The inflammation can cause aching, swelling, and redness in the lower portion of one leg. A blood clot in one of the veins of the leg can further increase swelling by blocking the flow of blood back to the heart. With nowhere else to go, the blood seeps out of the vein into the surrounding tissues, causing swelling. **Phlebitis requires immediate medical attention to keep a potential clot from moving into the heart or lungs.**

Congestive Heart Failure

Congestive heart failure occurs when the heart muscle is weakened, for example, by a heart attack, and is no longer able to pump blood well. Unlike phlebitis, congestive heart failure brings swelling in both legs at the same time and does not cause pain. When the heart is pumping inefficiently, the result is a backup of blood that leads to a buildup of fluids in the legs. The liver and lungs may also be affected, enlarging the liver and causing shortness of breath because fluid collects in the lungs. Raising the legs may relieve swelling, but if you have these symptoms, you should see your doctor.

Drugs

Drugs such as testosterone, estrogen, blood pressure drugs, birth control pills, and long-term corticosteroid use may also cause swelling in the legs. If you are on any of these drugs and have swelling, call your doctor.

Intermittent Claudication

Intermittent claudication is pain caused by narrowing of the arteries (atherosclerosis) that creates a buildup of fluid in the leg and keeps the lower leg muscles from getting enough oxygen. The condition usually occurs in older adults and heavy smokers. Activity may cause pain, as the working muscles fail to get the oxygen they need. The pain is relieved shortly after exercise or activity is stopped. If you have these symptoms, see your physician.

Other Causes of Lower-Leg Pain

Of course, overuse and trauma can also cause pain in the lower leg. The following conditions are among the most common.

Shin Splints

A shin splint causes aching at the front or inner side of the lower leg. Generally there is no swelling, redness, or bruising. The pain may begin suddenly or build slowly. A shin splint is an overuse injury that causes inflammation of the shin muscles, sometimes pulling muscle away from the bone. Tiny tears in the muscle may also contribute to the pain.

The most common causes of shin splints include:

- Muscle imbalance (calf muscle is much stronger than the shin muscles)
- Not enough shock absorption during high-impact exercise (from wearing worn-out shoes or shoes without enough padding)
- Running on the balls of the feet, without allowing the heel to touch the ground
- Flat feet
- Doing too much activity too fast (starting out jogging 5 miles instead of 2, or hiking in boots you're not used to)
- A tight Achilles tendon (the tendon at the back of the heel and ankle)

Shin splints are a common injury among runners and other athletes, store clerks, warehouse and factory workers, and others who are on their feet all day on hard concrete floors in shoes (especially high heels or cowboy boots) that don't provide good support.

Contusion and Anterior Compartment Syndrome

A strong blow to the shin can cause a painful bruise. After the skin color returns to normal, a bump as hard as bone may remain for as long as several months, but it usually goes away on its own with time.

But a blow to the front of the leg on the outside can cause more serious problems than bruising. Internal bleeding may cause swelling, which puts pressure on the nerves and blood vessels—a condition called **anterior compartment syndrome**. If not treated immediately with surgery to relieve pressure, the swelling may permanently damage the main nerve to the foot. When this happens, the

I've been jogging three times a week for the past several months. I usually jog along the paved paths in the city parks. Recently, I noticed a sharp pain in the middle of my shin every time I ran. By the next day, the pain was usually gone. So I would run again on my usual schedule. Each time I ran, the pain got worse. I tried icing it after each run and took some over-the-counter Aleve. But the problem kept getting worse. I finally saw my physician, who ordered X-rays and said I had a stress fracture exactly where I was feeling the pain—in the middle of my shin. The physician recommended the RICE method and said to switch to biking or swimming to stay in shape while the fracture healed. In about six weeks I was able to gradually return to my running schedule. The physician said the fracture probably started from worn out, improperly fitted running shoes. I spent the extra money to invest in a comfortable pair that fits my running style.

Cary

injured person is left with a condition known as "drop foot." The person loses the ability to lift his or her foot, which will seriously affect walking.

Symptoms of anterior compartment syndrome may begin with mild pain and swelling that builds to loss of color (pallor), feeling, and pulse; severe pain; paralysis; and swelling so bad that the skin turns shiny. If the latter symptoms appear, prompt treatment is crucial to prevent or lessen permanent nerve damage. **If you have these symptoms after a blow to the shin, apply ice and seek medical help immediately.**

Stress Fractures

Stress fractures can result from overuse, a blow, or twisting the lower leg. Stress fractures are common in high-impact activities. Stress fractures are hard to detect on X-rays until about 10 to 14 days after the fracture begins. You may notice a sudden spreading pain in your shin during or after exercise. In most cases, people with stress fractures can pinpoint exactly where the pain is coming from by pressing on the spot. Although a cast is

not needed, stress fractures should be checked with X-rays until fully healed, usually about 6 weeks. During this time, rest the leg by avoiding high-impact activities. Generally, low-impact activities, such as walking, bicycling, or swimming, are safe to do while a stress fracture heals.

SPECIAL CONCERNS FOR CHILDREN

Growing pains are not a myth, but a real problem in children between the ages of 6 and 12. The pains usually occur in the evening, often in the calves and thighs. Acetaminophen or ibuprofen, along with a heating pad set on "low" or soaking in a warm bath, will provide relief. Call a doctor if the pain is always in the same spot; if there is swelling, redness, tenderness to the touch, or fever; or if your child is limping.

SELF-CARE STEPS FOR LOWER-LEG PAIN

- As with most other injuries in the extremities, the RICE method and anti-inflammatory medications (p. 97) provide the core of treatment for shin splints, stress fractures, and contusions. For chronic swelling in both legs without pain, try raising your legs and call your doctor to see if he or she thinks you should be seen.

- For shin splints, rest the leg for 3 to 6 days, then do only low-impact activities (bicycling, walking, swimming) to keep up strength and prevent recurrence. After aching has gotten better, return slowly to your usual activities. You can also wrap the ankle and shin for support. Achilles tendon stretches and exercises to strengthen the

front of the leg may also be helpful. An ice massage four times a day is beneficial: freeze water in a paper cup; tear away the cup to expose the ice, and massage the ice over the painful area for 10 or 15 minutes.

- Wear shoes with good support and cushioning. Even if the outside of an athletic shoe looks fine, the cushioning in the sole may have lost its resiliency with wear and you may need a new pair. Also check to see if the heel counter (the part that supports your heel) is broken down and the bottoms are worn evenly.

- See your doctor if a shin splint does not get better after 2 to 3 weeks or if you feel numbness or tingling in your foot after a blow to the shin.

DECISION GUIDE FOR LOWER-LEG PAIN

SYMPTOMS/SIGNS	ACTION
Pain from overuse or blow; can bear weight	[bandage]
Chronic swelling, without pain	[bandage]
Blow to shin area, bruising, no swelling	[bandage]
Pain along the front or inner edge of the shin bone	[phone]
Shin splint does not get better within 2 to 3 weeks	[phone]
Gradual increase in shin or ankle pain; pain increases during or after activity	[phone]
Children: pain in legs, calves, or thighs at the end of the day or at night (see growing pains, p. 128)	[stethoscope]
Painful and sudden swelling and redness in only one leg (see phlebitis, p. 126)	[stethoscope]
Swelling and pain after a blow to the front of the leg (see anterior tibial compartment syndrome, p. 127)	[hospital]
Numbness or tingling in foot after a blow to the shin	[hospital]

[bandage] Use self-care   [stethoscope] See doctor

[phone] Call doctor's office for advice   [hospital] Seek help now

For more about the symbols, see p. 2.

NECK PAIN

The neck, or cervical spine, is the most flexible part of the spine, providing the greatest range of motion. But, because it is not well protected by muscles, it's also easy to injure. Daily stress, poor posture, trauma, and wear and tear from overuse and aging are the most common sources of neck pain.

Severe trauma to the neck may cause a fracture, creating risk for permanent paralysis. For possible neck or other spinal injuries from a severe blow or other trauma, **keep the injured person still.** *Do not move the person* without a back board or cervical collar *and* the help and direction of a trained paramedic or other medical professional.

A Bad Night's Rest

How you sleep at night can affect your neck during the day. A soft mattress, pillows that force your neck into awkward angles, and uncomfortable sleeping positions may be to blame if you awaken with a "crick in the neck." But the tossing and turning of a bad night's rest may be less to blame than awakening suddenly from a good sound sleep. A sudden jerk of the neck upon awakening can leave neck muscles tight and sore.

Body Mechanics

Poor sitting and standing posture—slumped shoulders, a "drooping" head, slouching or "rounding" of the lower back—can cause neck pain. But bad body mechanics are more than poor posture. Repeated tasks, such as holding the phone with your shoulder or always carrying a heavy briefcase or shoulder bag on the same side of the body, can also cause muscle stiffness or imbalance. Workstations, too, may force your body into less than the best positions.

I work a lot on a computer. Long hours at the computer often left me with a headache and pain in the neck. When our office moved last month, I got a new adjustable computer station and chair. A consultant who was setting up my workstation suggested I raise the computer screen higher so it would be at my eye level. I rarely get neck pain and headaches at work anymore. What a difference!

Mark

MUSCLES OF THE BACK OF THE HEAD AND NECK

Splenius capitis muscle

Sternocleido-mastoid muscle

Levator scapulae muscle

Trapezius muscle

Deltoid muscle

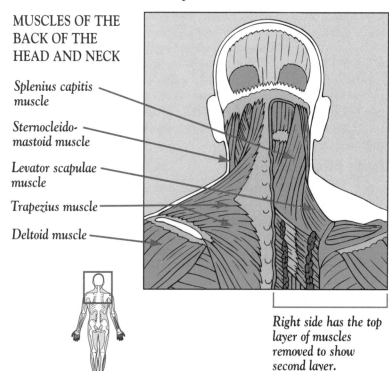

Right side has the top layer of muscles removed to show second layer.

Stress

The neck and upper back muscles are often among the first to become tense when a person is under emotional stress. Whenever these muscles remain tight for a long time, they may ache, become sore, and even cause headaches.

Neck Sprains and Strains

The term "whiplash" is often used to refer to neck sprains and strains that result when the neck is forced suddenly forward, backward, or both, such as from a rear-end car collision. But contact sports, a fall, or a sudden twist can cause similar injuries. Pain from neck sprains and strains may spread into the shoulders, upper back, and arms, and sometimes as far as the legs. Pain may remain for 6 weeks or longer, but generally improves with normal use. In some cases, physical therapy or special exercises may be helpful.

Degenerative Joint Disease (DJD)

Between each bone (vertebra) of the spine is a cartilage disc filled with a gelatin-like substance that provides cushioning. As we age, these discs become thinner, losing some of their capacity for absorbing shock. The joints of the neck may also become inflamed due to arthritis or bone spurs, or a disc may herniate (push outward) from its normal space and place pressure on the nerves. DJD usually occurs in people over the age of 40. DJD often causes painful muscle spasms in the neck and upper back, a dull aching in one arm, or numbness and tingling in the arm or fingers. A direct blow can also make discs bulge or break, causing similar problems to those of disc degeneration. Any pain, numbness, or tingling should be evaluated by a doctor.

Brachial Plexus Stretch

A brachial plexus stretch, often called a "burner" or "stinger," occurs when the neck and shoulder are twisted in opposite directions at the same time, stretching the brachial plexus nerves. The result is shooting, burning pain, weakness in the shoulder muscles, and loss of feeling in the shoulders, which require **an immediate visit to the doctor.** This type of injury tends to occur most often in contact sports.

Meningitis

Meningitis symptoms include a very stiff neck, fever, and headache. Because meningitis can be life threatening if not treated promptly with antibiotics, you should **see your doctor immediately** if you have these symptoms.

Neck pain can often be relieved or prevented with a few adjustments to the way we work and rest. Even if the pain is caused by an injury or a worsening condition, self-care can often provide relief.

SELF-CARE STEPS FOR NECK PAIN

• If you wake up often with a sore neck, consider sleeping in a different position, getting a new mattress and box spring, or putting a $^3/_4$-inch plywood board between the mattress and box spring for extra support.

• If you sleep on your side, choose a pillow that allows your head to rest comfortably centered between your shoulders. If you sleep on your back, choose a pillow that doesn't push your chin toward your chest. A special cervical-support pillow or a rolled towel pinned around your neck can also help you position your spine correctly. Avoid sleeping on your stomach.

• Learn to relax. If daily stress makes your neck and upper back muscles tense, take time out to relax (see Self-Care Steps for Stress, p. 199).

• If your neck or upper back muscles feel tight and sore, especially from stress, ask a friend to massage the area for a few minutes.

• The spine naturally curves in at the neck, out at the upper back, and in again at the lower back. An easy way to improve your posture is to focus on keeping the natural curve at the lower back. When you do this, the rest of the spine tends to pull into place, straightening your shoulders and head as well. Be sure, however, that your effort to "straighten up" doesn't cause your neck or abdomen to "stick out."

• Use a telephone headset if you spend a lot of time on the phone. Keep your briefcase or purse as light as possible and routinely switch carrying sides. When either is packed full, try to distribute the weight evenly on each side of your body by splitting the contents into two bags or briefcases. Hold reading materials and place computer screens at eye level; don't bend over your work. Type with your elbows, hips, and knees at 90-degree angles, and make sure you have good low-back support.

• Ice a sore neck 10 to 15 minutes several times a day to relieve pain and inflammation. A bag of frozen peas or corn makes a great cold pack for the neck. Switching between heat and ice may also work.

• A warm shower or heating pad on top of a moist warm towel can help loosen sore, tight muscles. Apply heat for 20 minutes, three times a day starting no sooner than 2 days after injury. But ice may be better for relieving pain even long after an injury, especially if muscle spasms are present. Follow with gentle stretching.

• Take anti-inflammatory drugs for pain. If pain persists, your doctor may prescribe other drugs.

• Take a load off. When pain is at its worst, rest. Lie flat on your back for an hour or so with a fairly flat pillow supporting your head. Extended bed rest, however, can make neck problems worse by allowing muscles to weaken from lack of use.

• Stretch! Working on the problem is especially important for the neck. Reduce stiffness and soreness by gaining motion and strength with the stretches shown below.

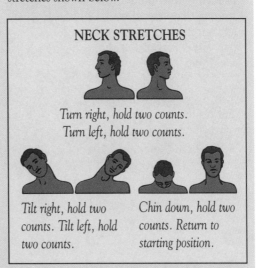

NECK STRETCHES

*Turn right, hold two counts.
Turn left, hold two counts.*

Tilt right, hold two counts. Tilt left, hold two counts.

Chin down, hold two counts. Return to starting position.

• After exercise, cool down in a healthy posture. One of the best—and easiest—times to assume a healthy posture is when your muscles and joints are loose after exercise.

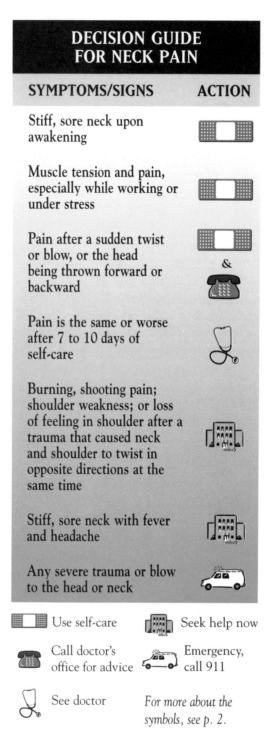

DECISION GUIDE FOR NECK PAIN

SYMPTOMS/SIGNS	ACTION
Stiff, sore neck upon awakening	Use self-care
Muscle tension and pain, especially while working or under stress	Use self-care
Pain after a sudden twist or blow, or the head being thrown forward or backward	Use self-care & Call doctor's office for advice
Pain is the same or worse after 7 to 10 days of self-care	See doctor
Burning, shooting pain; shoulder weakness; or loss of feeling in shoulder after a trauma that caused neck and shoulder to twist in opposite directions at the same time	Seek help now
Stiff, sore neck with fever and headache	Seek help now
Any severe trauma or blow to the head or neck	Emergency, call 911

Use self-care

Call doctor's office for advice

See doctor

Seek help now

Emergency, call 911

For more about the symbols, see p. 2.

SHOULDER PAIN

The shoulder is one of the most vulnerable joints in the body. Made for movement in all directions, the bones forming the shoulder joint give little in the way of stability. The shoulder is the junction of three bones: the upper-arm bone (humerus), the collarbone (clavicle), and the shoulder blade (scapula). But the smaller rotator cuff muscles, along with ligaments and other muscles and tissues, provide support and allow the shoulder a wide range of movement. Like other joints in the body, the shoulder can be injured by trauma (such as a fall or a blow) and overuse or repeated motions that add up over time.

Referred Pain

Sudden onset of shoulder pain without an injury can be a sign of other problems. When in the left shoulder, it may mean a possible heart attack, angina, or neck, spleen, liver, or lung problems. When in the right shoulder, it may mean gallbladder problems. When pain is referred from somewhere else, moving the arm will not increase the pain. **Call a physician or 911 immediately** if you have these symptoms or the symptoms of heart attack (p. 86).

Overuse Injuries

Three common overuse injuries include tendinitis, bursitis, and rotator cuff injuries (see Definitions of Common Muscle and Joint Problems, pgs. 98-99, for descriptions and treatments).

Trauma

A sudden twist, fall, or blow can lead to a sprain, shoulder dislocation (the upper arm bone comes "out of socket"), a partial dislocation, or broken bone. With any of these conditions, you may hear or feel popping, snapping, or tearing when the injury occurs. You may be unable to

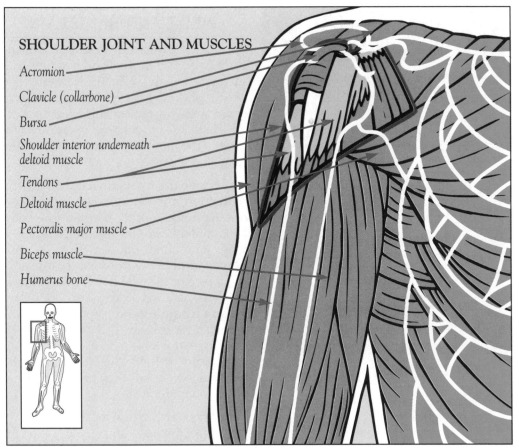

SHOULDER JOINT AND MUSCLES

Acromion

Clavicle (collarbone)

Bursa

Shoulder interior underneath deltoid muscle

Tendons

Deltoid muscle

Pectoralis major muscle

Biceps muscle

Humerus bone

I scraped and painted my entire garage in one weekend with no problems. Three days later, I noticed I had missed several spots on the eaves of the garage. It took less than an hour to get them done, but that night I had an awful pain in my shoulder. It was too late to call the doctor, so I tried icing the shoulder and took some aspirin. I got tired of holding the ice pack, so I wrapped it in place with an elastic bandage. When I called the doctor's office in the morning, the nurse said I had used the RICE method—exactly what I should have done. He said to keep doing it until the pain got better—which it did a few days later.

Jack

move your shoulder and, except for a sprain, there may be visible deformity of the shoulder. Although a sprain can be treated safely at home using the RICE method (p. 97), see your health care provider to make sure the shoulder isn't dislocated or fractured.

Another possible injury caused by falls or blows to the shoulder is an **acromioclavicular (AC) joint separation**. The AC joint is held together by ligaments, which connect the collarbone to a narrow part of the shoulder blade that extends to the front of the shoulder. AC separations can range from bruising the

joint to "stretching" or completely tearing the ligaments. With AC separations, a painful lump may form at the end of the collarbone, near the shoulder.

Muscle Imbalance

General muscle aches and tightness around the shoulder, upper back, or neck are often caused by muscle imbalance, which occurs when one side of the body is much stronger than the other side. Stretching and ice applications can help relieve the pain. But to keep it from happening again, weight training to strengthen the weaker side of the body is important.

SELF-CARE STEPS FOR SHOULDER PAIN

Although injuries should be seen by a doctor as soon as possible, overuse and muscle imbalance injuries can usually be treated with self-care. The RICE method (p. 97) and anti-inflammatory drugs, such as aspirin, ibuprofen, or naproxen, are the basics of self-care for shoulder injuries. Also, to keep it from happening again, you should work to strengthen the muscles around the joint. Your doctor's office or a physical therapist can suggest appropriate exercises.

DECISION GUIDE FOR SHOULDER PAIN

SYMPTOMS/SIGNS	ACTION
Shoulder pain after activity, limited to only certain movements	
Overuse injury still present or worse after 7 to 8 days, despite self-care	
Unable to raise arm	
Trauma with sudden pain; a pop, snap, or cracking sound or feeling; inability to move shoulder; a deformity or lump	
Sudden pain in right or left shoulder; no injury; and able to move arm without increasing pain	

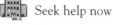 Use self-care

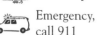 Call doctor's office for advice

See doctor

Seek help now

Emergency, call 911

For more about the symbols, see p. 2.

WRIST AND HAND PAIN

Together, the wrist and hand are composed of 29 bones: 19 in the hand and fingers, 8 in the wrist, and 2 in the forearm. The wrist, hand, and fingers are capable of a great variety of movements. But the forearm muscles are actually responsible for most of the movement and strength of the hand and fingers.

Because the wrist and hand have little protection, they are perhaps more likely to fracture than other bones in the body. Falls and blows are common causes of wrist and hand injuries. But, as with other joints, overuse and repeated motions can take their toll on the hand and wrist, causing a variety of conditions, such as tendinitis and carpal tunnel syndrome. The injuries listed below are by no means the only conditions that can cause pain or limit the function of the hand and wrist, but they are some of the more common ones.

Fractures and Sprains

Fractures and sprains of the wrist, hand, and fingers can be hard to pinpoint without an X-ray. Unless deformity, a change in feeling, or lack of motion is noticeable, you may start with self-care. However, you may want to call your doctor's office to ask if your injury should be seen by a health care provider. If pain or stiffness lasts more than 24 hours after injury, it should be seen. Children in obvious overnight discomfort should be seen right away.

When a wrist is fractured, the break often occurs at the end of the radius, one of the long bones of the forearm. These fractures require careful attention. Another fracture near the wrist—a navicular (a small wrist bone located at the base of the thumb) fracture—can cause long-term problems, is difficult to diagnose, and takes a long time to heal.

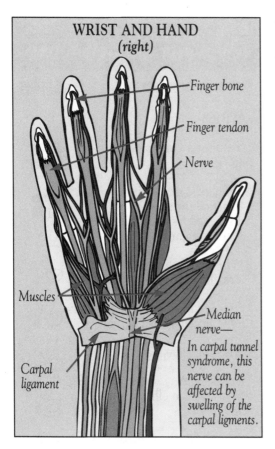

WRIST AND HAND
(right)

Finger bone

Finger tendon

Nerve

Muscles

Carpal ligament

Median nerve—

In carpal tunnel syndrome, this nerve can be affected by swelling of the carpal ligments.

Because the bone is so small and almost all of its surface touches other bones, an improperly healed fracture can cause the navicular to rub and scrape in places it shouldn't. The result is pain and loss of range of motion in the wrist.

If you fall on your outstretched hand, bending your wrist back, and the pain does not get better within a day, you should see your doctor and have an X-ray. If the X-ray shows no sign of fracture, but the pain is still present 1 week later, another X-ray is needed. Sometimes small fractures are easier to see by X-ray in 7 to 10 days.

Tendinitis

It is common for tendons in the wrist, hand, and fingers to become irritated from overuse or repeated motions, causing pain, swelling, and stiffness.

Tendinitis pain in the wrist may spread down to the fingers or up to the elbow. Tendinitis in the fingers may affect one or more fingers at the same time. Pain may be constant or felt only with certain movements. The area around the tendon may be tender. You may even notice a cracking sound or odd feeling when you bend or flex the finger or wrist.

Ganglion

Ganglions (see definition, p. 98) are harmless, may or may not cause pain or discomfort, and may go away eventually on their own. Rarely, if you find a ganglion bothersome, your doctor may drain it with a needle or remove it surgically. In most cases, the risks of surgery outweigh the benefits of removing the ganglion, so just watching for changes is preferred.

Carpal Tunnel Syndrome (CTS)

A condition caused by pressure on a large nerve in the wrist as it passes through a "tunnel" formed by tendons, CTS causes pain that may spread into the hand and forearm. There may be numbness and tingling in the fingers, especially your thumb, index, and middle finger, and loss of strength in the hand. You may find yourself dropping things often or even being awakened at night by tingling and numbness in your hand.

Mallet Finger

You reach to catch a ball and instead of landing in your palm, it smacks right into the end of your finger. The result: a mallet finger. Inside the finger, a tendon is partly torn. From the outside, you may see very little, but the finger cannot be fully straightened. An X-ray is recommended. With time, however, mallet fingers usually heal on their own.

Skier's Thumb

This often happens during a fall while skiing. The pole catches on the snow or ground and pulls the thumb away from the fingers. But any forceful motion that pulls the thumb in the wrong direction can cause "skier's thumb," a tear in the ligament connecting the thumb to the metacarpal bone of the hand. In bad cases, the ligament severs completely. This injury should be seen by a doctor.

There are some general self-care guidelines for handling wrist and hand pain. However, for specific injuries, treatment is needed.

SELF-CARE STEPS FOR WRIST AND HAND PAIN

- Apply ice immediately.
- Always remove rings before exercising or doing manual labor. If you are wearing rings and hurt your hand, remove them immediately before swelling has a chance to begin.

 Use self-care   See doctor

 Call doctor's office for advice   Seek help now

For more about the symbols, see p. 2.

DECISION GUIDE FOR WRIST AND HAND PAIN

SYMPTOMS/SIGNS	ACTION
WRIST	
Tendinitis symptoms (p. 135)	
Numbness or tingling in fingers during day or awakened by these symptoms at night	
Pain after falling on outstretched hand	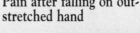
Fever or rapid swelling in joint, accompanied by pain	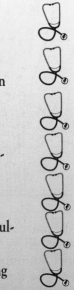
Shooting pains	
Pain spreading up from wrist to elbow/shoulder/neck	
Pain and neck stiffness	
Dropping objects or difficulty holding objects	
Clicking, popping, grinding	
Visible deformity after a fall	
HAND AND FINGERS	
Injury not affecting movement	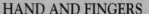
Symptoms not relieved after 4 to 8 hours of self-care	
Mallet finger (p. 136)	
Tender spot on shaft of finger bones (not at joint)	
Pain, swelling, and bruising after thumb is accidentally bent backward	

PROBLEMS OF SEXUALITY

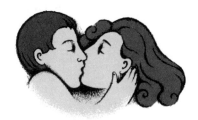

Not only can health problems related to sexuality have a devastating effect on you as an individual, such problems almost always affect others as well.

This section describes how to recognize and treat common sexual problems. Because sexually transmitted diseases are becoming more common, and the consequences of getting a sexually transmitted disease (STD) can be serious, this section offers specific advice on how to protect yourself and others through safer sex.

AIDS AND OTHER SEXUALLY TRANSMITTED DISEASES

Millions of Americans are affected by sexually transmitted diseases (STDs) of all kinds. Yet, since we first began hearing about the AIDS epidemic in the early 1980s, many people seem to have forgotten that other STDs are still alive and well. Although AIDS is the most deadly STD, other diseases such as syphilis, gonorrhea, genital herpes, hepatitis B, and chlamydia also pose serious health risks.

Acquired Immune Deficiency Syndrome (AIDS)

An estimated 1 million to 1.5 million Americans have **human immunodeficiency virus (HIV)**—the virus that leads to AIDS. The virus is spread through some types of sexual contact, shared intravenous (IV) needles, and introduction of infected blood or semen into the body. Once a person gets HIV, it can take years before AIDS actually develops. AIDS is usually fatal. Although drugs like zidovudine (formerly called AZT) can slow it down, at this point there is no cure. HIV can damage the immune system, allowing a person to get certain infections and cancers.

Even if an infected person is otherwise healthy and has not yet developed AIDS, *any time* after he or she "catches" HIV this person can spread it to other people. This can occur through unprotected sexual contact (intercourse without a condom) or shared IV drug needles.

Chlamydia

About 3 million to 4 million people in the United States have this bacterial infection. Those at high risk for chlamydia infections include sexually active young adults (under age 25, especially teenagers), those who have several sexual partners or a new sexual partner within the last two months, and those whose sexual partner has chlamydia. In women, chlamydia can cause inflammation of the cervix and pelvic inflammatory disease (PID)—a leading cause of ectopic pregnancies (when the fetus attaches and grows in the fallopian tubes instead of in the uterus) and infertility in American women. In men, it can cause inflammation of the urethra, the organ through which urine passes, and the epididymis, where sperm are stored. Fortunately, chlamydia is easily cured by taking antibiotics for a week.

Genital Herpes (Herpes Simplex Virus Type 2)

An estimated 20 million people in the United States have genital herpes. Herpes simplex virus type 2 causes painful sores on the genitals and around the mouth. Even after the initial outbreak of sores heals, an infected person may carry the virus for years, with new sores erupting from time to time. The herpes virus can be spread to other people through sexual contact whether sores are present or not. Although there is no cure for herpes, there are drugs that can reduce the length and pain of herpes outbreaks.

Gonorrhea

About 2 million Americans get gonorrhea each year. In men, the infection can cause inflammation of the genitals and rectum. In women, it can cause painful PID and complications during pregnancy. People who have several partners are at high risk for gonorrhea, but anyone can get infected. Fortunately, gonorrhea is easily treated with antibiotics.

Hepatitis B Virus (HBV)

HBV is a sexually transmitted disease that causes inflammation of the liver and can lead to cirrhosis and cancer of the liver. High-risk factors for getting HBV include IV drug abuse, having several sexual partners, or having a partner who is currently infected or a chronic carrier. If you think you have been exposed to HBV, your doctor may be able to give you hepatitis B immune globulin to prevent hepatitis from developing. (Also see Viral Hepatitis, p. 56).

Syphilis

In early stages, this bacterial infection causes painful sores of the genitals, rectum, and throat. If left untreated, it can produce warts in the genital area, contagious sores on other parts of the body, disease of the lymph nodes, and later problems with the nervous system and heart and mental illness. Unfortunately, the number of syphilis cases in America is now at its highest point since 1950. Syphilis, however, is easily treated with antibiotics.

Special Risks during Pregnancy

Sexually transmitted diseases pose special risks during pregnancy. All the STDs discussed above can be passed from mother to child during pregnancy, at birth, or shortly after. Often, STDs can lead to health problems for newborns. For example, chlamydia can cause pneumonia; gonorrhea causes blindness; syphilis causes genital herpes, and AIDS can kill. Many children who get hepatitis at or before birth become chronic carriers of the virus. Women who have syphilis, gonorrhea, or chlamydia can be treated with antibiotics during pregnancy to prevent complications for themselves and their babies. Women with active genital herpes sores may need to deliver by caesarean section to keep their babies from getting the virus. Women who are HIV positive should take the drug zidovudine (AZT) during pregnancy to reduce the risk of passing the virus to the baby.

PREVENTIVE STEPS

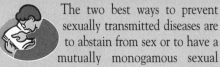

The two best ways to prevent sexually transmitted diseases are to abstain from sex or to have a mutually monogamous sexual relationship with someone who is uninfected. If neither option works for you, here are some other things you can do:

• Always use a latex condom and spermicidal gel. Choose latex condoms with receptacle tips rather than natural-membrane condoms, which may be more likely to break or to allow viruses and bacteria to pass through. The spermicide nonoxynol 9 has also been shown to provide added protection against HIV, HBV, and herpes simplex virus. It also reduces the risk of chlamydia and gonorrhea in women.

• Limit the number of sexual partners you have. Remember that when it comes to STDs, having sex outside of a mutually monogamous relationship puts you at the same risk as if you had sex with all your partner's partners. Thus, the more sexual partners you have, the greater your risk for STDs.

If you think you may have an STD, see your doctor. He or she can advise you on whether or not you should be tested, and treat you properly if you test positive.

Keep in mind that neither condoms nor spermicides offer foolproof protection. In fact, condoms fail at a rate of 10 to 15 percent as a result of flaws or improper use.

CONTRACEPTION

The decision to have or not have children is a very personal one for individuals and couples. For married couples and those in long-term relationships, the decision of whether or when to use birth control and the choice of method is best made jointly.

Birth control options range from natural methods, such as the rhythm method, to surgical sterilization (vasectomy for men, tubal ligation for women). In between are a variety of choices, some of which are more effective than others. The effectiveness of a contraceptive method is measured in terms of the number of pregnancies that can be expected if 100 couples used the method for 1 year. Thus, a 2 percent failure rate means that of those 100 couples, two could expect to become pregnant during the year using that method. Without any method of birth control, 85 of the 100 couples would conceive within the year. Below are descriptions of various birth control choices and their effectiveness rates.

Natural Methods
(20 percent failure rate)
These methods are called natural because they do not rely on devices, pills, or other products. The rhythm method involves abstaining from intercourse during the time a woman is fertile. The woman calculates her fertile period by one of four methods: by calendar, basal body temperature, ovulation (monitoring changes in vaginal mucus to identify when ovulation occurs), and symptothermal (a combination of basal body temperature and ovulation methods). The calendar method, which relies simply on predicting ovulation mathematically based on the average number of days between periods, has a very high failure rate. When used diligently and correctly, the latter three rhythm methods can have failure rates as low as 5 percent. On average, however, they fail 20 percent of the time.

The other "natural" method is withdrawal. Using this method, the man withdraws his penis from the woman's vagina before ejaculation. Withdrawal requires a great degree of control and flawless timing on the man's part. The failure rate of this method is quite high.

Spermicides
(18 percent failure rate)

Spermicides kill sperm before they can enter the uterus. They come in foams, jellies, suppositories, creams, and foaming tablets, which are inserted into the vagina before intercourse, providing protection for up to 2 hours. When used with condoms or diaphragms, spermicides provide added protection against pregnancy and even some STDs. Occasionally, a man or a woman may be allergic to spermicides.

Barrier Methods
(12 to 18 percent failure rate)

Condoms and diaphragms fall into this category. **Condoms** can be bought over the counter and do not cost much. Worn over the erect penis, condoms can fail if they break or if the penis remains in the vagina after it is no longer erect and the condom slips off (see How to Put on a Condom, p. 142). Condoms used without spermicide fail to prevent pregnancy 12 percent of the time. Condoms with reservoir tips, spermicide, or both are safer in preventing pregnancy. When using a condom, the penis should be withdrawn from the vagina immediately after ejaculation, before the penis becomes soft.

A **diaphragm** is a saucer-shaped piece of rubber with a flexible metal rim. It is inserted into the vagina where it sits snugly against the cervix, or entrance to the uterus. Although the diaphragm is a partial physical barrier against sperm, the real protective agent is the tablespoon of spermicidal cream or jelly it holds against the cervix. Diaphragms must be fitted by a doctor or nurse practitioner. When used with spermicide, they fail to prevent pregnancy 18 percent of the time.

Intrauterine Devices
(2 percent failure rate)

Intrauterine devices (IUDs) are small devices placed inside the uterus. They may be made of plastic and may contain copper or hormones. No one knows exactly how they work. They are thought to keep the fertilized eggs from implanting in the uterine lining, possibly by causing changes in the lining itself. The copper or ParaGard IUD also kills sperm as they approach the IUD, thereby preventing fertilization. Depending on the device and the woman, an IUD can be worn for up to 10 years. Fertility returns as soon as the device is removed. IUDs must be put in and removed by a doctor or nurse practitioner. They are best for women who have had children and want to space pregnancies, but are not ready for permanent sterilization.

Birth Control Pills
(1 to 3 percent failure rate)

Birth control pills, or "the pill," work mainly by preventing ovulation and changing cervical mucus and the lining of the uterus. Birth control pills are available only by prescription. They contain synthetic versions of the female hormones estrogen and progesterone, or just progesterone. Side effects of one pill are often resolved by switching to another. The pill is convenient and highly effective.

Implants
(less than 1 percent failure rate)

Norplant is the only implant now available in the United States. Like the pill, it contains hormones. A local anesthetic is used to surgically place the implants under the skin on the inner side of the upper arm. Implants can provide contraceptive protection for 5 years. Irregular bleeding and weight gain are common side effects of contraceptive implants.

METHODS OF CONTRACEPTION

Spermicides *are inserted into the vagina before intercourse. They come in foams, jellies, suppositories, creams, and foaming tablets. They provide protection for up to 2 hours. They have an 18 percent failure rate.*

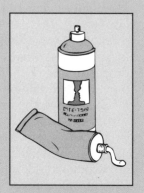

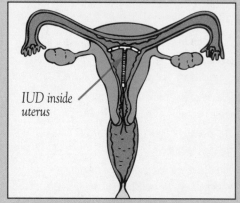

IUD inside uterus

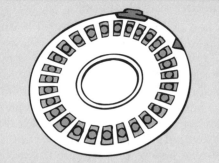

Birth control pills *work by preventing ovulation. They come in various formulations of the female hormones estrogen and progesterone, as well as a progesterone-only formulation. They have a 1 to 3 percent failure rate.*

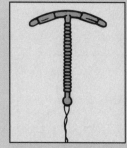

Intrauterine devices *are small devices, usually made of plastic, that are placed inside the uterus. They can be worn for up to 10 years. They have a 2 percent failure rate.*

Barrier methods *include condoms and diaphragms. Condoms are worn over the penis and prevent semen from entering the vagina.*

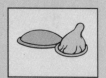

Diaphragms are inserted into the vagina where they fit snugly against the cervix, or entrance to the uterus. They have a 12 to 18 percent failure rate.

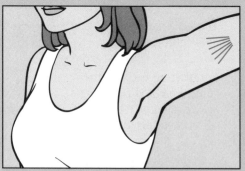

Implants *are placed surgically under the skin on the arm. They provide up to 5 years of protection. They have a less than 1 percent failure rate.*

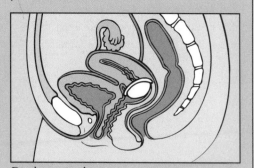

Diaphragm in place

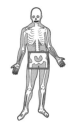

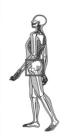

HOW TO PUT ON A CONDOM

1. Make sure the condom has a reservoir or leave at least a half-inch extra space at the top for semen.

2. Put on the condom when the penis is fully erect. Squeeze the reservoir end free of air and roll condom down to the base of the penis.

3. Withdraw the penis soon after ejaculation while the penis is still erect. Hold on to the base of the condom while withdrawing, to avoid spilling the semen.

You can use a lubricant to help keep the condom from tearing. Be sure to use only water-base lubricants. Oil-base lubricants like petroleum jelly or baby oil can damage condoms and can cause them to break.

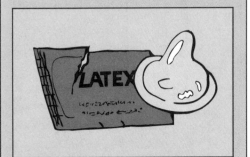

Use only latex condoms and follow instructions. *Condoms made of other materials have tiny holes that can let sexually transmitted diseases through. Check the expiration date on the condom package. Do not use the condom if the expiration date has passed. Store condoms in a cool, dark, dry place. Heat can harm them.*

Progesterone Injections
(less than 1 percent failure rate)

Progesterone injection, or Depo-Provera, given once every 3 months prevents ovulation. It also prevents implantation, should an egg be fertilized, by keeping the lining of the uterus from building up. Proper timing of the injections is important for maintaining contraceptive protection. When the first injection is given within the first 5 days of a normal menstrual cycle, protection from pregnancy is immediate. Infrequent or irregular periods are a common side effect of Depo-Provera. Weight gain can also be a side effect.

Making the Decision

When choosing a birth control method, you and your spouse or partner may wish to talk with your doctor, nurse practitioner, or other clinic staff to discuss the options and decide which is most suited to your needs. A health care professional can help you weigh the risks and benefits of the options you are considering and tell you how to properly use the method you choose.

DECISION GUIDE FOR CONTRACEPTION

SYMPTOMS/SIGNS	ACTION
You need more information on a contraceptive	
You wish to use a birth-control method requiring a prescription or would like surgical sterilization	
If a woman suspects she is pregnant	

 Call doctor's office for advice   See doctor

For more about the symbols, see p. 2.

SEXUAL PROBLEMS

The "right way" to make love and the "right" frequency for sex are simply what work best and are most satisfying for each couple. Unfortunately, however, anxiety and physical, emotional, or relationship issues can sometimes interfere with a person's or couple's ability to enjoy or participate fully in sex.

Simply growing older, too, brings changes in sexual function for both men and women. Most people don't have the same level of sexual desire at age 55 that they had when they were 20. Interest in sex usually declines slowly with age, though it seldom disappears totally. Similarly, as people grow older, they usually need more time and more direct genital stimulation before reaching orgasm.

In older men, erections are usually not as firm as they once were and more time (days, as opposed to hours) may be needed after ejaculation before they are able to have another. In postmenopausal women, vaginal dryness may cause discomfort during intercourse. Water-soluble lubricants, however, are available to help this problem (see Menopause, p. 182, and Vaginal Discharge, p. 186).

Unfortunately, without knowing that such changes are a normal part of aging, many people worry that something is wrong with them sexually or with their relationships.

Common sexual problems that can occur at any age include differing or decrease in sexual desire, erection problems, rapid ejaculation, and problems with orgasm. Often these problems are caused by a combination of physical and psychological or relationship issues.

The first of these issues, differing sexual desire, is problematic only if a couple cannot find a mutually satisfying compromise. Sexual desire naturally varies from person to person. Some may want sex three times a day; others, three times a year. There is no "right" or "normal" level of desire.

Diminished desire is common in both men and women in times of stress, when ill or recovering from an illness, or when tension exists in their relationship. Alcohol and certain drugs—birth control pills, antihistamines, and blood pressure medications, among others—can also cause a loss of desire. These same factors can cause temporary erection problems (impotence) and inhibit orgasm in both men and women.

At some time in life, most men will have temporary erection problems, during which they are unable to achieve or keep enough of an erection for intercourse. About 30 million American men, however, have a long-term problem that could benefit from medical treatment, counseling, or both. Of all long-term sexual problems, 50 to 75 percent have a physical cause, such as diabetes, vascular problems, or drug side effects.

Early ejaculation (when semen is released before you or your partner have time to achieve climax) and delayed ejaculation often can be relieved by making adjustments in lovemaking (see Self-Care Steps, p. 144).

For both men and women, there's more to sex than intercourse. Touching, kissing, caresses, massage, even holding hands and talking are all as important to intimacy and sexual pleasure as intercourse. In women, orgasm is achieved by stimulating the clitoris. A very high percentage of women do not have orgasms during intercourse. Orgasm from oral or manual stimulation of the clitoris, however, is just as satisfying as vaginal orgasm. In men, stimulating the head of the penis brings orgasm. As men age, they often need more direct stimula-

Several months ago, I realized that my husband and I hadn't had intercourse or any sexual contact in more than 2 months. I became afraid that maybe he was mad at me or no longer found me attractive. At first I tried starting sex, but he was always "tired" or "busy." I felt lonely and rejected. The tension got so bad we finally had to talk. It wasn't an easy discussion by any means. But we were able to begin to clear up some issues both in and out of bed. It seemed we both needed to make changes in the way we made love and in the way we treated each other the rest of the time.

Anne

tion of the penis to achieve an erection or orgasm. But foreplay that focuses only on the genitals doesn't always give either partner time to become mentally and emotionally aroused for sex—an important step to orgasm. Whole-body massage and caresses can help arouse and prepare a man or woman for more direct genital stimulation.

Couples and individuals can often fix sexual problems on their own, but sometimes need medical help or counseling. Your doctor can recommend a qualified counselor or a doctor specializing in sexual health, and the Self-Care Steps below list some things to try on your own.

DECISION GUIDE FOR SEXUAL PROBLEMS

SYMPTOMS/SIGNS	ACTION
Loss of sexual desire, erection, ejaculation, or orgasm problems	
Sexual problems continue or worsen despite self-care	
Physical problem or medical condition (such as diabetes or heart disease) may be causing sexual problem	

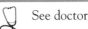 Use self-care   See doctor

Call doctor's office for advice   *For more about the symbols, see p. 2*

SELF-CARE STEPS FOR SEXUAL PROBLEMS

• Talk. Good communication is the key to good sex and a good relationship. Tell and show your partner how you like to be touched. Talk through other problems and tensions in your relationship as they arise. If you aren't getting along well the rest of the day, you'll be less likely to get along in bed.

• Focus on your senses. This can help reduce sexual anxiety and heighten responsiveness for men and women. Agree not to have intercourse for at least a month. During that time, set aside an hour or two each day to massage each other. While naked, explore and massage all parts of each other's body, except the genitals and breasts. Once you are fully comfortable with this, begin to include the breasts and the genitals, but do not have intercourse.

Finally, when you are both more relaxed, start having intercourse. Continue to use whole-body sensuality in your foreplay.

• Pause, change positions, or think about something else. If fast ejaculation is a problem, doing any one of these three things at the first sensation of ejaculation can allow a man to hold onto an erection longer.

• Remember, good sex is possible even without intercourse. An erection is not a requirement for either person to have an orgasm.

• Avoid alcohol and drugs that warn "may cause drowsiness." If you are having sexual problems, ask your doctor if any drugs you are taking could be a cause.

SKIN AND HAIR PROBLEMS

Your skin offers the most visible indication of your overall health. This section describes common problems of hair and skin, and suggests ways to take care of nonurgent conditions at home.

Your primary care doctor (pediatrician, family practitioner, or internal medicine specialist) can offer advice and treatment for many skin and hair problems. If your condition is especially difficult to handle, your primary care doctor may involve other medical providers who specialize in the care of skin—such as dermatologists or allergists. *This information cannot replace care by your health care providers.*

Use the Decision Guides to see if your symptoms warrant medical attention or if they can be handled with self-care. However, you need to consider your own medical history and your current health when deciding if self-care is right for you. If you have any conditions that do not seem to be healing normally, or if self-care steps do not seem helpful, call your health care provider.

ACNE

Who among us has not looked in the mirror and seen the blemish we were sure would ruin our day, if not our life? Three out of four teenagers have some acne, and some adults continue to have acne into their twenties, thirties, and forties.

When hair follicles in the skin become plugged with a combination of sebum (fat) and cellular material, a pimple results.

In teenagers, acne is linked to hormonal activity and often occurs on the face, back, chest, and upper arms. Adult acne shows up mainly on the face. An especially problematic form of adult acne, called **rosacea**, affects the skin of the nose, forehead, and cheeks. Acne rosacea usually responds well to medical treatment.

The good news is: acne eventually goes away. The bad news is: it doesn't go away overnight. A regular skin care regimen, perhaps combined with prescription medicine recommended by a health care provider, can help avoid outbreaks and potential scarring.

I'm 34 years old and I'm sick and tired of having pimples. This has been going on since I was 17. I can't seem to point to any one thing that makes my acne flare up, but antibiotics and Retin-A help contain it.
Betsy

A primary care doctor or other provider may recommend a topical medicine, oral antibiotics, or both. Lotions, creams, or gels containing vitamin A acid (tretinoin—commonly called Retin-A) help stop pimples from forming by preventing dead skin cells from sticking to the wall of the hair follicle. Antibiotics work by keeping bacteria from forming and reducing inflammation. Severe cases of acne can be treated with a pill containing vitamin A called isotretinoin (Accutane). Accutane does have side effects, however, and cannot be taken by pregnant women.

The aftereffect of acne—scarring—also can be treated by a doctor, although it is costly. Collagen may be injected into scars to "fill them up." This treatment is expensive and temporary, lasting only 4 to 6 months. Surgery involving skin grafts is an option for deeper scars.

Although acne is not life threatening, its effects on self-esteem and self-confidence should not be downplayed.

HOW ACNE DEVELOPS

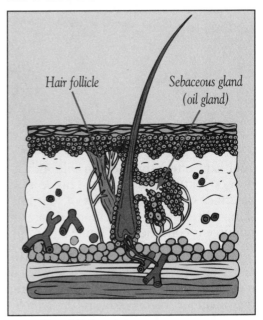

Normal hair follicle and skin structure

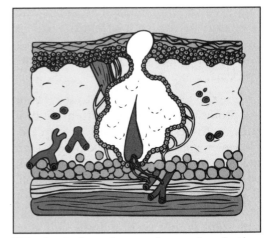

Whiteheads *form when pores become clogged with oily secretions and hair follicles break down.*

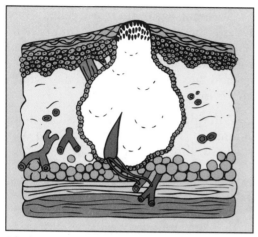

Blackheads form when the clogged pore is invaded by bacteria and pus. Blackheads should not be squeezed because this can cause further spreading of the bacteria.

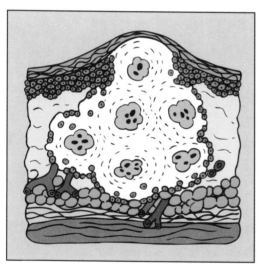

Acne or pimples form when the hair follicle walls rupture. Acne can then spread. Squeezing the pimple can cause the infection to spread further.

SELF-CARE STEPS FOR ACNE

• Wash your face once or twice daily with the cleanser of your choice.

• Use an "acne" cream or lotion. Start with over-the-counter lotions that contain benzoyl peroxide, sulfur, resorcinol, or salicylic acid as the main ingredient.

• Use a moisturizer labeled noncomedogenic (this has been tested and found not to cause pimples).

• Don't open your pimples unless your health care provider has given you instructions on how to do it correctly.

DECISION GUIDE FOR ACNE

SYMPTOMS/SIGNS	ACTION
Mild acne	
No improvement or worsens after 6 to 8 weeks of self-care	
Large red sore bumps that last longer than 3 days	
Lowered self-esteem because of appearance	
Tendency to scar	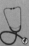

 Use self-care

 Call doctor's office

See doctor

 For more about the symbols, see p. 2.

When my daughter was diagnosed with asthma, I was terrified until I replaced fear with facts. I've learned to control house dust mites and molds. She knows what to do in an asthma attack. In fact, she got an "A" for a speech she presented to her class about her asthma inhaler.

Jolene

In my 15 years as a practicing allergist, treatments have improved greatly. Immunotherapy (allergy injections) produces results that can usually be seen in a year or less. It's remarkable how effective modern drugs are for allergy sufferers.

Allergy Specialist

ALLERGIC REACTIONS

For Hives, see p. 158; for Poison Ivy/Poison Oak/Poison Sumac, see p. 164; for Rashes, see p. 166.

Over 40 million Americans are allergic to pollens, molds, drugs, insect bites, animals, cosmetics, foods, dusts, and other substances. These substances are called allergens. Symptoms may be seasonal or year round.

Suspect allergies if you have:

- Sneezing or a runny nose
- Hives or rashes
- Itchy throat and eyes
- A sore throat or a dry cough
- Wheezing
- A family history of allergies

Allergic rashes *See Rashes, p. 166.*

Asthma *See Asthma, p. 207.*

Insect stings *See Insect Bites, p. 29.*

Life-threatening allergic insect sting symptoms include dizziness, nausea, stomach cramps, diarrhea, weakness, difficulty in breathing, a drop in blood pressure, shock, or unconsciousness (see Insect Bites, p. 29).

Seasonal nasal allergies, called "hay fever," are caused by molds and pollens of trees, grasses, and weeds. Sneezing, runny nose, itchy eyelids, and nasal congestion are common symptoms, which last as long as the exposure.

Allergic skin reactions include eczema (p. 156), hives (p. 158), and skin tissue swelling (edema).

MEDICAL MANAGEMENT

Your doctor will ask you questions about your allergy symptoms and allergies in your family. An exam of your nose, mouth, and chest will be performed. Treatment options include avoiding exposure to allergens, drugs such as antihistamine/decongestants and prescription nasal sprays, and sometimes allergy shots, which boost your resistance to allergens. If you do not respond to common treatment, referral to an allergist for special testing may be suggested. Allergy shots require several office visits over a period of months or years to raise dosages for boosting your resistance to allergens.

SELF-CARE STEPS FOR ALLERGIC REACTIONS

- Avoid exposure to allergens.
- Wash pets regularly.
- Vacuum your home carefully twice weekly to control dust.
- Consider installing air conditioning and air cleaning devices in your home. Have heating and cooling systems professionally cleaned twice a year.
- Remove unnecessary carpeting, paper, and cloth materials from your home.
- Use nonprescription antihistamines carefully.
- Lubricate your nasal passages with nasal saline rinses.
- Wear a medical alert bracelet warning of severe allergies (especially allergies to drugs).

DECISION GUIDE FOR ALLERGIC REACTIONS

SYMPTOMS/SIGNS	ACTION
Mild allergic reaction that resembles a cold	
Rash accompanies the allergy	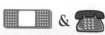
Runny nose, watery eyes, and sneezing lasts longer than 10 to 14 days	
Allergic reaction includes chest tightness, wheezing, and a hivelike rash	
Choking or difficulty swallowing*	
Swelling of lips, tongue, or throat*	
Rapid pulse, flushed face or skin, bluish color around lips*	
Severe gastrointestinal symptoms, like vomiting or diarrhea*	
Insect sting causes a widespread rash *(also see Insect Bites, p. 29)	
Severe asthma flare-up	

*If these symptoms occur within 1 to 15 minutes after exposure to allergen, remember: *Allergic reactions are potentially emergency conditions; if you are concerned, call your doctor immediately or go to urgent care or the emergency room.*

ATHLETE'S FOOT

You don't have to be an athlete to get athlete's foot, a common fungal skin infection that thrives in hot, moist conditions.

Caused by the same infection as ringworm and jock itch, athlete's foot usually shows up between the toes. Symptoms include red scaling and peeling or dead skin. The affected area may itch and develop a musty odor.

Although annoying, athlete's foot usually responds to prompt treatment. Left unchecked, however, it can spread to the toenails, causing nails to thicken and discolor.

SELF-CARE STEPS FOR ATHLETE'S FOOT

- Wash feet often and dry thoroughly, especially between toes.
- A hair dryer, set on the coolest setting, can dry skin fast and well.
- After drying, apply an antifungal product such as clotrimazole (Lotrimin) or tolnaftate (Tinactin).

Note: Powders help keep the area dry, which adds to comfort and may prevent spread of infection. Lotions and creams can attack the infection more directly.

DECISION GUIDE FOR ATHLETE'S FOOT

SYMPTOMS/SIGNS	ACTION
Athlete's foot responds promptly to self-care	
Self-care doesn't clear up the problem in about a week	

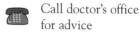 Use self-care

 Call doctor's office for advice

Seek help now

For more about the symbols, see p. 2.

BLISTERS

Blisters are usually caused by repeated rubbing or friction on tender skin until fluid collects under the outer layer of skin. Blisters often form on hands unaccustomed to physical labor and feet exposed to ill-fitting shoes. However, blisters can also be caused by burns, allergic reaction, and chemical irritation.

Blisters can also signal other health problems. Blisters that appear on the genitals can be herpes simplex virus type 2 (see AIDS and Other Sexually Transmitted Diseases, p. 137). Blisters that form a ring on the scalp or body can be ringworm (p. 167). Unusual blisters should be seen by your health care provider.

To keep common blisters from developing, wear work gloves when doing physical labor. Extra socks, a bandage, or petroleum jelly on a foot likely to blister can reduce friction and prevent a blister.

Hiking precautions include good shoes, thin inner socks, and changing socks. Use moleskin for any areas of skin that feel hot, one of the first signs of a blister.

SELF-CARE STEPS FOR BLISTERS

• Friction blisters are best left unbroken if skin irritation can be avoided until the fluid disappears.

• For blisters on the feet use "second skin," an over-the-counter product, to help when walking.

• If the blister breaks open, treat it like an open wound. Wash it with soap and warm water. Apply an antibacterial ointment and cover with a clean bandage. Watch for signs of infection—redness, pain, swelling, or red streaks leading toward the body. Call your health care provider if the wound becomes infected.

DECISION GUIDE FOR BLISTERS

SYMPTOMS/SIGNS	ACTION
Minor blister	
Common blister infection	
Unusual blister appears without warning	

 Use self-care    See doctor

Call doctor's office for advice   *For more about the symbols, see p. 2.*

BOILS

When skin bacteria, called *staphylococci*, invade a hair follicle, a boil results. Skin tissue swells, and a tender and red, pus-filled lump emerges (see color photo p. 309). The pus contains white blood cells fighting the infection. Until the boil opens and the pus is released, the boil will be painful and tender to the touch.

Boils can range in size from a pea to a walnut. Although boils may be found anywhere on the body, they most commonly occur in areas where there is hair and chafing, such as the neck, armpits, genitals, breasts, face, and buttocks.

Boils can be a bit contagious. Scratching can spread the infection to other areas of the body. Keep the boil area clean and always wash hands after touching it.

SELF-CARE STEPS FOR BOILS

- Apply warm compresses to relieve pain and bring the boil to a head.

- Keep the area clean to prevent the spread of bacteria.

- Take a pain reliever to reduce pain and inflammation.

- When the boil opens, carefully wipe away the pus.

- Wash gently and cover with thick, absorbent gauze.

Note: Do not squeeze the boil or attempt to drain it before it clearly comes to a head. Squeezing it before this happens may succeed only in driving the infection deeper into the skin.

Carbuncles are extremely large boils or a series of boils usually deeper and more painful than regular boils. Always check with a doctor if you suspect a carbuncle because the infection can get into the bloodstream and antibiotics will be required.

DECISION GUIDE FOR BOILS

SYMPTOMS/SIGNS	ACTION
Boil responding well to self-care	
Boil not coming to a head or improving after 3 days of self-care	
Temperature of 101° F or higher	
Boil above the lips, on the nose, or in the ear	
Red streaks leading away from the boil	
Person also has diabetes	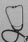

Note: Your doctor may lance the boil by making a small incision with a surgical blade so that the pus can drain. *Never attempt to lance a boil yourself without approval from your doctor.*

 Use self-care   See doctor

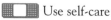 Call doctor's office for advice   *For more about the symbols, see p. 2.*

I think of myself as a tough guy with a high pain threshold, but when I got a boil on my buttocks, I thought I'd go through the roof every time I sat down. It got so my co-workers noticed me eyeing the chairs in the conference room, trying to decide which might be most comfortable. When my boil finally went away, I was the happiest man alive.

Andy

I had a nasty boil above my lip. Not only did it hurt so much that I could hardly eat or talk, it also looked terrible. Finally, a friend convinced me to see a doctor. He lanced it and I felt a lot better fast.

Sharon

I went to my niece's birthday party on a Sunday afternoon. The next day my sister called with the bad news: The birthday girl had come down with chicken pox Sunday evening. At least I had some warning. Like clockwork, my first red spots appeared 15 days after Claire's birthday.

Jarod

CHICKEN POX

A very contagious viral disease, chicken pox can be memorable for everyone involved. Many adults still vividly recall their childhood bout with the illness—those dramatic bumps that suddenly covered the body and the itching that seemed to go on forever. Any parent who nurses a child through chicken pox is not likely to forget it, either.

Despite all the drama, chicken pox is normally a mild disease of childhood. (It affects 4 million American children each year.) Adults who have never had the disease can get chicken pox, although only 4 percent of adults have not had the disease. Symptoms tend to be worse in adults, and the risk of complications is higher.

The early symptoms of chicken pox are cold symptoms, fever, abdominal pain, headache, and a general feeling of illness. These can come with the rash or before it by a day or two. The fever may be higher the first few days after the rash appears (see color photo p. 309).

The rash appears as small, itchy, red bumps and spots on the face, scalp, shoulders, chest, and back. It is also normal for it to appear inside the mouth, on the eyelids, and in the genital area. Some people may have just a few bumps, while others are covered with them.

The early bumps are usually flat, red marks with a central clear blister. The blisters quickly break open and become dry crusts or scabs, which fall off within 2 weeks (see color photo p. 309). New sores will continue to appear for the first 4 to 5 days, so all stages of the rash may be there at the same time.

SELF-CARE STEPS FOR CHICKEN POX

Relieve the itching
Scratching the scabs off chicken pox sores can lead to more itching and/or infection. These steps will help reduce the urge to scratch:

- Take cool baths every 3 to 4 hours.

- Add Aveeno oatmeal (follow directions) or baking soda (about a half cup) to tub water to reduce itchiness.

- Give nonaspirin (acetaminophen) cold or pain medicine up to four times a day if symptoms are very bothersome.

- Keep fingernails trimmed short and wash hands often.

- Wear clean, cotton gloves to bed to reduce the danger of scratching while asleep.

- Apply calamine lotion and/or hydrocortisone products to itchy areas. Caladryl is helpful, too, but on occasion people develop an allergy to it.

Manage other symptoms
- Drink plenty of cold fluids.

- To reduce fever, take acetaminophen (Tylenol, Tempra, or a generic). Do not use aspirin.

- For mouth ulcers, eat a soft, bland diet. Avoid salty foods and citrus fruits and juices.

- Gargle with a mouthwash of cold tea or an antacid solution after meals and before bed.

- For painful or itchy pox in the genital area, apply petroleum-based A&D ointment or an over-the-counter local anesthetic.

- If a sore seems to be infected, wash with antibacterial soap and apply antibacterial ointment.

Chicken pox is usually spread by breathing in droplets coughed, sneezed, or breathed out by an infected person. Between exposure to the disease and the appearance of symptoms, there is an incubation period of 10 to 21 days. Usually a person develops the symptoms 14 to 16 days after exposure.

A person can spread the disease to others before he or she even has any symptoms of chicken pox. The contagious period begins about 2 days before the rash appears and continues until new sores stop appearing. Once all the sores have turned to scabs, the contagious period is over.

If you've been exposed to chicken pox, there is nothing you can do during the incubation period to prevent the disease if you aren't already immune to it. (*Note*: Pregnant women and high-risk people may be candidates for a shot to prevent or lessen the severity of chicken pox.)

It is rare for a person to have more than one case of chicken pox in a lifetime. But, although a case of the pox causes immunity to the virus, the virus may lay quiet and later be reactivated in some adults. This rash, called **shingles** (or **herpes zoster**), is more common in people over 60 years old. It also happens to people with weakened immune systems. Shingles rarely occurs from direct exposure to a person with chicken pox.

Chicken pox is a serious health concern in people with weak immune systems, such as people with AIDS; people having radiation or chemotherapy; and people with leukemia, kidney transplants, or any other transplant. **Encephalitis**, a viral infection of the brain, is a very rare complication of chicken pox. Still, it's wise to be alert to its symptoms: fever, mental confusion, forgetfulness, tiredness, and a stiff neck. Take the person to the doctor's office or emergency room **at once** if you see these symptoms.

Chicken pox may leave permanent scars, especially in teenagers and young adults. Temporary marks may remain for 6 months to a year before fading away.

A vaccine for chicken pox is used in several other countries, and has been approved for general use in the United States. It is recommended for children over 12 months of age who have not had chicken pox (see Chicken Pox Vaccine, p. 242). The vaccine may be given to children with weakened immune systems who have been exposed to chicken pox.

A drug called acyclovir may speed up a bout with chicken pox and make it less severe. It must be given very soon after symptoms appear—preferably within the first 24 hours. Several pediatric associations do not recommend the use of the drug routinely in otherwise healthy children because it may only speed up the disease by 1 day and because children who take it may not develop immunity to the chicken pox, which is more serious in an adult.

The worst part about chicken pox is the itching. The other bad part is that I can't see my friends or go anywhere because people who haven't had it before could catch it. The best part is that I've probably given it to my brother already and he doesn't even know it.

Kristine, age 8

SPECIAL CONCERNS FOR CHILDREN

Children and teenagers with chicken pox should not take aspirin because it may be linked to Reye's syndrome, a dangerous condition of the liver and brain. Reye's syndrome sometimes develops as a complication of viral illnesses such as influenza and chicken pox. Although it is uncommon, it is seen more often in children who have been treated with aspirin for flu or chicken pox.

Children don't have to stay in bed, but should be kept cool and quiet.

Children may return to school or day care when they have no fever and all sores are crusted over.

DECISION GUIDE FOR CHICKEN POX

SYMPTOMS/SIGNS	ACTION
Normal chicken pox symptoms, including rash, fever, and itching	
Temperature is higher than 101° F for more than 4 days	
Lymph nodes become larger or more painful to the touch	
Itching does not respond to treatment, lasts more than 2 weeks	
Pain with urination	
Suspicion that several sores are infected (pus drains from sore)	
Sore in or near the eye, causing redness, drainage, pain, or changes in eyesight	
Blistery, red rash and confusion, delirium, forgetfulness, or other mental changes	
Hard to awaken, very tired	
Stiff neck and very bad headache, difficulty breathing	

PREVENTIVE STEPS

• Avoid contact with others during the contagious period—until all sores have turned to scabs. That means anyone with chicken pox should not be at work, school, or day care while contagious. If other people may have been exposed to the disease, be sure to call and tell them to watch out for spots about 2 weeks from the date of exposure.

• It's nearly impossible to prevent the spread of chicken pox within a household. Some studies find that nine times out of ten, siblings of a chicken pox patient will get the disease.

• If you need to take the patient to the doctor's office, call ahead and tell the staff that you suspect chicken pox so arrangements can be made to avoid spreading the disease to other clinic patients. In most cases, chicken pox patients don't need to come to the clinic. The condition can be successfully handled at home, with calls to the doctor's office for advice.

SPECIAL CONCERNS DURING PREGNANCY

Call your doctor if you get chicken pox during pregnancy. Pregnant women are more at risk for a type of pneumonia.

There is a slightly higher risk of birth defects in children born to women who had chicken pox in their first or second trimesters of pregnancy. A doctor should be actively involved in the birth of a child to a woman with a current outbreak of chicken pox. You will not give chicken pox to your fetus if you are exposed to the virus but have already had chicken pox.

 Use self-care

 See doctor

 Call doctor's office for advice

Seek help now

For more about the symbols, see p. 2.

CRADLE CAP

New mothers dislike cradle cap more than their infants do. Cradle cap is oily, yellowish scales or crusts that appear on babies' heads—behind the ears, on eyebrows, and along the lash line—and occasionally, in the groin area (see color photo p. 310).

Common in children less than 1 year old, cradle cap may be a mild form of dermatitis. Cradle cap doesn't cause the baby any discomfort, but a new mother may be unhappy with the baby's appearance. Fortunately, it's easy to treat at home.

SELF-CARE STEPS FOR CRADLE CAP

• Soften the crusty scales with baby or mineral oil and leave on the baby's head for about 15 minutes.

• Use a soft brush to loosen the scales after soaking in oil.

• Gently rub difficult areas with a washcloth or gauze dipped in oil to remove scales.

• Shampoo the baby's head.

• Don't use dandruff shampoos on your infant without checking with your doctor.

DECISION GUIDE FOR CRADLE CAP

SYMPTOMS/SIGNS	ACTION
Quick response to self-care	
No signs of improvement after 2 weeks of self-care	
Spreads beyond the scalp	

DANDRUFF

The stigma attached to dandruff is far worse than the condition warrants. Everyone can get dandruff. The skin all over your body, including your scalp, sheds dead cells all the time. Dead skin cells on the scalp may stick together and become visible white flakes.

Dandruff is not contagious and is a very common problem. It affects about 20 percent of adults in the U.S., men and women alike. Although there's no cure for dandruff, it's fairly easy to control.

SELF-CARE STEPS FOR DANDRUFF

• Gently brush hair before each washing.

• Wash hair every day, which may be enough to keep mild dandruff under control.

• Use antidandruff shampoos if the scalp is red and scales are obvious.

• Follow shampoo directions: most say to lather and let it sit for at least 5 minutes before rinsing.

• If a dandruff shampoo seems to lose its effectiveness after several weeks, try another.

• Try not to scratch or brush the scalp hard. Too much scratching may cause more dandruff.

DECISION GUIDE FOR DANDRUFF

SYMPTOMS/SIGNS	ACTION
Responds to self-care	
No improvement after several weeks of self-care	
Constant irritation or itchiness	
Thick scales, yellowish crusts, or red patches	

When my baby got cradle cap, I thought it meant I was a bad mother. Wasn't I keeping her clean enough? Fortunately, the doctor reassured me that cradle cap is fairly common. A little oil and a soft scrub brush helped clear up the cradle cap quickly.

Monica

It was the classic scene right out of the TV commercials. I was wearing a black sweater and my friend came up to me, brushed off my shoulders, and said, "You really ought to try a dandruff shampoo." I was mortified. I did start using a dandruff shampoo, however, and it has really helped.

Marsha

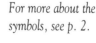 Use self-care

Call doctor's office for advice

For more about the symbols, see p. 2.

ECZEMA

If you're scratching patches of reddened skin that look flaky or scaly, the doctor may say you have eczema or "dermatitis." Both terms mean an inflammation of the skin. There are several different types of eczema or dermatitis.

Atopic dermatitis usually develops in childhood and may last into adulthood, although an adult can develop atopic dermatitis without a previous history of it. People with atopic dermatitis have a greater chance of having hay fever or asthma than other people (see color photo p. 310).

In babies, atopic dermatitis takes the form of a rash around the mouth and cheeks. In older children, rashes may appear behind the knees, in the creases of the elbows, and on the neck. In atopic dermatitis, the skin is extremely itchy and usually dry.

Contact dermatitis results from an allergy or exposure to an irritant (see Rashes, p. 166). When the skin touches something to which it is allergic or that it finds irritating, it becomes itchy and red (see color photo p. 310). Common types of contact dermatitis include diaper rash and poison ivy. Allergic reactions can be caused by hair dyes, jewelry containing nickel, and some rubber compounds. Irritant contact dermatitis may be caused by repeated use of soaps, solvents, and detergents.

Itch-scratch-itch cycle dermatitis develops when an itchy area is scratched or rubbed repeatedly. The skin becomes harder and annoyingly itchy. Scratching makes this worse. It may be hard to break the itch-scratch-itch cycle.

Seborrheic dermatitis is red, flaky, slightly itchy skin on an adult's scalp and face (for infants, see Cradle Cap, p. 155, color photo, p. 310). The area from the side of the nose to the corner of the mouth may be affected, as well as the scalp and eyebrows. The person often has dandruff (p. 155), too, which may be treated with a variety of antidandruff shampoos (see color photo p. 310).

DECISION GUIDE FOR ECZEMA

SYMPTOMS/SIGNS	ACTION
Dermatitis responds promptly to self-care	
Self-care is not providing relief after 2 weeks	
Sores are crusting or weeping or itching is very bad	

 Use self-care

 Call doctor's office for advice

For more about the symbols, see p. 2.

SELF-CARE STEPS FOR ECZEMA

- Wash the skin gently in cool or warm water, not hot, and don't bathe too often if you tend to have dry skin.

- Use mild soaps or cleansers and moisturize skin with bath oil after each bath or shower.

- Keep nails short to reduce damage to the skin by scratching.

- Dress lightly and wear soft, nonscratchy clothes.

- Apply a cold compress for temporary relief of itching.

- Apply over-the-counter 1 percent hydrocortisone creams to relieve itching.

- Protect the skin from contact with harsh chemicals and substances to which you are allergic; use latex gloves and wear protective clothing, if possible.

HAIR LOSS

Everyone loses between 50 and 100 hairs per day. The average lifespan of hair is 3 to 4 years. Ninety percent of the hairs on your head are actively growing. The other 10 percent are resting, a stage that lasts between 2 and 6 months, after which the hairs fall out.

Losing more than 50 to 100 hairs a day has a variety of causes. Hereditary balding is the most common cause of hair loss. Despite common myth, hereditary balding can be inherited from either the mother's or father's side. Hereditary balding affects both men and women, although in different ways. Men's hairlines recede and eventually join bald spots on the top and back of the head. Some women notice a slow or episodic thinning on the front of the head. Bad news: the earlier the thinning starts, the worse it's likely to be.

Prescription drugs can cause hair loss in some people. (Some blood pressure medicines, anticoagulants, antidepressants, antiarthritic, and antigout drugs can cause reversible hair loss.) Radiation and chemotherapy used to treat cancer can cause people to lose up to 90 percent of their hair. Birth control pills can cause increased hair loss while they are taken or for 2 to 3 months thereafter.

Rising and dipping hormone levels can be hair loss culprits in women. Many women may lose hair after childbirth, and a few have hair loss during menopause (p. 182) or during post-menopausal hormone therapy.

Crash diets have been implicated in hair loss, and ringworm (p. 167), a fungal infection, can cause scaly bald spots.

Alopecia areata is a disease that causes hair to fall out in smooth, round patches. Most of the scalp is normal.

Thyroid disease and lupus can cause thinning hair. Major surgery, infection, or high fever can make hair shed up to 3 months afterward.

Hairstyle traction baldness can occur in those who wear tight braids or ponytails.

My dad has a receding hairline, my older brother has a receding hairline, my younger brother has a receding hairline. My mother's hair is even thinning. In my family, losing one's hair is part of our heritage. You look at family pictures and everyone has a glint off the top of their heads— or they're wearing hats.

Brad

SELF-CARE STEPS FOR HAIR LOSS

Although there's no cure for hereditary baldness, there are some remedies if your appearance bothers you:

• Use toupees, wigs, or hairpieces to cover thinning or bald areas.

• Do what the hairdressers do: color or perm your hair, but avoid overbleaching, which causes hair breakage; use a hair dryer for more volume; wash daily with a gentle shampoo; use mousse.

• If you suspect your hairstyle is causing your hair to fall out, avoid curlers, braiding, ponytails—anything that puts traction on the hair.

When the baby was about 4 months old, I was combing my hair one day and a lot of it came out in my hand. My hair got really nice and thick when I was pregnant and even though I was prepared for hair loss after I had the baby, I still was shocked when it happened.

Sandy

MEDICAL HELP

- Hair transplants, which move hair from other parts of your body to your scalp, sometimes a hair at a time, have been chosen by some balding people. Total cost can be several thousand dollars, which rarely is covered by health insurance.

- Treatment for alopecia areata can speed its end, but it often will resolve itself. If not, a potent steroid lotion may be prescribed by a doctor.

- Minoxidil, a prescription hair restorer, is successful in producing fine, downy hair in about one-third of the people who try it. The newly grown hair falls out, however, when the drug is no longer taken.

DECISION GUIDE FOR HAIR LOSS

SYMPTOMS/SIGNS	ACTION
Gradual hair thinning or loss	
Occurs 2 to 3 months after surgery, major illness, or childbirth	
Sudden hair loss with scabs or scales on scalp, pain, soreness, or tenderness	
Bald spots suddenly appear, rather than slow symmetrical thinning	
Scalp has rash or scales, in addition to hair loss	
Suspicion that a drug may be causing hair loss	
Bald spots and scaly spots, pus, or scabs (see Ringworm, p. 167)	

 Use self-care

 Call doctor's office for advice

See doctor

For more about the symbols, see p. 2.

HIVES

Why does a person taking penicillin suddenly break out in itchy pink lumps? The person is having an allergic reaction called *hives* (see Allergic Reactions, p. 148).

Hives occur when something prompts cells to release histamine, a chemical found in the skin. The histamine causes nearby blood vessels to dilate (open up). Fluid leaks out and collects under the skin in a raised, flushed, itchy bump called a wheal or hive. Some wheals look like mosquito bites. Wheals often come in groups and may be as small as pencil erasers or as large as 2 or 3 inches across (see color photo p. 311).

Some people know that certain foods or drugs give them hives. For most others, the causes may not be obvious.

"Acute" hives (hives that are a reaction to a removable stimulus such as a drug) can last for hours or days. Chronic hives (often of unknown cause) can last for weeks or months.

Some foods that occasionally cause hives are peanuts (and other nuts), eggs, beans, chocolate, strawberries (and other berries), tomatoes, seasonings (mustard, ketchup, mayonnaise, spices), fresh fruits (especially citrus fruits), corn, fish (both freshwater fish and shellfish), milk, wheat, and cheese.

Drugs that have been known to cause hives include penicillin, sulfa antibiotics, and codeine.

Some extensive hives outbreaks can be very serious, such as when hives form on the lips and in the throat, interfering with breathing and swallowing. Shock—in which severe swelling, dizziness, and even loss of consciousness occur—can accompany widespread hives (see Shock, p. 36).

SELF-CARE STEPS FOR HIVES

- Take an oral antihistamine such as Benadryl or Chlor-Trimeton, but this may also make you drowsy.

- Topical anti-itch treatments seldom help but are an option.

- Rub ice directly over hives or take a cool shower for temporary relief from itching.

- Soak in a lukewarm or cool bath with 1 cup of baking soda or an oatmeal product such as Aveeno.

- If hives develop after a bee sting or other insect bite, see your health care provider. You may need a prescription kit to carry with you. EpiPen and Ana-Kit are two types of kits, both of which contain an injectable dose of epinephrine.

DECISION GUIDE FOR HIVES

SYMPTOMS/SIGNS	ACTION
Hives respond well to self-care	
Don't know what's causing hives	
No response to self-care after a few weeks	
Hives develop shortly after you begin taking a new drug. If this occurs, stop taking the drug right away.	
Hives cause very bad discomfort	
Big hive develops at bite site or after bee or other insect sting (see Insect Bites, p. 29)	
Widespread hives over body	
Difficulty breathing	
Extensive hives with swelling around the face and in the throat and mouth	

 Use self-care

 Call doctor's office for advice

 See doctor

 Seek help now

Emergency, call 911

For more about the symbols, see p. 2.

I don't know what causes my hives, which makes it hard to avoid the problem. Sometimes I'll go for weeks without any problems, and sometimes it's every day for weeks at a time. I suspect I'm overly sensitive to changes in routine and temperature.

Sally

I was concerned when Adrianne got impetigo. She had a cold and had gotten a sore between her nose and upper lip. She said it itched and kept rubbing it. Soon it was really red, and then it started to weep a gold liquid. I called the doctor and followed her directions faithfully. I was so relieved to see Adrianne get better after a couple of days.

Carole

I hadn't had impetigo since I was a kid, so I was really surprised when an annoying sore on my cheek started to ooze and crust. "Uh-oh," I thought, "I remember this symptom." I just called up Mom and she remembered how to treat it. A couple days of washing and soaking off the crust and I was back to normal. I didn't have to deal with shaving when I was a kid, though.

Mike

IMPETIGO

As children, our parents often told us not to scratch sores or insect bites. There's a good reason for this. Impetigo is a contagious bacterial infection most often seen at the site of broken skin. Red sores start to ooze a straw- or honey-colored liquid, which, when partially dried, becomes a crust or scab (see color photo p. 311). Touching or picking the sores can spread bacteria to other parts of the body—or other people.

With quick and careful home treatment, impetigo can be brought under control in several days. A rare kidney problem called **glomerulonephritis** is a complication of impetigo. Its symptoms are red or cola-colored urine, headache, and raised blood pressure. See a doctor immediately if these symptoms occur.

In Children and Infants

Impetigo in infants starts with a small blister containing yellowish or white pus surrounded by reddened skin. The blister breaks easily, leaving a small raw spot that may not crust over as with older children. Impetigo in infants is most often found in moist areas, such as the diaper edge, groin, or armpit.

SELF-CARE STEPS FOR IMPETIGO

• Gently and frequently clean sores with antibacterial soap and water or hydrogen peroxide.

• Apply an antibiotic ointment using a Q-tip.

• Don't cover the area with a Band-Aid unless the sore is in an area where the scab may rub off. If needed, for example, to keep children from scratching, cover with a dry gauze pad and keep the tape as far from the sore as possible.

• Wash your hands well with antibacterial soap and water after cleaning sores and applying ointment.

• Make sure everyone in the household uses separate towels, washcloths, and bath water.

• For facial sores, men should shave around sores, not over them. Don't use a shaving brush, as it may spread infection. Replace the razor blade every day.

DECISION GUIDE FOR IMPETIGO

SYMPTOMS/SIGNS	ACTION
Mild impetigo	
Self-care does not control or clear up the problem in 3 days (oral antibiotics may be needed)	
Infant has small, pus-filled blisters that break easily and leave a raw spot behind	
Large blisters develop	
Blisters show other signs of infection such as warmth, redness, or tenderness	
Urine turns red or cola-colored, and a headache occurs (signs of glomerulonephritis, a rare kidney problem)	

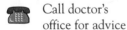 Use self-care

 Seek help now

 Call doctor's office for advice

For more about the symbols, see p. 2.

JOCK ITCH

Jock itch is one of the most descriptive names for an ailment. Jock itch is a fungal skin infection in the groin that mainly affects men. Men with jock itch also often have athlete's foot (p. 149).

Jock itch thrives in the warm, moist area of the groin. Fortunately, in most cases, self-care will clear up the red, raised, itchy areas on the skin in 1 to 2 weeks.

SELF-CARE STEPS FOR JOCK ITCH

- Wash the groin daily with a mild soap; rinse and dry thoroughly.

- After drying, try an over-the-counter antifungal cream (such as Lotrimin or MicaTin), then powder with talc or baby powder to reduce moisture and friction.

- If the rash clears, keep the area as dry as possible and, as a preventive measure, apply an antifungal powder daily to prevent flareups.

- See your doctor if self-care does not improve the problem or infection worsens within 2 weeks.

I felt I had failed as a mother when the note came home from my daughter's day care that head lice was going around. To be on the safe side, the day care asked all of us to wash our children's heads with special head lice shampoo, and wash their bedding and pillows in hot water. I don't think my daughter had head lice, but I do think quick action kept it from spreading.

Jennifer

I went to a foreign country to do some research in the countryside. Foolishly, I was careless about where I slept and by the time I came home, I had lice all over my body. Thank goodness for Kwell! I dipped myself in it. Then I washed everything I had ever touched in hot water. I got rid of the lice but I didn't feel clean for months.

Leah

LICE

We all itch from time to time, but if you're infested with head lice, pubic lice, or body lice, you'll know. Lice make you itch constantly. Lice can be spread by shared bedding, hats, or even combs, but having lice is no longer believed to be a sign of poor hygiene or squalid living standards.

Lice feed on human blood. As they burrow into the skin, their saliva causes intense itching. Adult lice are the size of a pinpoint. Their eggs, which they cement to hair shafts with a gluelike substance, are easier to spot (see color photo p. 311). The eggs, called nits, are white and shaped like footballs or cattails. A female louse can lay up to six eggs a day, and between 50 and 100 in her lifetime. Left untreated, lice are annoying and easily spread.

Head Lice

More than 6 million cases of head lice are reported among school-age children, and the infestation can easily spread to other family members. When diagnosed, head lice should be treated promptly and steps taken to prevent their spread to others.

A case of head lice is often mistaken for dandruff (p. 155). Symptoms include itching, white nits on hair shafts that aren't dislodged with regular shampooing, and red bite marks along the nape of the neck and around the ears.

Pubic Lice

Pubic lice also are known as "crabs." They attach themselves to pubic hair and itch like crazy. Pubic lice are spread through sexual contact or contact with lice-infested bedding or clothing (see color photo p. 311). Thus, it's important to tell your sexual partner if you have crabs so he or she also can be treated. Likewise, it's important to thoroughly wash all household bedding.

Body Lice

Body lice are not very common in this country. Body lice are hard to spot because they burrow into the skin. Instead, look in the seams of underwear. Body lice actually live in clothing and invade the skin only to eat, leaving behind that telltale itch (see color photo p. 312).

SELF-CARE STEPS FOR LICE

• To kill lice, you must use a shampoo just for that purpose. Several are sold over-the-counter. There also are shampoos available with a doctor's prescription. Follow the directions on the box, including leaving the shampoo on the affected area for several minutes. This gives the medicine time to work.

• After shampooing, use a rinse made of equal parts white vinegar and water. This will help remove stubborn nits.

• Combing hair with a fine-toothed comb also will help remove nits after shampooing.

• Wash everything that has touched the affected area. Bedding and clothing must be washed in hot water for at least 10 minutes and machine dried at the hottest setting for at least 20 minutes. Vacuum furry toys, carpets, drapes, mattresses, and upholstery, including fabric-covered car seats and headrests. Soak all combs, brushes, and hair accessories in hot water or alcohol for at least 10 minutes.

• If you have pubic lice, make sure your sexual partner is treated also.

• See your doctor if over-the-counter remedies aren't working or the lice have infested your eyelashes.

LYME DISEASE/DEER TICKS

Ticks probably spread a larger variety of diseases to humans and domestic animals than all other pests. The tick's bite is relatively painless; the real dangers are the viruses, bacteria, and other organisms that the tick may have.

Humans usually pick up ticks from woodsy underbrush, tall grass, and the fur of outdoor pets. Once on a host, the tick bites the skin, embeds its head, and taps into a blood source—a small vein or capillary (see color photo p. 312).

One of the diseases often spread by deer ticks is Lyme disease. It is an infection that can affect the skin, joints, brain, and heart, as well as other organs. It was identified in 1975 in the woodlands around Lyme, Connecticut. It is caused by a previously unknown bacteria. This disease is spread by deer ticks only, not the common dog tick or wood tick. Deer ticks are smaller and have different markings than those of dog ticks or wood ticks. Lyme disease symptoms can vary greatly from person to person; however, three phases have been identified.

Phase One

Between three and 30 days after being bitten by an infected tick, a small red bump may appear at the site. The bump is sur-rounded by a bull's eye rash that slowly grows for several days before fading (see color photo p. 312). Flu-like symptoms—fatigue, headache, chills, joint and muscle aches, and a low fever—may occur during this period. However, one-third of those who get Lyme disease never get a rash.

Phase Two

Weeks or months after the bite, about 20 percent of untreated victims have neurological or cardiac disorders, ranging from poor coordination to abnormal heart rhythm. Skin lesions develop in about half of those who are untreated. These symptoms also disappear, usually within a few weeks.

Phase Three

Up to 60 percent of untreated victims may develop recurring or chronic arthritis after a period of up to 2 years. The arthritis mainly affects large joints, most often the knees.

Lyme disease can be treated and nearly always cured—especially in its early stages. The bacteria that cause Lyme disease are sensitive to antibiotics such as tetracycline, penicillin, and erythromycin. If you see or have had the bull's eye rash, see your health care provider right away.

Lyme disease can be a serious illness. It is caused by the bite of a deer tick. One early sign is a rash that rapidly expands. It often looks like an expanding pink circle. If you develop such a rash and have been where deer may have been present, call your doctor.

Infectious Disease Specialist

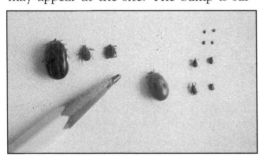

Dog ticks are many times larger than deer ticks. To the left of the pencil are dog ticks in engorged (left) and unengorged (right) states. To the right of the pencil are deer ticks in (clockwise from upper left) larval, nymph, adult, and engorged stages.

PREVENTIVE STEPS

When in woodsy areas, check yourself for ticks twice daily. Wear long pants, long-sleeved shirts, and shoes. Tuck your shirt into your pants and your pants into your shoes or boots to help prevent ticks from attaching themselves to your skin. Apply insect repellent containing no more than 30 percent DEET to your pants, socks, and shoes. Higher concentrations of DEET are not recommended, especially for young children and those with sensitive skin.

SELF-CARE STEPS FOR TICK BITES

• If you discover a tick on your skin or clothing, remove it immediately. The sooner you remove it, the less your chance of picking up infectious organisms. If the head of the tick is attached to your skin, don't try to remove it with your bare fingers. Use a pair of fine-tipped tweezers instead.

• To remove a tick, grip it close to your skin and pull it straight away until it releases its hold. Avoid twisting the head or squeezing the body because this may cause bacteria to be injected into your skin. Wash hands and affected skin with soap and water.

DECISION GUIDE FOR LYME DISEASE/DEER TICKS

SYMPTOMS/SIGNS	ACTION
Tick not attached	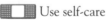
Tick attached	
Rash or infection	
Arthritic symptoms	

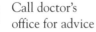 Use self-care    See doctor

Call doctor's office for advice

For more about the symbols, see p. 2.

POISON IVY/POISON OAK/POISON SUMAC

A simple walk through the woods shouldn't make you miserable. If you touch poison ivy, poison oak, or poison sumac, however, you may get an allergic reaction to these plants (see Allergic Reactions, p. 148).

The poison trio contain an almost invisible clear-to-slightly-yellow oil called *urushiol*, which comes from any cut or crushed part of the leaves, stem, or vine crawling on the ground. When the oil touches skin, it penetrates within minutes. In 12 to 48 hours, a red, itchy rash and tiny, weeping blisters may appear (see color photo p. 312). The oil can be carried on paws or fur of cats and dogs, on shoes or clothing, or on garden tools.

Poison ivy usually grows east of the Rocky Mountains as a vine or shrub. Its leaves are in clusters of three, and it has yellowish-white berries. It grows very easily and is widespread both inside and outside "city limits."

Poison oak grows west of the Rockies as a shrub, small tree, or, less often, a vine. It has greenish-white berries and has leaves in clusters of three, similar to those of poison ivy.

Poison sumac is found in swampy, boggy areas in the South and northern wetlands. It's a tall shrub with 7 to 13 pointed, small leaves per branch and cream-colored berries.

Your best defense against the poison trio is twofold: learn to identify them by sight, and watch what you are handling when gardening or cleaning up around the yard.

The most common exposures to poison ivy occur when pulling weeds or "cleaning up" at the cabin, gardening around the edges of the lawn, and gathering or exploring in wooded areas.

DECISION GUIDE FOR POISON IVY/POISON OAK/ POISON SUMAC

SYMPTOMS/SIGNS	ACTION
Mild itching; self-care effective in treating discomfort	
Rash covers a large area or involves the face or eyes	
Very bad swelling from rash	
Rash may be infected; however, this is rare	
Temperature of 101° F or higher	

Note: Your doctor may treat a very bad reaction with cortisone by injection or in pill form.

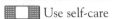 Use self-care

See doctor

 Call doctor's office for advice

For more about the symbols, see p. 2.

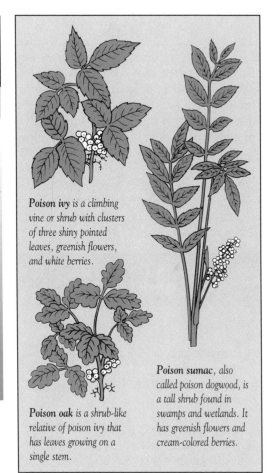

Poison ivy is a climbing vine or shrub with clusters of three shiny pointed leaves, greenish flowers, and white berries.

Poison oak is a shrub-like relative of poison ivy that has leaves growing on a single stem.

Poison sumac, also called poison dogwood, is a tall shrub found in swamps and wetlands. It has greenish flowers and cream-colored berries.

SELF-CARE STEPS FOR POISON IVY/POISON OAK/POISON SUMAC

• Wear rubber gloves if you're allergic and have to work near infested areas.

• Wash suspected areas of contact with soap and water as quickly as you can.

• If water isn't available, wipe affected areas with rubbing alcohol.

• Use water to rinse off pets, clothes, shoes, and camping or gardening gear if you or your pets have been in infested areas.

• Calamine lotion may relieve initial itching and help dry the rash.

• Over-the-counter antihistamine pills may help relieve itching and help avoid an allergic reaction.

• A soak in lukewarm water mixed with oatmeal or baking powder may soothe irritated skin and dry oozing blisters.

The size and spot of the rash may give a clue to its cause. For example, it may appear only where an elastic waistband touches your skin. Once you determine the cause of the rash, you need to avoid further contact with the offending agent. Most rashes will clear up on their own within a week or two.

Dermatologist

Diaper rash is pretty predictable in my kids if their skin comes in contact with urine or feces for any length of time. Keeping the diaper area clean and dry is the best treatment for diaper rash. Leaving the area exposed to air is helpful, too. If your child has diaper rash, change diapers often and don't use plastic pants.

Linda, Mother of two

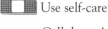 Use self-care

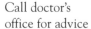 Call doctor's office for advice

 See doctor

For more about the symbols, see p. 2.

RASHES

Most of us have had skin rashes at one time or another. One form of skin rash is called **contact dermatitis**. Symptoms include red swollen patches, raised red dots, itching, burning, and blisters that may weep or ooze. The rash develops when the skin comes into contact with an irritating chemical. Poison ivy (p. 164), cosmetics, deodorants, soaps, metals, and dozens of other natural and artificial substances can cause contact dermatitis (see Allergic Reactions, p. 148).

DECISION GUIDE FOR RASHES

SYMPTOMS/SIGNS	ACTION
Tolerable pain or itching	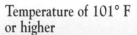
Temperature of 101° F or higher	📞
Lasts longer than 2 weeks	📞
Rash in diaper area that is bright red, raw, or sore-looking; has blisters or crusty patches	📞
Red streaks leading away from the rash	
Reddened, sunburned-looking skin that feels like sandpaper	🩺
Swollen joints, chills, dizziness, nausea	🩺
Burning eyes and nose, weeping blisters	🩺
Swollen glands in groin	🩺
Expanding circular rash	🩺

Rashes can also be caused by infections such as chicken pox, measles, strep, insect bites (p. 29; also see Lyme disease, p. 163), and fungal infections (see Athlete's Foot, p. 149; Jock Itch, p. 161; Ringworm, p. 167).

Prickly Heat Rash

Prickly heat rash is very common among infants. It's caused by perspiration when babies are overdressed and overheated. The rash appears as small red dots on an infant's head, neck, and shoulders. The baby may be overdressed if the skin is hot or moist between the shoulder blades. Once the hot, humid conditions are removed, the rash usually goes away.

Eczema

See p. 156.

SELF-CARE STEPS FOR RASHES

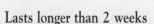 The first step in treating a rash is to find out what may have caused it. **Ask yourself these questions:**

- Have I started a new drug?

- Have I changed soaps, shampoos, deodorants, cosmetics, or hair dyes lately?

- Does the rash appear on a part of the body where clothes are worn?

- Have I worn any new jewelry or used new handcream or nail polish?

- Have I been near plants such as poison oak, poison ivy, or poison sumac?

If you suspect any of these substances may have caused the rash try to avoid them.

Second, follow these self-care steps to treat the rash:

- Gently wash the affected area with mild soap and water.

- Relieve itching by using calamine lotion or over-the-counter hydrocortisone cream.

- Watch the rash for 24 hours to see if it spreads or changes.

RINGWORM

Ringworm is an outdated term for a fungal skin infection. The name "ringworm"—going back to the early fifteenth century—comes from the idea that the skin infection was caused by a burrowing worm. Fungal skin infections, like athlete's foot and jock itch, are caused by tiny fungal organisms that can be seen only under microscopes. Fungal infection is no longer believed to be a sign of poor hygiene or squalid living standards.

The fungal infection starts as a small spot, then spreads or radiates out in a ringlike pattern (see color photo p. 313). It can infect most surfaces of the body, including the nails. On the scalp, it may show up as areas of hair loss.

Fungal infections are contagious, and some kinds can be spread to humans by cats and dogs.

DECISION GUIDE FOR FUNGAL INFECTION

SYMPTOMS/SIGNS	ACTION
Fungal infections on the feet and groin (see Athlete's Foot, p. 149, and Jock Itch, p. 161)	
Fairly small affected area	
Improvement within 1 to 2 weeks with over-the-counter remedies	
Fungal infection of the scalp, face, or fingernails	
More than one affected area or the infection is spreading	

 Use self-care   See doctor

For more about the symbols, see p. 2.

SELF-CARE STEPS FOR FUNGAL INFECTION

• Over-the-counter antifungal creams work well for fungal infections on the feet. However, groin and body lesions do not respond as well to these creams. Try tolnaftates (Tinactin, Aftate), clotrimazoles (Lotrimin AF, Mycelex), or miconazoles (MicaTin, Monistat) on small patches, especially for areas other than the feet. Apply twice a day for at least 2 weeks.

• Keep moist areas dry. Use powder after bathing. Try drying the affected area with a hair dryer set on cool.

• Thoroughly clean combs and hats.

• If your pets develop scaly, hairless skin lesions, have the animals checked for fungal infection by a veterinarian.

I couldn't figure out what was causing Jessica's itching. I thought it might be chicken pox so I took her to the doctor. I was mortified to discover she had scabies—which meant her brother probably had it, too. Luckily, the treatment was quick and effective.

Judy

SCABIES

For unknown reasons, the incidence of scabies is on the rise. Like head lice, scabies can occur in any family, in any neighborhood. It is no longer believed to be a sign of poor hygiene or squalid living standards.

The tiny mites that cause scabies are passed easily from one person to another. The mites burrow into the skin where the females lay eggs, which hatch in about 5 days. The cycle then begins anew (see color photo p. 313).

Scabies causes very tiny bumps that itch a lot, especially at night. The itching doesn't begin until several weeks after the mites have taken up residence in the skin (see color photo p. 313).

Scabies most often appears in the finger webs and around the wrists, but itchy areas may occur anywhere. It often affects the male genital area. The burrowing of these mites leaves very tiny grooves and tunnels on the skin that may look somewhat like white splinters.

When someone in the household has scabies, the entire household should be treated at the same time.

DECISION GUIDE FOR SCABIES

SYMPTOMS/SIGNS	ACTION
Very itchy gray lines or red patches appear on the body	
Criss-crossing, itchy lines or tunnels in the skin	
Fairly certain that the rash and itching are caused by scabies	
Side effects from insecticide lotion	
Constant itching and rash of an unknown cause	

 Call doctor's office for advice   See doctor

For more about the symbols, see p. 2.

SELF-CARE STEPS FOR SCABIES

• Call your doctor to discuss the problem. If the symptoms clearly are from scabies—or if you know you were in contact with someone infested by scabies—the doctor can call your pharmacy with a prescription for a lotion that will kill the mites. The doctor will also give you specific instructions to halt the infestation. This may need to be repeated a week later.

• Apply the insecticide lotion to all members of the household according to package directions.

• Wash all bedding and clothing used before or during treatment.

SKIN CANCER

The good news: skin cancer can be cured in 95 percent of cases. The bad news: cases of skin cancer are increasing, and Americans are getting skin cancer at ever-younger ages.

Skin cancer may or may not be easily identified. It will be easier for you to see changes in your skin, however, if you perform a skin self-exam once a month.

After your shower or bath, start by noticing where birthmarks, moles, and blemishes are and what they look like. Be sure to check your entire body, including back, scalp, buttocks, and genitals. Use a mirror to check hard-to-see areas. Giving yourself the once-over once a month will help you notice changes that may signal one of the three most common forms of skin cancer.

Basal cell cancer is the most common skin cancer in the United States, accounting for more than 90 percent of all cases. It is slow-growing and seldom spreads (metastasizes) to other parts of the body. Basal cell cancers may look like pearly or waxy nodules that sometimes have depressions in the middle. As the cancer grows, the center becomes more ulcerated and looks "gnawed." Because of the gnawed appearance, the term "rodent ulcer" sometimes is applied to basal cell cancers (see color photo p. 313).

Squamous cell cancer is raised or lumpy-looking bumps with rough, scaly surfaces on a reddish base. Often, the border is irregular. Squamous cell cancers tend to bleed, but seldom spread to other parts of the body, although this happens more often than with basal cell cancer (see color photo p. 314).

Malignant melanoma may appear as a mole that changes size, color, surface, shape, or border. The faster these changes occur, the more suspicious the lesion. Look for an irregular border with different colors in the same mole and some black color. Most melanomas are not raised (not a bump). In the early stage, most resemble a very dark and larger-than-normal freckle (see color photo p. 314). Melanomas are most often found on the back in men and on the back, thighs, and calves in women. If not detected early, malignant melanoma can spread to other areas of the body, mainly the lymph nodes, liver, lungs, and central nervous system, and can be lethal.

Actinic keratosis (pre-skin cancer) appears as scaly areas on sun-exposed parts of the body, particularly the ears, face, scalp, and hands (see color photo p. 314). The scaly areas may be easier to feel than to see. They may be premalignant and should be treated.

Most skin cancer is caused by sun damage of the skin. Light-skinned, light-eyed people are at greatest risk for skin cancer, while dark-skinned people have less risk. People who live in areas with higher levels of ultraviolet (UV) radiation from the sun, such as the southern United States, South Africa, or Australia, are more likely to develop skin cancer than those from areas where the UV radiation is less intense, such as the northern United States, Canada, or Norway.

Your best defense against developing skin cancer is protecting your skin from the sun consistently and at an early age. Apply sunscreen with a sun protection factor (SPF) of at least 15 before you go out, and reapply every hour or two. Wear loose-fitting, light-colored clothing, and a hat. Most common skin cancers hit the skin right where the sun does—on the backs of the hands and neck, the face, the tops of the ears, and the scalps of bald or balding people.

All forms of UV contribute to a person's lifetime total exposure. Using sunscreen reduces the amount of exposure, but doesn't ensure against skin cancer. Tanning beds are deceptive because they don't burn, but they provide a large dose of UV, which can contribute to cancer.

DECISION GUIDE FOR SKIN CANCER

SYMPTOMS/SIGNS	ACTION
Regular exposure to intense sunlight	▨▢
Any signs of skin cancer, such as skin growths or bumps that grow and/or change shape or color	🩺
Rough, scaly areas on sun-exposed parts of the body	🩺

▨▢ Use self-care

🩺 See doctor

For more about the symbols, see p. 2.

SKIN TRAUMA

Also see Scrapes and Abrasions, p. 35.

Human beings are truly imaginative in finding ways to harm themselves. Bruises, bumps, and rashes cause trauma to the skin. Most skin trauma can be treated with self-care, but it's important not to minimize skin injury. Prompt medical attention, if needed, can ensure quick healing and reduce the possibility of scars.

Bruises

Bruises, commonly referred to as "black-and-blue marks," are caused when blood cells seep from veins into surrounding skin tissue. They are like a sore that doesn't break the skin, usually caused by a hard knock or being hit by something. New bruises are dark. As they heal, they turn green and yellow. Some drugs such as anticoagulants and aspirin can cause people to bruise more easily.

Bumps and Rashes

Many different conditions can be responsible for bumps and rashes on the skin. See Acne (p. 145), Athlete's Foot (p. 149), Boils (p. 151), Eczema (p. 156), Hives (p. 158), Lice (p. 162), Jock Itch (p. 161), Poison Ivy/Poison Oak/Poison Sumac (p. 164), Ringworm (p. 167), and Skin Cancer (p. 169) for descriptions of different bumps and rashes.

SELF-CARE STEPS FOR BRUISES

• Apply ice as quickly as possible. This helps veins constrict, reducing the flow of blood into the skin tissue and helping to minimize the bruise.

• Raise and rest the bruised area.

DECISION GUIDE FOR SKIN TRAUMA

SYMPTOMS/SIGNS	ACTION
Medication makes you more likely to bruise	
Pain from a bruise becomes increasingly bad	
Temperature of 101° F or higher	

 Call doctor's office for advice

For more about the symbols, see p. 2.

 See doctor

SUNBURN

Sunburn results from overexposure to ultraviolet (UV) radiation from the sun. In a first-degree burn, symptoms include redness, sensitivity, and pain. If you have a sunburn, stay out of the sun until the skin recovers. Long exposure can lead to the swelling and blistering of a second-degree burn.

Sunburn can be prevented by avoiding too much sun, particularly between 10 a.m. and 2 p.m. and in midsummer. Sunscreens and sun-blocking lotions protect by filtering out the UV rays that cause sunburn. The higher the sun protection factor (SPF), the greater the protection against sunburn. A sunscreen of at least SPF 15 is recommended.

Sunburn is uncomfortable, usually for 24 to 48 hours. Frequent overexposure to the sun can cause long-term damage to the skin, resulting in premature aging, wrinkling, and skin cancer (p. 169). Although most skin cancer is curable, malignant melanomas may be fatal.

Some drugs can make you more sun-sensitive, causing you to burn with little exposure to the sun. Before starting a drug, ask your health care provider or pharmacist about the possible reactions to sunlight. Drugs that react to sunlight include tetracycline and sulfa antibiotics.

We always thought you had to get red first to get a really good tan, so we'd spend hours in the sun the first day we went out. Oh, we suffered for days afterward, but we thought we were suffering for beauty. Little did we know those dark tans we craved would come back to haunt us 30 years later.

Kathy

SELF-CARE STEPS FOR SUNBURN

• The best treatment for sunburn is to soak the affected area in cold water (**not ice water**) or apply cold compresses for 15 minutes. This will reduce swelling and provide quick pain relief. Do not apply greasy lotions such as baby oil or ointment to sunburned areas. They can make the burn worse by sealing in the heat.

• If sunburn affects large areas of your body, soak in a cool bath. A half cup of cornstarch, oatmeal, or baking soda in the bath will help reduce inflammation and soothe sunburned skin.

• Adults who do not have stomach problems or a history of allergy to aspirin products can take aspirin to reduce inflammation.

• For the most protection from sunburn, apply sunscreen 45 minutes before exposure to sunlight. Reapply sunscreen often during extended exposure. Apply to dry skin after swimming or strenuous activities that cause heavy perspiration.

• The sun's rays are more intense at higher altitudes, nearer the equator, and on the water and in the snow. Protect yourself with sunscreen. Zinc oxide products block all the sun's rays and are good for the nose and lips.

DECISION GUIDE FOR SUNBURN

SYMPTOMS/SIGNS	ACTION
Minor sunburn	
Blistering, painful sunburn	
Sunburn and purple blotches, skin discoloration, or blisters	
Fluid-filled blisters	
Chills, nausea, temperature of 102° F or higher, faintness, dizziness, or vision problems	

 Use self-care

 See doctor

 Call doctor's office for advice

Seek help now

For more about the symbols, see p. 2.

SPECIAL CONCERNS FOR MEN

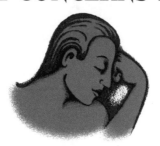

Although current news has focused on the special health concerns of women, men have some unique problems as well. For example, annual death rates for men with prostate cancer are similar to the rates of breast cancer deaths in women. There may be more of a stigma in talking about men's health issues, but progress in treating men's health problems will be hard until men are encouraged to deal with their health concerns openly.

This section describes common problems for men and how to take care of nonurgent conditions at home. Your primary care doctor (pediatrician, family practitioner, or internal medicine specialist) can offer advice and treatment for most gender-related problems you may encounter. If your condition is especially hard to handle, your primary care doctor may involve other medical providers who specialize in diagnosing and treating men's diseases. *This information cannot replace care by your health care providers.*

Use the Decision Guides to see if your symptoms warrant medical attention or if they can be handled with self-care. However, you need to consider your own medical history and your current health when deciding if self-care is right for you. If you have any conditions that do not seem to be healing normally or if self-care steps do not seem helpful, call your health care provider.

HERNIAS

Although hernias occur in men and women, they are far more common in men.

Inguinal Hernias

An inguinal (groin) hernia occurs when the lining of the abdominal cavity weakens, allowing part of the intestine to balloon out. These hernias are common in older adults as a result of strained or weak abdominal muscles. In infants, hernias are in the muscle layer.

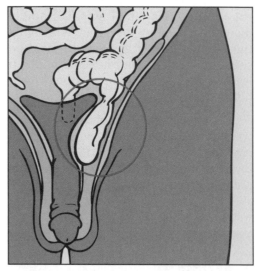
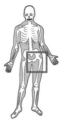

In the above inguinal hernia, the intestine has bulged through the passage where the testicle descends into the scrotum.

The chief cause of these hernias is too much abdominal pressure caused by heavy lifting or straining during bowel movements. Correct lifting (using your legs and keeping the back straight) can reduce your risk of hernia.

Hernia symptoms and pain may start slowly or you may one day feel that something isn't quite right. Symptoms include:

- A gurgling feeling
- Aches and pain in the abdomen that start and stop
- A feeling of pressure or weakness in the groin
- Visible bulges slightly above or within the scrotum
- Pain and tenderness in the lower abdomen and scrotum

Strangulated hernias occur when hernias are so pinched by the abdominal wall that the blood supply is cut off and the tissue dies and swells. Rapidly increasing pain in the groin is a signal that the hernia is strangulated. The dead tissue quickly becomes infected and can lead to a life-or-death situation within hours.

If you have these symptoms or suspect you have a hernia, call your health care provider for a full diagnosis. Treatment includes surgery to repair the abdominal wall or, if the patient is not uncomfortable, simply living with the hernia and watching that it doesn't get worse.

SELF-CARE STEPS FOR INGUINAL HERNIAS

- Avoid activities such as heavy lifting that cause straining and more abdominal pressure.
- Use correct lifting techniques.
- Don't strain during bowel movements.

Hiatal Hernias

A hernia at the spot where the esophagus passes through the diaphragm to the stomach is called a hiatal hernia or hernia of the diaphragm. This hernia is caused by a weak spot in the diaphragm muscle that allows the stomach to push up through the diaphragm.

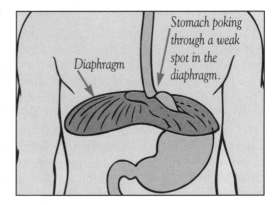

Diaphragm

Stomach poking through a weak spot in the diaphragm.

These hernias are usually not painful by themselves. However, food or acid may pass back into the esophagus, causing heartburn, indigestion, chest pains, hiccuping, and belching following meals.

SELF-CARE STEPS FOR HIATAL HERNIAS

- Treatments for hiatal hernias include taking antacids, avoiding irritating foods, and raising the head of the bed several inches to help prevent stomach contents from flowing back into the esophagus.

- Other treatments that can offer relief include avoiding going to sleep or lying down shortly after eating and eating small, frequent meals. Surgery to tighten the hiatal opening is a last resort if other measures fail to provide relief. See your health care provider if you suspect you have a hernia.

TESTICULAR PAIN

Suddenly painful testes can be a very serious medical condition. Because this pain can have several causes, correct diagnosis requires medical expertise. See your health care provider right away if you feel sudden, sharp pain, or swelling in the testes. Prompt medical attention can prevent the unnecessary loss of the testicle.

Lumps within the scrotum are usually benign, and are often a cyst or other inflammation. A scrotal lump, whether or not it is painful, should always be checked by your health care provider to be sure that it is not a tumor.

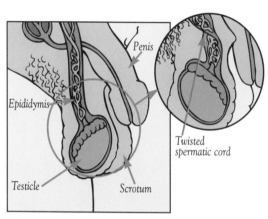

Testicular torsion occurs when a testicle gets twisted in the spermatic cord from which it is suspended within the scrotum. This unusual condition can occur spontaneously—even while the victim sleeps—or after strenuous activity at any age. (The most common age for this ailment is 11.) It can strangle the blood supply to the testicle and, without immediate treatment, can cause permanent damage.

Sudden pain, severe enough to cause vomiting and nausea, is the main symptom of testicular torsion. Although your health care provider may be able to carefully shift the testicle back into its normal position, surgery to securely anchor

it in place is usually performed within several hours.

Epididymitis is the inflammation of the long, coiled tube (epididymis) that carries sperm from the testicle to the vas deferens. It is often caused by a bacterial or chlamydial infection traveling from the urinary duct to the sperm duct. Epididymitis is usually treated with antibiotics.

Orchitis is an infection of the testicle that often occurs with epididymitis. Orchitis can also be a viral infection connected to the mumps. Although this condition is rare, it can cause infertility and irreversible damage to the testes.

If you feel sudden pain in your testes or find a scrotal lump, see your health care provider right away.

SELF-CARE STEPS FOR TESTICULAR PAIN

 •Men between the ages of 13 and 45 should do testicular self-examinations monthly. After a warm shower or bath, gently roll each testicle between your thumb and index finger. Check all areas of the testicle, feeling for lumps or hard bumps.

DECISION GUIDE FOR TESTICULAR PAIN

SYMPTOMS/SIGNS	ACTION
Scrotal lump	See doctor
Sudden, painful swelling in testes	Seek help now

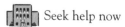

See doctor

Seek help now

For more about the symbols, see p. 2.

SPECIAL CONCERNS FOR WOMEN

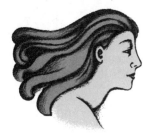

Research on women's health concerns has long been neglected. Most of the major studies in understanding disease have been conducted on men. But recently there has been a new emphasis on the unique health concerns of women.

This section describes common problems related to women's health and suggests ways to take care of nonurgent conditions at home. Your primary care doctor (family practitioner or internal medicine specialist) can offer advice and treatment for most gender-related problems. If your condition is especially hard to handle, your primary care doctor may involve other medical providers who specialize in women's health, such as gynecologists or nurse practitioners. *This information cannot replace care by your health care providers.*

Use the Decision Guides to see if your symptoms warrant medical attention or if they can be handled with self-care. However, you need to consider your own medical history and your current health when deciding if self-care is right for you. If you have any conditions that do not seem to be healing normally or if self-care steps do not seem helpful, you should call your health care provider.

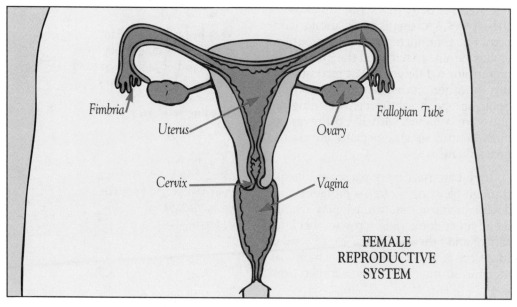

Fimbria

Uterus

Cervix

Ovary

Fallopian Tube

Vagina

FEMALE REPRODUCTIVE SYSTEM

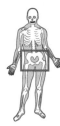

I'm 46 years old and have rarely had problems with my menstrual cycle. It's always been fairly regular, with about 28 days from the start of one period to the next. But in the last 6 months I've had bleeding in the middle of the month about four times. The first two times it was just spotting for 2 days—enough to need a pantiliner, but not much more. Still, I was concerned. I decided to start a diary to record the days I had bleeding, how heavy or light the flow was, and what other things were happening at that time.

The third month, the bleeding lasted as long and the flow was as heavy as my periods usually are. After the bleeding stopped, I went to see my doctor. I showed her the diary. After examining me, she said I was probably nearing menopause and that irregular periods and spotting are common among premenopausal women.

Not knowing when spotting or a full-fledged period might start is still a nuisance. But I feel better knowing that nothing is wrong.

Virginia

BLEEDING BETWEEN PERIODS

Bleeding between periods can be inconvenient and annoying. In most cases, however, it is nothing to worry about. In fact, most women have spotting, breakthrough bleeding, or irregular periods at some point in their lives. But, because bleeding between periods can also be a sign of more serious problems, such as ectopic pregnancy or cancer, it merits a call or visit to your doctor or nurse practitioner if it happens more than 2 months in a row.

Spotting (light bleeding) or breakthrough bleeding (heavier bleeding) between periods usually lasts 1 or 2 days. About 10 percent of women regularly have spotting around the time of ovulation. Bleeding between periods is also common when hormones are fluctuating (rising and falling) the most—during the first few years of menstruation and again as women approach menopause.

Spotting is very common in women with intrauterine devices (IUDs). It may also occur if the hormone levels in the birth control pills a woman is taking are not well-suited to her body. In most of these cases, spotting is not cause for concern, but your doctor or nurse practitioner may be able to help end the problem by prescribing a different pill or recommending another form of birth control. Spotting and breakthrough bleeding are also very common with Depo-Provera (a birth control shot), especially during the first 3 months.

If you are near menopause and breakthrough bleeding is often a problem, your doctor or nurse practitioner may recommend an endometrial biopsy to check for cancer and other problems. Or a D and C (dilation and curettage), in which the uterine lining is gently scraped and cleaned away, may be suggested. For some women, that will end the problem.

If you are having spotting or breakthrough bleeding that is accompanied by pain, lasts 3 days or more, is very heavy, or happens more than 2 months in a row, you should see your doctor or nurse practitioner. Also, if pregnancy is a possibility and you are spotting, you should see your health care provider.

DECISION GUIDE FOR BLEEDING BETWEEN PERIODS	
SYMPTOMS/SIGNS	**ACTION**
Occasional spotting or breakthrough bleeding	🩹
Spotting or breakthrough bleeding occurring 1 or 2 months	☎
Bleeding between periods lasts 3 or more days	☎
Menstrual pattern doesn't return to normal by the third month	☎
Very heavy bleeding (for example, bleeding enough to soak a pad or tampon an hour for 2 to 3 hours in a row)	🩺
Bleeding between periods and pain	🩺
Over 40 years old and more than 6 months since your last period and irregular bleeding is now occurring	🩺

🩹 Use self-care   🩺 See doctor

☎ Call doctor's office for advice   *For more about the symbols, see p. 2.*

SELF-CARE STEPS FOR BLEEDING BETWEEN PERIODS

• After a while, most women take their menstrual cycles in stride. Many find it difficult to remember the exact date of the first day of their last period, let alone dates a few months earlier. That's why it's important to keep a menstrual diary if you begin having bleeding that is unusual for you. Keep a written record of the dates of your periods and any bleeding between periods. Also note how long the bleeding lasted and how heavy the flow was. This diary can help your doctor or nurse practitioner find the possible cause and decide whether the between-period bleeding is anything to be concerned about.

• Wear a pad or tampon to protect your clothing while you are bleeding, just as you would during a regular period.

• Avoid aspirin while you are bleeding. It may increase the flow.

• Relax. In most instances, spotting and breakthrough bleeding are nothing to worry about.

BREASTFEEDING PROBLEMS

Breast milk has several advantages for newborn babies: It contains all the essential nutrients in their ideal proportions and provides natural protection against infection. Very few new mothers are physically unable to breastfeed. Some of the most common problems—pain, engorged breasts, or a low milk supply—can be overcome with persistence and support from your doctor and family.

Engorgement (overly full, hard breasts) occurs when the milk first comes in. It may also make the breasts feel sore in between feedings. Mild swelling and tenderness is normal for 24 to 48 hours. More severe engorgement is usually caused by not feeding correctly or often enough.

Nipple pain is most often caused by the baby latching on to the nipple incorrectly.

PREVENTIVE STEPS

• Hold the baby close to your breast (nose and chin should lightly touch your breast) to reduce tugging.

• Encourage letdown before feedings by gently massaging the breasts from the fleshy part down to the nipple.

• Try to get the baby to open wide and take a portion of the areola (the darkened area around the nipple), not just the tip of the nipple.

• Make sure the baby eats at least eight times in 24 hours.

• Vary the baby's nursing positions.

• Wear a supportive bra.

After reading about the benefits of breastfeeding, I was determined to make it work for my baby and me. Instead, I was frustrated and in pain. My nipples were sore and cracked and my left breast became inflamed. I felt like I had the flu and could barely get out of bed, much less feed my baby.

Kim

If a breast infection (a localized "abscess" or generalized "mastitis") is diagnosed, an antibiotic will be prescribed. Breastfeeding can continue normally without danger from the infection or the antibiotic. It usually becomes less painful and more enjoyable with time.

Family Practitioner

DECISION GUIDE FOR BREASTFEEDING PROBLEMS

SYMPTOMS/SIGNS	ACTION
Normal engorgement, short-term nipple pain	
Engorgement lasts longer than 48 hours	
Unable to get baby to nurse at least eight times in 24 hours	
Nipple tenderness at latch-on does not get better after the first minute when the baby begins to swallow	
Nipple pain lasts beyond 1 week; cracked or bleeding nipples	
Part or all of one breast becomes inflamed, or painful lump in one breast	
Temperature of over 100.5° F and feeling ill	

 Use self-care

 Call doctor or breastfeeding specialist for advice

For more about the symbols, see p. 2.

SELF-CARE STEPS FOR BREASTFEEDING PROBLEMS

For engorgement
- Apply warm compresses to breasts for a few minutes to help the milk start to flow (called letdown).

- Do gentle breast massage.

- Encourage frequent feedings (every 1 to 3 hours).

- Use cold compresses after feedings for up to 10 minutes for comfort and to reduce swelling.

- Acetaminophen or ibuprofen may be used for pain relief; follow the manufacturer's instructions.

For sore nipples
- Do gentle breast massage to assist letdown.

- Begin feedings on the least tender nipple.

- Encourage frequent feedings limited to 10 to 15 minutes per breast.

- Apply a drop or two of expressed breast milk to the nipples after feedings to ease nipple discomfort.

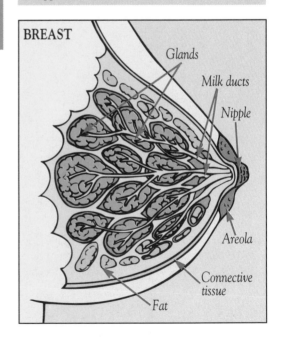

BREAST

Glands

Milk ducts

Nipple

Areola

Connective tissue

Fat

DIFFICULT PERIODS

Menstrual periods are different from woman to woman. For some, they may last only 3 days, and for others, they are as long as 7 days. The flow may be light or heavy, and cycles from the start of one period to the start of the next can be anywhere from 21 to 40 days. Over the years, a woman's menstrual pattern is likely to change. In the early years, it may be irregular and heavy. As time goes by, it may come like clockwork. The amount of flow may change over time as well.

All these variations are normal. For most women, menstruation comes and goes each month with ease. But for others—or at various times in a woman's childbearing years—periods are complicated by pain (**dysmenorrhea**) or premenstrual symptoms.

Menstrual cramps are most common between the ages of 15 and 24 years and among women who have not given birth. Pain can be mild or so bad that it sends the woman to bed for 1 to 3 days. Very bad cramps may be accompanied by diarrhea, nausea, and headache.

One type of painful period seems to run in families. Researchers in the 1970s and 1980s discovered higher than average levels of **prostaglandin**—fatty acids in the body that act much like hormones—in the menstrual fluid of women who suffered from cramps. Prostaglandins serve many functions in the body, but too much can cause pain from uterine irritability or contractions.

Another type of painful period may be caused by **fibroids** (noncancerous growths) in the uterus, infection, or **endometriosis** (uterine lining growing outside of the uterus). If your periods become more painful or begin to last longer than they used to, you should see your doctor or nurse practitioner. Intrauterine contraceptive devices (IUDs) may also cause pain during menstruation.

Premenstrual Syndrome

Some women feel irritable or depressed, retain fluid or have bloating, and have headaches beginning a few days before their periods. Usually these premenstrual symptoms go away as soon as the menstrual flow begins. About 5 percent of women have more severe symptoms of premenstrual syndrome (PMS), including a monthly cycle of anxiety, depression, and sometimes changes in behavior.

DECISION GUIDE FOR DIFFICULT PERIODS

SYMPTOMS/SIGNS	ACTION
Painful periods or cramps that can be relieved	
Mild to moderate premenstrual symptoms	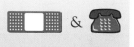
Pain during period is worse than it used to be	
More than your usual amount of menstrual flow	
Very heavy bleeding (enough to soak a pad or tampon an hour for 2 to 3 hours in a row)	
Severe depression, anxiety, or other premenstrual symptoms that are not relieved with self-care	

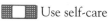 Use self-care

 Call doctor's office for advice

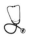 See doctor

For more about the symbols, see p. 2.

My periods were never easy. Other women barely seemed to notice theirs, but I was having such bloating before and awful cramps during my periods that I'd come to dread them. My first semester at college, I missed 1 or 2 days of class each month because of menstrual cramps. The nurse on campus told me to start taking ibuprofen or aspirin the day before I expected my period, to head off the cramps. It worked! I still had some pain, but it wasn't nearly as bad. I was able to attend classes. She also said to avoid salt and increase the amount of fluids I drink to relieve the bloating and fluid retention. Knowing what to do has made a big difference. I don't dread my periods like I used to!

Karen

SELF-CARE STEPS FOR DIFFICULT PERIODS

For painful periods

• Use aspirin, ibuprofen, or prescription pain relievers. Aspirin usually relieves mild to moderate menstrual pain. Ibuprofen (Advil, Motrin) is often effective when the pain is worse. If you do not get enough relief from these over-the-counter drugs, your doctor or nurse practitioner may be able to prescribe a higher dose of ibuprofen or a prescription nonsteroidal anti-inflammatory drug. Begin taking the drug at the first sign of symptoms, whether menstrual bleeding has actually begun or not.

• Apply heat. A heating pad or hot-water bottle placed on the lower abdomen will ease the pain.

• Raise your hips. If you find yourself in bed because of cramps, try lying on your back with your hips elevated above the level of your shoulders. Put your feet up on the footboard of the bed or the arm of the couch and place pillows under your hips. Firm massaging of the lower back may also help.

For premenstrual symptoms or syndrome

• Avoid salt and caffeine, and drink plenty of fluids to relieve water retention and bloating.

• Exercise regularly and eat a well-balanced diet, low in sugar and high in protein and fiber.

• Daily vitamin B_6 supplements (50 milligrams a day) may help relieve premenstrual symptoms.

MENOPAUSE

The years leading up to menopause, when ovulation and menstruation stop, are different from woman to woman. Some women menstruate regularly until their periods suddenly stop. Others may see changes in the amount of menstrual flow or the length of time between periods. Still others have missed periods or bleeding between periods. Although irregular periods are often a normal part of the years leading up to menopause, irregular vaginal bleeding can also be a warning sign of cancer. If your periods become irregular or you have bleeding between periods, keep a menstrual diary and check with your doctor or nurse practitioner. He or she may decide to check for uterine cancer with a procedure called an endometrial biopsy. (See also Missed Periods, p. 185 and Bleeding between Periods, p. 178.)

As many as 80 percent of women have hot flashes as they near menopause. Some women may have them before periods stop. **Hot flashes**—a flushed feeling that usually begins around the chest and spreads to the neck, face and arms—usually last 3 to 4 minutes and can occur as often as once an hour. Often hot flashes are followed by sweating and then chills. They can happen any time of day—or night—and may last for up to 5 years, as the woman's body adjusts to the ovaries' much lower production of the hormones estrogen and progesterone. Hot flashes rarely last longer than 5 years.

Increasingly, researchers have come to believe that lack of adequate sleep as a result of nighttime hot flashes is to blame for moodiness and other psychological symptoms linked with menopause. Scientific studies have yet to prove a relationship between lower estrogen levels and depression, moodiness, irritability, fatigue, or other psychological symptoms commonly felt during menopause. Lack of adequate sleep, however, can cause any number of these symptoms, making nighttime hot flashes a likely culprit. Other life issues happening along with menopause may also add to depression or other symptoms. Examples include career issues, children leaving home, caring for aging parents, or, possibly, struggling with what it means to be growing older or no longer being able to bear children.

Reduced estrogen levels in the body do, however, contribute to vaginal dryness and urinary problems, both of which can continue to be problems well beyond menopause. With much less estrogen in the body, the vaginal walls lose elasticity, thin, and secrete less fluid. A drier, less elastic vagina can mean discomfort or pain during or after intercourse. Surprisingly, avoiding intercourse can make the problem worse, while continued sexual activity improves blood circulation and suppleness of the vagina, thus reducing or stopping discomfort during intercourse.

Hormone replacement therapy (HRT) can relieve vaginal dryness, reduce or end hot flashes, help bladder symptoms, prevent osteoporosis, and may reduce cardiovascular disease risk. In the 1960s, estrogen was often given alone, and some women later developed a low-grade endometrial (uterine) cancer. When both estrogen and progesterone are given for HRT, however, the risk of endometrial cancer is actually less than if the woman is taking no estrogen at all. For this reason, combined estrogen and progesterone is recommended for women who have not had a hysterectomy. Estrogen alone is recommended for those who have had a hysterectomy.

Many women and health care providers worry that estrogen replacement therapy may increase the risk of breast cancer. The largest and most carefully done studies, however, show no convincing evidence that this is true.

I knew I was going through "the change" when I started waking at night with hot flashes. I've always had trouble getting back to sleep once awakened. But I found that lowering the thermostat and putting a few layers of thin blankets on the bed helped. That way I could easily uncover to cool off or cover up to warm up without getting out of bed or waking up fully. When I started exercising regularly and stopped drinking so much coffee, the hot flashes seemed to let up a bit and I slept better all the way around.

Thelma

SELF-CARE STEPS FOR MENOPAUSE

- Dress in layers and wear loose clothing.

- Set the thermostat at 68° F or lower.

- Drink plenty of water. Six to eight glasses a day is about right.

- Exercise regularly. Thirty minutes of moderate, weight-bearing exercise (such as walking) 3 days a week can help reduce hot flashes and guard against osteoporosis by building stronger bones. Non-weight-bearing exercise, such as swimming or bicycling, will also help with hot flashes and benefit your heart, but is not helpful in preventing osteoporosis.

- Avoid caffeine and alcohol, which can intensify hot flashes and cause insomnia.

- Use a water-soluble lubricant (K-Y Jelly, Astroglide, Replens, Surgilube) to relieve vaginal dryness. Don't use petroleum jelly products, such as Vaseline.

- Allow yourself time to become aroused before having intercourse. Menopause does not cause you to lose your sex drive. By savoring the moment, intercourse can be even more enjoyable, and less uncomfortable if you suffer from vaginal dryness.

- Eat a balanced diet that includes 1,200 to 1,500 milligrams of calcium—the equivalent of four to six 8-ounce glasses of milk. If dairy products don't agree with you, a calcium supplement such as Tums E-X may be used. A supplement of vitamin D (400 IU each day) will help your body absorb the calcium, whether from your diet or a supplement.

Furthermore, estrogen has been shown to lower the risk of cardiovascular disease and osteoporosis. Most experts today agree that the benefits of HRT far outweigh any potential risks.

About 10 percent of women receiving HRT have minor side effects, such as breast tenderness, nausea, headaches, fluid retention, or irregular vaginal bleeding. For most women, however, these side effects do not interfere with continuing the hormone therapy.

Some women should not use HRT (such as those with a history of breast cancer), but other drugs are available to help relieve menopausal symptoms. The decision to use or not to use HRT is best made jointly by each woman and her health care provider.

Whether you choose to use HRT or not, there are some nonhormonal measures you can use to help relieve menopausal symptoms.

DECISION GUIDE FOR MENOPAUSE

SYMPTOMS/SIGNS	ACTION
Hot flashes, vaginal dryness, or irregular periods	
Symptoms not relieved by self-care	
Irregular periods that don't return to normal within 3 months (i.e., periods less than 20 days from the start of one to the start of the next cycle; cycles longer than 90 days apart; bleeding longer than 8 days)	
Bleeding between periods or bleeding heavy enough to soak a pad or tampon an hour for 2 to 3 hours in a row	
Any vaginal bleeding after no periods for 6 months or longer	
Pain or burning during urination	
Vaginal bleeding after intercourse	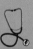

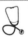 Use self-care   See doctor

Call doctor's office for advice

For more about the symbols, see p. 2.

MISSED PERIODS

For most women, the first thing to come to mind when a menstrual period is missed is pregnancy. Although pregnancy is the most common cause of missed periods, there are many other factors that can cause a woman not to menstruate (**amenorrhea**). Stress, being very overweight or underweight, birth control pills, regular hard exercise, and the approach of menopause are all common causes of amenorrhea. Menstrual periods may not resume for several months after a woman gives birth or while she is breastfeeding. Diseases that affect the body's hormonal system can also lead to missed periods, but this is rare.

Periods usually begin between the ages of 11 and 14, although some girls begin earlier and others later. But if a girl has not started to menstruate by age 16, she may have one type of amenorrhea. Hormone imbalances or problems with the ovaries, uterus, or vagina may be at fault. If menstruation hasn't begun by age 16, it is wise for the girl to see a doctor.

Although birth control pills are sometimes prescribed to regulate irregular periods, they can also have the opposite effect, causing no periods. If your periods stop while you are taking one type of pill, switching to another birth control pill may solve the problem. If you are on the pill and your periods stop, talk with your doctor or nurse practitioner. Going off the pill after being on it for a while may also disrupt your menstrual cycle for a few months while your body adjusts to the change in hormones.

The first thing to rule out if you miss a period is pregnancy. Home pregnancy tests on the market today are fairly accurate beginning about 2 weeks after the missed period was supposed to begin. Better pregnancy tests available through a doctor's office are accurate within days after the period should have started.

If you are sure you are not pregnant, it's time to consider other possible causes—many of which you can do something about yourself.

My periods have always been regular. I could predict almost to the day when they would start. But a few months ago I had a big scare. My husband and I had just moved to Minneapolis from Chicago. He was settling into a new job. I was still looking—without success. I took a waitressing job nights to keep cash coming in and looked during the day for a job in my profession. In the midst of all this, what should happen? My period doesn't come. I was in a panic.

I waited 2 weeks in fear and then broke down and bought a home pregnancy test kit. It was negative. But that still didn't explain why I missed my period. I'd heard that stress can sometimes cause amenorrhea. I knew I was stressed out! I'd even begun to lose weight. I decided to try taking time out to relax and find ways to ease the stress I was feeling. By the next month, my period returned—back on its usual schedule.

Linnea

SELF-CARE STEPS FOR MISSED PERIODS

- If you are in your 40s or 50s, a missed period may mean you are starting menopause. Before your periods stop entirely, they may be irregular for a time (see Menopause, p. 182).

- For some women, a good bout of the flu or stress at work or home can throw their menstrual cycles off. If you are under stress, find ways to relieve it. Take time out daily to meditate, listen to soothing music, or read a book. Regular exercise and getting enough sleep each night can also reduce stress.

- Rapid weight loss or being very overweight or underweight can also cause amenorrhea. If you are trying to lose weight, make sure you are eating at least 1,200 calories a day from a well-balanced variety of foods. If you are underweight, eat a well-balanced diet that provides about 2,000 calories a day. Whether you are overweight, underweight, or dieting, your doctor, nurse practitioner, or a dietitian may be able to help you set up a healthy diet and exercise plan. (See also Lifestyle Choices, p. 265).

- Very hard training and exercise are another cause of amenorrhea. If you are in training and missing periods, easing up may return your periods to normal. If you are an endurance athlete, ask your doctor or nurse practitioner if hormone therapy or calcium supplements might be right for you to help prevent osteoporosis.

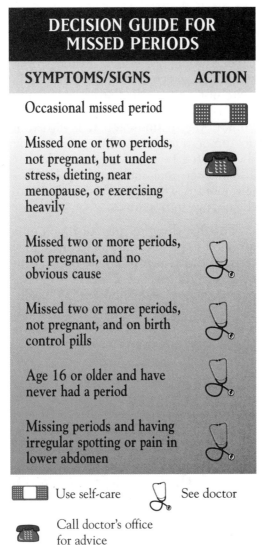

DECISION GUIDE FOR MISSED PERIODS

SYMPTOMS/SIGNS	ACTION
Occasional missed period	🩹
Missed one or two periods, not pregnant, but under stress, dieting, near menopause, or exercising heavily	☎
Missed two or more periods, not pregnant, and no obvious cause	🩺
Missed two or more periods, not pregnant, and on birth control pills	🩺
Age 16 or older and have never had a period	🩺
Missing periods and having irregular spotting or pain in lower abdomen	🩺

🩹 Use self-care   🩺 See doctor

☎ Call doctor's office for advice

For more about the symbols, see p. 2.

VAGINAL DISCHARGE AND IRRITATION

Although makers of feminine hygiene sprays and douches would like you to believe otherwise, a healthy vagina cleans itself naturally. A clear or opaque vaginal discharge is part of this cleaning process.

But several conditions can cause irritation around the vagina and changes in the color, smell, amount, or consistency of the vaginal discharge. These include vaginal yeast infections, nonspecific vaginitis, trichomoniasis, and sexually transmitted diseases, such as the herpes simplex virus type 2 (see AIDS and Other Sexually Transmitted Diseases, p. 137).

Yeast infections are usually marked by a thick, white discharge like cottage cheese, although sometimes it is clear. The vagina and labia (the lips of the vagina) may be red and swollen. Yeast infections also cause intense itching and burning in the genital area. An overgrowth of normal vaginal flora, *Candida albicans (Monilia)*, is the usual culprit. This type of infection is more likely during pregnancy, after taking antibiotics, when using birth control pills, or if you have diabetes. Spreading it through sex is rare, but if your partner has genital itching, an over-the-counter antifungal cream may be used topically.

Bacteria-caused vaginal infections include **Gardnerella**. Symptoms include a yellow or white vaginal discharge, itching, burning during urination, and pain in the vaginal area following intercourse. If you think you may have Gardnerella, see your doctor or nurse practitioner for treatment to keep the infection from spreading to the uterus and Fallopian tubes. Bacterial vaginal infection is usually treated with specific prescription antibiotics.

Trichomoniasis is caused by a tiny organism. Symptoms include a yellow-green frothy discharge from the vagina, itching, and sometimes pain. The discharge may have a bad odor, but doesn't always. Because the *Trichomonas* parasite can live in the male prostate gland, your partner should also be treated to prevent reinfection. See your doctor or nurse practitioner if you have symptoms of *Trichomonas* infection. He or she can prescribe drugs which you will need to take for the full time prescribed—even if your symptoms seem to be gone.

Sexually transmitted diseases (STDs) can also cause vaginal irritation, and some cause an abnormal vaginal discharge. (For more information on STDs and their prevention, see p. 137.)

Although other vaginal infections usually require examination and treatment by a doctor or nurse practitioner, yeast infections can usually be treated safely and well at home.

PREVENTIVE STEPS

- Clean perineal area daily with water.

- Wear cotton underwear.

- Avoid tight-fitting jeans and pantyhose.

- Avoid deodorant tampons or frequent douches.

- Avoid a high-carbohydrate diet.

- Use adequate lubrication during intercourse.

- Avoid scented or deodorant soaps, laundry detergents, or fabric softeners that cause irritation.

I'd never had a vaginal yeast infection before, but I had heard about them. And I was pretty sure all the symptoms I was having fit. The itching and discharge were driving me crazy! Because this was the first time I'd had these symptoms, I called the doctor's office to make sure. The nurse recommended a nonprescription vaginal cream and gave me some "recipes" for cool compresses to soothe the itching. What a relief!
Sonya

SELF-CARE STEPS FOR VAGINAL DISCHARGE AND IRRITATION

- An antiyeast antibiotic taken by mouth just once is a very effective treatment for vaginal infections. This must be prescribed by a doctor.

- Use an over-the-counter antifungal vaginal cream or suppository (such as Monistat, Gyne-Lotrimin, Mycelex). Follow the package directions and be sure to use all the medicine. Don't stop treatment just because the symptoms are gone.

- Expose the area to air.

- Apply cool compresses to the perineal area (area between the vagina and rectum) or soak in an oatmeal bath product (Aveeno bath treatment).

- Avoid bubble baths, vaginal sprays, and douching (unless prescribed). Soaking in a tub of plain, lukewarm water, however, is helpful.

- Avoid sexual intercourse until you finish the medicine to prevent further irritation.

- If home treatment doesn't relieve your symptoms, or if symptoms get worse, see your doctor or nurse practitioner.

DECISION GUIDE FOR VAGINAL DISCHARGE AND IRRITATION

SYMPTOMS/SIGNS	ACTION
Itching; white, cottage-cheese-like discharge; redness and swelling around vagina and labia	
Self-care fails to relieve symptoms, or symptoms worsen	
More than three yeast infections a year	
Yellow or greenish vaginal discharge with itching, burning during urination, or pain during or after intercourse	
Sores in the genital area	
Lower abdominal pain	

Use self-care

Call doctor's office for advice

See doctor

For more about the symbols, see p. 2.

STRESS-RELATED PROBLEMS

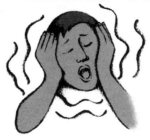

Your body is often the first to let you know when you are crumbling under the stress of modern living. Juggling family and career, elbowing through crowds, and dealing with conflict have all become commonplace. Coping with a hurried and harried lifestyle can take its toll both emotionally and physically.

This section describes common problems related to stress, such as headaches and fatigue, and suggests ways to take care of nonurgent problems at home. Your primary care doctor (pediatrician, family practitioner, or internal medicine specialist) can offer advice and treatment for most stress or fatigue problems. If your condition is especially hard to handle, your primary care doctor may involve other medical providers who specialize in diagnosing and treating these problems, such as psychiatrists, psychologists, neurologists, or infectious disease specialists. *This information cannot replace care by your health care providers.*

Use the Decision Guides to see if your symptoms warrant medical attention or if they can be handled with self-care. However, you need to consider your own medical history and your current health when deciding if self-care is right for you. If you have any conditions that do not seem to be healing normally or if self-care steps do not seem helpful, you should call your health care provider.

ATTENTION DEFICIT AND HYPERACTIVITY

Almost all children have times when they don't seem to pay attention, can't sit still, or just have more energy than they can burn. For some children, however, difficulty concentrating or very high physical energy levels (hyperactivity) interfere with social and academic tasks right for their ages.

A child with true attention deficit/hyperactivity disorder (ADHD) may have problems paying attention or being impulsive, be hyperactive, or have some combination of these. Such a child may talk constantly, be unable to wait turns in groups, and pay little attention to details, with schoolwork being messy or filled with careless mistakes. He or she may be easily distracted, act before thinking, or have trouble sitting still.

In some ways, a diagnosis of ADHD is a "relative" diagnosis, meaning that a child with the disorder has far more difficulty with attention or controlling impulses or activity than do most other children. But not all children with ADHD have big problems with hyperactivity and impulsivity. For some, inattention is the primary problem. Likewise, some children who are clearly hyperactive are able to concentrate if they can just sit still long enough. Children with ADHD may also face the added problem of having difficulty controlling anger.

Our second child, Michael, has always been very active. Even before he was born, he was always moving. We thought he would grow out of it, but when he got to school, he couldn't sit still and had trouble finishing tasks and paying attention. His kindergarten teacher seemed to think Michael was just another "bad" kid. His first grade teacher, however, was great. She recommended that Michael be assessed for ADHD. Our doctor and the school professionals agreed that Michael showed signs of ADHD. The doctor prescribed drugs for him to take on school days, and a child guidance specialist began working with Michael and us to help him find ways to control his behavior and concentrate. Michael still has problems, but he's doing much better and getting good grades.

Margaret

Because there is no scientific "blood" test for ADHD, the disorder can be difficult to tell from age-appropriate behaviors in active children. And symptoms like those of ADHD may be brought on by grief (over the death of a parent or a divorce); depression; post-traumatic stress (after physical or sexual abuse); or other physical, emotional, or psychological problems.

Symptoms usually subside in late adolescence and early adulthood. But some teenagers and adults may continue to have feelings of restlessness or difficulty engaging in quiet, sedentary activities.

The exact cause of ADHD is unknown. Popular theories that sugar, food dyes, or other food additives contribute to hyperactivity or that the condition is caused by minute levels of brain damage have not been proven. But a controlled environment, special training for the child, and drugs, such as methylphenidate (Ritalin) or antidepressants, have been helpful in dealing with—but not curing—ADHD.

DEPRESSION

Depression is a "whole-body" illness that affects a person's body, feelings, thoughts, and behavior. Depression is not a passing blue mood. It is not a sign of personal weakness or a condition that can be willed or wished away. People with depression cannot merely "pull themselves together" and get better. It is a set of painful symptoms that can last for months, and sometimes years.

If you think you are depressed, or if the symptoms of depression seem to be lasting, see your doctor. There are several tests or mental health assessments that can help tell if you are depressed.

What are the symptoms of depression?

- Inability to enjoy life
- Tiredness (see Fatigue, p. 193)
- Sleep disturbances (see Insomnia, p. 197), early morning waking, or oversleeping)
- Eating disturbances (loss of appetite, weight loss, or weight gain)

SELF-CARE STEPS FOR ADHD

- Get an evaluation. A careful evaluation will look at how your child functions intellectually, socially, emotionally, physically, and academically. Ideally, the professional(s) doing the evaluation should observe your child during normal daily activities in more than one setting (at home and at school) and at different times of the day.

- Stick to a routine and set firm limits at home and school.

- Make sure schoolwork matches your child's abilities. A class that's not suited to your child's academic skills can lead to inattention, boredom, and frustration.

- Provide outlets for your child's physical energy.

- Find ways to cope yourself. Parenting a hyperactive child can be challenging. Avoid becoming very critical, controlling, or angry at your child. Remember—and let your child know—you don't like the behavior, but you love the child.

- Use other resources. Ask your doctor or your child's school for information on help available in your community.

- Poor concentration
- Feelings of guilt, worthlessness, or helplessness
- General irritability
- Thoughts of death or suicide; suicide attempt
- Vague physical aches and pains
- A lot of crying

The causes of depression are not always known. Consider the following:

- Research shows the tendency to develop depression may be inherited.
- An uneven balance of mood-influencing chemicals in the brain can play a role.
- People who have a poor self-image, who view themselves negatively, or who are easily overwhelmed by life challenges may be more likely than others to experience depression.
- A serious loss, chronic illness, difficult relationship, or any unwelcome change can trigger depression.

FACTS ABOUT DEPRESSION

- Major depression is a medical illness, not a character defect.
- Over 11 million Americans suffer from depression.
- About twice as many women as men suffer from depression.
- With treatment, recovery is the rule—not the exception.
- The aim of treatment is not just getting better, but staying well.

SELF-CARE STEPS FOR DEPRESSION

- Share your treatment plan with people close to you. Talk to friends and relatives and explain what you are going through.
- Take drugs as instructed. You may be tempted to stop taking your drugs too soon. However, it is important to keep taking them until your doctor says to stop, even if you begin feeling better.
- Report any unusual drug side effects to your doctor, especially if the side effects interfere with your functioning.
- Keep all follow-up appointments you have with your doctor. Do not miss an appointment, even if you are feeling better that day.

- Set realistic goals. Do not set hard goals for yourself or take on a great deal of responsibility.
- Divide your workload. Break large tasks into small ones, set priorities, and don't be hard on yourself if you are unable to get everything finished.
- Do activities that make you feel better. You might want to try moderate exercise, go to movies, or join in social activities.
- Do not expect to immediately "snap out" of your depression. People rarely get better overnight. Instead, help yourself as much as you can, and do not blame yourself for not being up to par.

When I began taking blood pressure medication, I started feeling very odd. I'd have episodes when it seemed like everything around me was moving around and spinning. I'd close my eyes and it felt like I was falling over. I had to sit still with my head between my knees until the feeling passed. I called the clinic, and they recognized it as a side effect of the drug right away. She gave me a prescription for a different drug, and I've never had the problem since.

Dennis

I awoke yesterday morning with a spinning feeling. I found I could not walk to the telephone, and then I noticed double images in my vision. My speech seemed slurred when I called my doctor. He told me to go to the emergency room because I might be having a warning stroke.

Elsa, age 70

DIZZINESS

Popular songs would have us believe that love is a major cause of dizziness. Emotions have been medically linked to episodes of unsteadiness, but stress and anxiety, not love, are usually the cause. A variety of other conditions—all rather unromantic—can also cause dizziness.

Dizziness is feeling lightheaded, faint, or giddy. It can be caused by drugs or viral infections like colds and flu, as well as by stress and anxiety.

Some people feel dizzy for a moment when they quickly get up from a sitting or reclining position. This dizziness, called **postural hypotension**, is considered harmless unless it leads to fainting spells or blackouts. However, if you are taking drugs for high blood pressure, report dizziness to your health care provider. If you are dizzy and have black stools or any other illness, you should also call the doctor's office.

Most dizziness is usually mild, temporary, and harmless. When coupled with other symptoms, however, it may be a sign of a serious health problem or even an emergency. For example, dizziness with chest pain can signal a heart attack. See a doctor immediately if you have this combination of symptoms.

Vertigo is another form of dizziness that may be a more serious condition. Vertigo is marked by a feeling of movement. You or the objects around you seem to be spinning. People who experience vertigo may be unable to walk in a straight line.

Vertigo can be caused by a condition called labyrinthitis, an inflammation of the inner ear. Involuntary movements of the eyes, nausea, and vomiting may accompany the vertigo. Sometimes symptoms only appear when the head is held in a specific position. Vertigo can signal as serious and rare a condition as a brain tumor or as benign a problem as earwax buildup.

SELF-CARE STEPS FOR DIZZINESS

- Avoid positions that cause dizziness.

- Take your time getting up if you get dizzy spells when you rise quickly from sitting or lying positions. Sit on the edge of the bed for a few minutes in the morning before standing up.

- When dizziness or vertigo strikes, slowly move to a sitting or reclining position. You'll be less likely to fall and injure yourself. If you feel faint or your vision begins to go dark, sit with your head between your knees.

- Drink more fluids.

- Avoid driving.

- Avoid caffeine, alcohol, smoking, and illegal drugs.

- Change positions slowly.

- Use relaxation techniques to combat anxiety. Breathe deeply and slowly.

- If you feel vertigo, keeping your eyes open and focused on a stationary object may lessen the symptoms.

- Take aspirin, acetaminophen (Tylenol or a generic), or ibuprofen (Advil or a generic) for pain or fever. Do not give aspirin to children or teenagers.

Ménière's disease is another common cause of vertigo. Symptoms of this condition include attacks of vertigo, muffled hearing, a ringing in one or both ears, nausea, and vomiting. Ménière's disease may be related to excess fluid in the inner ear. The disease can start and stop throughout life, and although there is no cure, symptoms can be relieved.

All dizziness needs to be discussed with and/or evaluated by your health care provider to find the cause.

DECISION GUIDE FOR DIZZINESS

SYMPTOMS/SIGNS	ACTION
Occasionally light-headed or dizzy when first standing up or getting out of bed	
Dizziness or vertigo with vomiting, nausea, fainting, or black stools (see Black or Bloody Stools, p. 43; Vomiting, p. 58)	
Dizziness lasts for 3 or more days or with ear pain, buzzing, or pounding sensation	
Dizziness with temperature of 101° F or higher	
Trauma, head injury (p. 23), or severe headache	
Weakness in extremities, or tingling in any body part	
Sudden loss of hearing, sudden blurred, double vision, slurred speech, or difficulty swallowing	
Symptoms of shock (p. 36)	
Chest pain (p. 85) or pressure	
Loss of bladder or bowel control	

FATIGUE

Frustrated. Apathetic. Tense and tired. Irritable. Grumpy. Unmotivated. Energyless and exhausted. These are feelings of fatigue, and everyone has had them at some time or another. They are a normal part of life. What most people refer to as fatigue is brought on by hard work or exertion and can be remedied by sleep. When sleep and rest do not help, though, your body is sending you a signal that something else may be wrong.

Depression (p. 190) and anxiety are common, treatable causes of fatigue. Symptoms of anxiety disorder or depression may include a depressed mood, feelings of apprehension, eating or sleeping disturbances, or not being able to experience joy. See your health care provider if you are unable to enjoy life because of a depressed mood.

Fatigue is an overwhelming sense of tiredness that makes your body feel weak. Fatigue lasts 6 weeks or longer, and can be an early symptom of many types of serious illness, although usually it is not. These illnesses include anemia, cancer, diabetes, hepatitis, heart disease, hypoglycemia, hypothyroidism, mononucleosis, rheumatoid arthritis, obesity, alcoholism, sleep disorders, or low-grade urinary tract infection.

Fatigue can also be traced back to drugs and prescriptions you may be taking. Many of these can rob you of energy. Chief among the over-the-counter culprits are pain relievers, cough and cold medicines, antihistamines and allergy remedies, sleeping pills, and motion sickness pills. Energy-sapping prescriptions include tranquilizers, muscle relaxants, sedatives, birth control pills, and blood pressure reducers.

 Use self-care

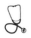 See doctor

Seek help now

For more about the symbols, see p. 2.

Too much stress can harm your health, but if there are not enough changes in your day, you will become unmotivated—and weary from boredom. Changing parts of your lifestyle may help you recharge your internal batteries.

A pattern of serious fatigue could be a sign of a disabling condition known as **chronic fatigue syndrome**. Causing flu-like symptoms, such as fever, sore throat, and muscle pain, this debilitating illness affects more women than men.

Confusion, sleep problems, and depression sometimes go hand in hand with chronic fatigue syndrome. In fact, more than two-thirds of those with the illness also suffer from depression. Antidepressant drugs are often used in treatment. Researchers have not linked any virus or other disease to chronic fatigue syndrome and are investigating other possible causes, including infection, stress, and impaired hormone production.

SELF-CARE STEPS FOR FATIGUE

• Organize your time. Get up a few minutes earlier, so that you won't have to start your day feeling rushed and tired. Learn to delegate—and how to say "no" when you have enough responsibilities and activities in your life.

• Exercise regularly. You should exercise three to five times a week, for 20 to 30 minutes—and move around as much as possible during the day. Also, avoid late-night activities, as they can disrupt your regular sleeping habits and make you tired in the morning.

• Get the right amount of sleep. Most people need 6 to 8 hours of sleep each night. Shortchanging yourself on sleep will leave you exhausted, and getting too much sleep will make you feel groggy. Older people who tend to sleep less soundly and younger people with hectic schedules may also need naps during the day.

• Breathe deeply and slowly. Shallow, rapid breathing often leads to fatigue because the body gets less oxygen.

• Quit smoking. Smoking steals some of your body's oxygen supply, replacing it with useless carbon dioxide. Because nicotine is a stimulant, going through the consequent withdrawal symptoms can cause temporary tiredness.

• Lose weight. Stick to well-balanced meals and avoid crash diets. When your calorie intake is too restricted, it's very stressful for the body. One of the many symptoms of this type of stress is fatigue.

• Drink less caffeine and alcohol. Alcohol is a depressant and will make you feel tired, not boost your energy. Likewise, caffeine will give you a temporary boost of energy, but when the effect wears off, your energy level will drop drastically.

• Find your lunch style. Some people function best after eating a lighter lunch, while others need to eat their largest meal of the day at lunch. In either case, avoid high-fat foods. Because fats burn off slower than carbohydrates, they will slow you down.

• Take a break. Interrupt your workday with periodic breaks. And if you haven't gone on a vacation in a while, take that dreamed-of trip or unplug the phone and refresh at home.

• Watch less TV. If you depend on television to relax, you may find yourself relaxed into a state of lethargy. Try something more stimulating, such as reading or taking a walk.

• Find ways to calm yourself. Listen to music or relaxation tapes. Say a word, phrase, or prayer that gives you a sense of peace. Imagine yourself on a beach, at the mountains, or in your favorite spot.

HEADACHES

Headaches are one of the most common health complaints. They have many different causes including tension, infection, injury, and changes in the flow of blood within the head. Most headaches occur when the muscles of the head or neck become tense and contract.

Contrary to popular belief, aspirin is not a cure-all for headaches. In fact, occasionally aspirin will mask symptoms that might aid diagnosis, and continued overuse can cause side effects. Fortunately, most headaches that occur without other symptoms respond well to self-care.

Nearly 90 percent of all headaches are caused by tension or stress and can be controlled. Unusual or very bad headaches can be a symptom of a serious health problem. If you suffer from these types of headaches, seek medical help.

Headaches can be classified into three general categories: tension, cluster, and migraine.

Tension headaches (also known as *muscle contraction headaches*) are often caused by the tightening of muscles of the back and shoulders in reaction to emotional and physical stress. A tension headache may occur as pain all over the head, as a feeling of pressure, or as a band around the head.

Tension headaches are believed to be the most common cause of head pain. Although they may be caused by poor posture or working in awkward conditions, the most common triggers are

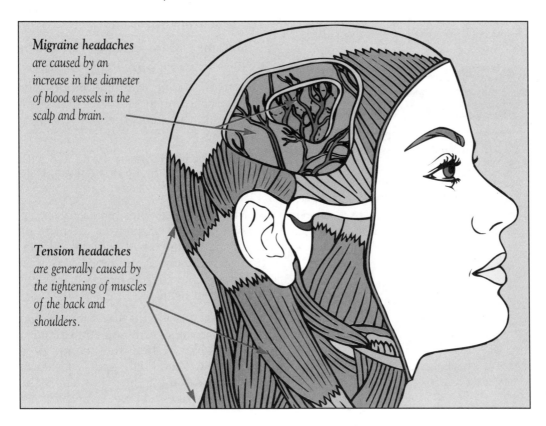

Migraine headaches are caused by an increase in the diameter of blood vessels in the scalp and brain.

Tension headaches are generally caused by the tightening of muscles of the back and shoulders.

stress, anxiety, and depression. Tension headaches that occur two or more times weekly for several months or longer are considered chronic, and you should consult your health care provider.

The symptoms of a tension headache include:

- Steady pain that doesn't pulse

- A tightness, fullness, or pressure over the top of the head or back of the neck

- Occasional nausea or vomiting

Home treatment of tension headaches is often successful. Aspirin or acetaminophen may relieve the pain; however, frequent use should be avoided. Taking a hot or cold shower, massaging the neck muscles or lying down in a dark room may provide relief. Learning to relax using biofeedback, meditation, music, visualization, hypnosis or taking a stress management class may also be helpful.

SELF-CARE STEPS FOR HEADACHES

- Lifestyle plays an important role with headaches. Eating and sleeping habits, stress, and exercise can all be factors in triggering occasional and more frequent headaches. Generally, over-the-counter pain relievers such as aspirin, acetaminophen, or ibuprofen can control a headache.

- For recurring headaches, a "headache calendar" may help to identify possible triggers. A headache calendar should record everything you eat, your sleep and exercise patterns, and work and home activities. Women should also record their menstrual cycles because headaches can be triggered by hormonal changes.

Cluster headaches are very painful and occur mainly in middle-aged men. A cluster headache lasts 30 minutes to 2 hours, before recurring (hence the name). There is no signal before a cluster headache begins, nor any sign it is going to end.

The pain from a cluster headache rapidly worsens in several minutes to a peak that often lasts for 30 minutes to 2 hours. Lying down during an attack generally makes the pain worse. Victims of cluster headaches are encouraged to keep a diary of patterns that may help identify a personal trigger.

Due to the rapid start of cluster headaches, over-the-counter pain relievers are of little use because they take effect too slowly. Inhaling 100 percent oxygen often brings relief. And, although prescription drugs provide relief, side effects may limit their use.

Symptoms of a cluster headache include:

- A steady, boring pain in or around one eye, occurring in episodes that often begin at the same time each day or evening

- Watering and redness of one eye with nasal congestion on the same side of the face

Migraine headaches have very specific symptoms. The pain of a migraine headache is caused by the increased dilation or widening of the blood vessels in the head. These headaches occur suddenly and often recur.

Because the victim may become nauseated, migraines are sometimes called *sick headaches*. Often the victim of a migraine will see bright spots, flashes of light, or areas of blindness just before the headache strikes. These symptoms are called an aura. Some victims have great bursts of energy and activity just before a migraine starts.

DECISION GUIDE FOR HEADACHES

SYMPTOMS/SIGNS	ACTION
Occasional headaches, causing minor discomfort	🩹
Recurring headaches, causing loss of function	☎
Nausea and vomiting	🩺
Convulsions	🏥
Weakness, numbness, or tingling in arms or legs	🏥
Sudden, disabling pain	🏥

🩹 Use self-care 🩺 See doctor

☎ Call doctor's office for advice 🏥 Seek help now

For more about the symbols, see p. 2.

A mild migraine headache may pass quickly if you go immediately to a darkened room and lie down. Place a cool, damp cloth on your forehead. Relax your entire body, focusing on the eyes, the forehead, the jaw and neck muscles, and working down to the toes.

Symptoms of migraine headache include:

• Throbbing pain

• Pain more often on one side of the head

• An aura, or preheadache phase, that can include flashes of light, bright spots, distorted vision, abdominal pain, and nausea

Possible triggers of migraine headache include hunger, fatigue, bright light, alcohol, caffeine, excitement or stress, birth control pills, and certain foods.

Most migraine headaches require professional diagnosis and treatment. See your health care provider to discuss appropriate treatment.

INSOMNIA

Insomnia is an occasional problem for almost everyone, but it is a chronic problem for 15 million to 20 million Americans. It sends many people to the doctor, often to get sleeping pills. Yet, most doctors believe that sleeping pills should be avoided whenever possible. Many nonprescription sleep aids rely on what doctors call the "placebo effect," which means they work only if you think they are going to. And prescription drugs are likely to really knock you out, rather than producing a natural, restful sleep.

For many people, insomnia is an occasional response to excitement or anxiety from good and bad events in life that keep you awake and thinking late at night. Others develop poor sleep schedules, sleeping late into the morning or napping during the day. This makes sleep at night more difficult.

Insomnia may be a symptom of depression. If you do not feel well, think you may be depressed (see Depression, p. 190), or are waking unusually early, you should discuss these symptoms with your doctor. There are helpful treatments for depression that may cure your insomnia if the two problems are related.

It may take several weeks or longer to establish a new, natural sleeping routine. If you are unable to make progress after giving the Self-Care Steps listed on the next page an honest try, call your health care provider for professional help.

SELF-CARE STEPS FOR INSOMNIA

• Avoid drinking alcohol in the evening. Although alcohol is a short-term sedative, and may quickly bring on sleep, it interferes with deep sleep, so that you may wake up suddenly after its depressant effect has worn off.

• Avoid or reduce caffeine. Caffeine stays in your system for up to 12 to 24 hours. Remember that in addition to coffee, caffeine is present in chocolate and many colas and teas. If you suspect caffeine is contributing to your sleeplessness, don't use any caffeinated products for at least 12 hours before you go to bed.

• Be aware of other drugs that may affect your sleeping patterns. Many widely used over-the-counter decongestants (including Sudafed) and products containing phenylpropanolamine can be as stimulating as caffeine. Before starting a drug, ask your pharmacist if it might keep you awake and if another product can be substituted.

• Break your chain of thought before turning in. Try setting aside 30 minutes before bedtime to work on problems that might keep you up later. Make lists and diagram strategies to attack your problems. You'll sleep better knowing you've taken steps to address those issues.

• Avoid eating large meals just before going to bed. The uncomfortable feeling of having a full stomach may delay sleep. Try a light snack instead. This will satisfy your hunger without interfering with your sleep. Many people swear by the virtues of a glass of warm or cold milk. Try adding a touch of honey, cinnamon, or vanilla to this bedtime standby.

• Take a warm bath an hour or two before bedtime. This can soothe tense muscles and help make you sleepy. However, taking a bath *immediately* before going to bed may be too stimulating and keep you awake. Experiment with the timing to see what works best for you.

• Exercise regularly. This will help relieve tension and clear your head. It will also tire you out, so you can sleep more soundly. Avoid strenuous physical activity for several hours before going to bed. It may stimulate you and interfere with falling asleep.

• Your bedroom should be quiet and dark. If noise is a problem, try ear plugs or "white noise." Many people like the reassuring sound of a fan or air conditioner as they drift off to sleep. A cool room temperature—between 60° and 65° F—is best for sleeping. A firm, comfortable mattress is also important for a good night's sleep.

• Avoid long, late afternoon naps. Short "catnaps," lasting no more than 20 minutes, can be surprisingly refreshing. Longer naps and those taken later than 4:00 p.m. may disrupt normal sleep patterns and contribute to insomnia.

• Read in bed for a few minutes before turning out the light. This helps you relax and can increase feelings of drowsiness.

• Counting sheep is not recommended. Counting requires focusing the brain on a specific activity. Instead, try picturing yourself in a pleasant place, and use your imagination to hear relaxing sounds as you drift off to sleep.

• Stick to a routine. Your body's internal clock responds best to a regular schedule. Try going to bed and getting up in the morning at the same time each day, including weekends.

STRESS

"I can't cope with all this stress." "I'm all stressed out." "I need to go to a desert island and get away from all this stress." Sound familiar? All of us have had these thoughts—and we have all needed that desert island. But if we really lived where there was absolutely no stress—no competition, no risks to take, no inspiration to try just a little bit harder—we would be completely bored. Sometimes stress adds just the amount of challenge and motivation we need to have a happy life—in fact, to stay alive.

It's when there are too many challenges confronting us and we lose our ability to juggle them all that the stresses in our lives cause us distress. Everyday hassles can cause as much stress as larger events, such as money worries, arguments, a divorce, a death in the family, losing a job, buying a house—or simply anticipating these things. Stress is unavoidable, but that doesn't mean it's unmanageable. A walk around the block, a nutritious meal, and a good night's sleep will usually give you the energy and strength to face another day. That changes when occasional stress turns into chronic stress.

Chronic stress cracks your emotional foundation—making you angry, apathetic, irritable, anxious, or even depressed. You may quit eating or eat too much. You find it hard to concentrate. You may start smoking. Too much stress may even make you more accident-prone, lead to alcohol or drug abuse, and weaken your body, increasing vulnerability to certain diseases.

SELF-CARE STEPS FOR STRESS

• Identify the things in your life that bring you stress. Try to avoid them, but if you can't, have a Plan A and B for dealing with them. You may have to learn how to be assertive.

• Share some of your responsibilities. A shared burden is lighter to carry—and you may develop a new friendship or learn another way of problem solving.

• Exercise regularly. Stretches and walking are especially helpful.

• Find some crumb of humor (to the point of absurdity) in even the worst situation—even when you have to force yourself.

• Organize your time and don't procrastinate. Focus on the individual steps for getting a job done so that you don't feel overwhelmed.

• Talk with a friend or family member. Sharing your thoughts and fears will make them less overwhelming and easier to handle.

• Get a pet and love it.

• Practice breathing deeply, from your diaphragm. Hold each breath for a few seconds, then exhale slowly.

• Tense and then relax every muscle in your body. Begin with your head and neck, and work your way down to your toes.

• Sit quietly and repeat to yourself a "cue" word that will make you feel calm, such as "peace."

• Listen to relaxation tapes or music.

• Relax in a warm bath.

• Avoid caffeine.

• Help other people. The sense of well-being you receive will help you put life's events in better perspective.

• Balance life (work, relationships, play, spirituality).

• Play. Join in athletics or take up a new hobby.

• Take time to focus on the spiritual (nature, religion).

So how do you regain control? Research has found that people who effectively manage the stress in their lives have three things in common:

- They consider life a challenge, not a series of hassles.

- They have a mission or purpose in life and are committed to fulfilling that.

- They do not feel victimized by life, but believe instead that despite temporary setbacks, they have control over their lives.

If worry is causing you a lot of distress or disability, you may become depressed (see Depression, p. 190). Anxiety is a normal part of life, but serious stress that depresses your mood or ruins your ability to experience joy may be the result of an anxiety disorder or depression. If these conditions are present and/or you experience these feelings, see your health care provider for an evaluation.

SECTION THREE
LIVING WITH CHRONIC
HEALTH PROBLEMS

When it comes to living with chronic health problems—those that can last a long time—it is often more important to know what type of person has the disease than it is to know the usual course of the disease. That's because a person's responses can play such a vital role in how the disease progresses or doesn't progress and what effect the disease has on lifestyle. If you have a chronic health problem, you know the kind of demands, both physical and emotional, that having a long-term disease can create. You may not realize that the decisions you make about your lifestyle and the amount of effort you bring to your own therapy can have a very big impact on the long-term effects of your illness. This section contains current guidelines for managing some of the most common chronic health problems.

Experts who treat particular chronic conditions know that there is an important body of knowledge that is unique to each disease. For example, someone with arthritis will benefit from learning a great deal about his or her particular form of the disease, how it can be treated, and how to prevent complications. This information will be very different from the information needed by someone with hypertension. Your primary care doctor is your best resource for helping you understand how to manage your condition and can refer you to a doctor who specializes in treating your condi-

tion if you have unusual problems that need more attention.

Although each chronic disease requires special knowledge and behaviors from the patient and the health care provider, there are many health practices that will help any chronic condition. Whether you have diabetes or high cholesterol, for example, getting and staying fit is a key to your self-care. Eating a healthy diet is a universal health strategy. A dietitian with special training in your chronic disease can design a meal plan that is safe given your present condition and help you change your eating habits to promote your health for the long run.

Living with a chronic health problem can take its toll emotionally. Learning skills to deal with stress is beneficial, no matter what disease you have. If you are part of a family, coping with a disease can disrupt former routines and can require special skills in resolving unexpected problems. You may benefit from family counseling or other approaches to good communication and conflict resolution.

When you are diagnosed with a chronic condition, you will benefit from becoming a central member of your health care team. Expressing your personal needs and interests will make you the central figure in the decisions that will affect your health.

ANGINA, CHRONIC STABLE

Angina is a heart condition that occurs when the arteries that bring oxygen-rich blood to the heart muscle are clogged with a fatty substance called plaque. Angina is a warning signal that the heart isn't getting the oxygen it needs. A person with chronic stable angina often experiences pressure or pain in the heart that comes and goes. Resting usually relieves this type of pain.

The pain of angina and a true heart attack can feel very similar. However, unlike a heart attack, the pain from angina usually goes away in 15 minutes or less with rest or the use of **nitroglycerin**. A person may need to use up to two or three nitroglycerin tablets under the tongue before angina pain is relieved. The pain is often brought on by exertion, a large meal, emotional upsets, smoking, or other triggers, although it may occur when resting.

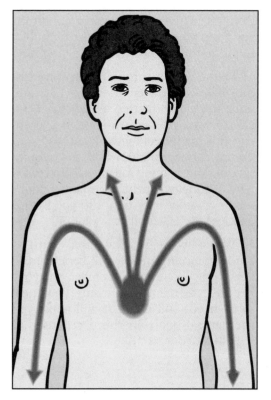

Know the Signs of Angina

Any of these symptoms can be caused by angina:

- A crushing, squeezing, burning pain in the chest
- Feeling of pressure in the chest
- Pain radiating to jaw, arms, neck and/or back

If you feel any or a combination of the symptoms above and the pain goes away with 15 minutes of rest, you may have angina. If you've never had this type of pain before, don't try to diagnose yourself. *Call your doctor or local hospital emergency room for advice.* If the doctor wants to see you right away, ask a friend or relative to drive you there.

If you have a history of angina, take your medicine as directed. Call the doctor's office if you have attacks of angina that are more frequent, longer lasting, or different or more painful than normal or if chest pain wakes you from sleep. Also, if angina symptoms occur with less activity than usual, discuss this with your doctor.

Use Medicine Effectively

If you take medicine for high blood pressure or angina, be sure you understand the possible side effects and what to do about them. Don't allow yourself to run out of the medicine. Keep nitroglycerin tablets in their original container. Check to be sure nitroglycerin tablets are not outdated. Bottle expiration dates are normally 4 to 5 years after the tablets are bottled.

Angina—pressure or pain in the chest that may be brought on by physical activity and is relieved by rest. Angina is a warning signal that the heart isn't getting the oxygen it needs. Pain radiates to jaw, arms, neck and/or back.

ARTHRITIS, CHRONIC

One in seven Americans has arthritis, making it the leading chronic illness for those over age 45.

Joint pain, also called rheumatic pain, is a common medical problem, ranking among the most frequent reasons why people visit their doctors. When pain occurs, most people's first reaction is to think the symptoms are arthritis. Although this is a natural response, often joint or muscle pain is due to something other than arthritis. Other structures that surround the joint—such as the tendon, bursa, or muscle—are often the source of the pain.

What Is Arthritis?

See Acute Arthritis, p. 100, for a detailed discussion on evaluating joint pain.

When Is Joint Pain Serious?

If joint pain occurs with fever and sudden, significant swelling, or if you feel severe pain, you should call your doctor. If you feel pain without swelling or fever, it is generally safe to wait and see what happens. Constant pain that affects normal activities, however, is a reason to see your doctor for an exam. Because each person's pain threshold is different, the decision to see your doctor should be based upon how significantly the pain is affecting your life.

What Type of Doctor Should I See?

A doctor who specializes in diagnosing and treating diseases of joints and muscles is called a rheumatologist. Orthopedic surgeons also specialize in diseases of bone and joints, but they focus mostly on surgical treatment of these conditions. Although it is often necessary and appropriate to see either the rheumatologist or the orthopedist for a particular problem, it may not be necessary. Primary care doctors are well qualified to evaluate and treat less complicated rheumatic problems. You should see your primary care doctor first, and then, if referrals are needed, follow his or her advice and see a rheumatologist or orthopedist.

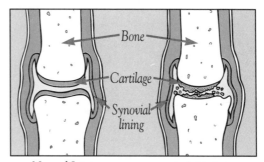

Normal Joint   *Arthritic Joint*

Arthritis is the inflammation of a joint. The illustration on the right is typical of osteoarthritis, where the protective cartilage cushion on the bone breaks down, and the bones of the joint rub against one another.

SELF-CARE STEPS FOR CHRONIC ARTHRITIS

OVER-THE-COUNTER MEDICINES

Frequently, over-the-counter medicines are the first treatment choice for arthritic pain. Two main types of medicines are used to treat arthritis: simple pain relievers and nonsteroidal anti-inflammatory medicines (NSAIDs), which relieve pain inflammation. Neither type is perfect for all situations. When used correctly, however, both can be very beneficial.

Pain Relievers

Pain relievers such as acetaminophen (Tylenol) very effectively control pain. Acetaminophen, like any medicine, must be taken over time to determine its effectiveness. Therapeutic doses may be as high as two extra-strength tablets three to four times daily. This dose may need to be used for several days before determining whether it will be effective for long-term treatment.

Acetaminophen's advantage is that most people can tolerate it. It is known for being gentle to the stomach. Acetaminophen does not cause gastrointestinal problems. It is not without risks, however. People with underlying liver disease or those who drink alcohol heavily may suffer liver problems as a result of taking acetaminophen.

NSAIDs

Medicines that relieve pain and decrease inflammation are called nonsteroidal anti-inflammatory drugs (NSAIDs). These include aspirin, ibuprofen (such as Motrin), and naproxen sodium (Naprosyn), all of which are available over the counter. Many other NSAIDs are available by prescription. NSAIDs are effective pain relievers and have the added advantage of decreasing modest levels of inflammation, which usually helps decrease pain.

Unfortunately, NSAIDs have more serious side effects than simple pain relievers. The biggest concern is ulcers or bleeding from the stomach. These problems occur more frequently in patients with a history of ulcers, elderly patients, those with other underlying illnesses, or those who are also taking other medicines. NSAIDs may also cause stomach upset. Fortunately, these side effects are relatively uncommon, especially the more serious ones.

Another concern with NSAIDs is the possibility of harming kidney function. This is a potentially serious problem; however, it is rare. The most important single risk factor is underlying kidney disease. Other, less risky, factors include having underlying liver disease, being elderly, and taking other types of medicine, particularly "water pills" or diuretics. If you have any of these risk factors, you should discuss using these medicines with your doctor before taking them.

Like acetaminophen, NSAIDs' effectiveness may not be evident right away. These medicines may need to be taken for a week or more before their best effect can be determined.

It is impossible to predict which NSAID will work best for each patient. Therefore, patients are often directed to choose one, use it regularly, and, if it is not effective, choose another. Use only one drug at a time, since using multiple NSAIDs together might increase the chance of side effects.

SELF-CARE STEPS FOR CHRONIC ARTHRITIS

OTHER HELPFUL PRODUCTS

Other products useful in treating arthritis are available in most drugstores. Products such as aspirin in cream form and capsaicin ointment have achieved limited success. Products that create heat where you apply them may give short-term pain relief.

Devices

Some assistive devices support painful areas or improve function in affected joints. The range of options is very broad. Wrist splints cut down wrist movement, which often relieves pain caused by arthritis, tendinitis, or carpal tunnel syndrome. Tennis elbow straps often decrease pain by altering the mechanical stresses of the injured tendon, and padded arch supports and heel pads decrease various kinds of foot pain. Examples of other devices include doorknob extenders, enlarged handle grips for silverware, adjustable canes, and special pillows to support the neck while sleeping.

Nutrition

Many people are interested in using diet to control disease. A well-balanced diet like those supported by the American Heart Association, the American Diabetes Association, and the American Cancer Society is the cornerstone of any dietary program. Following their guidelines makes it less likely that other illnesses will create problems that could complicate your arthritis.

Maintaining your ideal body weight is also a key to better health and can be very useful to treat arthritis. Carrying extra pounds increases the wear and strain on painful arthritic joints.

Also, some foods may affect arthritis symptoms. Fish oils can cut down on inflammation that often comes with rheumatoid arthritis. Studies suggest that fairly high doses are needed to achieve this effect, and inflammation is only modestly reduced; however, the effects are real. As a practical matter, substituting fish for meat is sensible. Fish oil pills also are available. If you choose to supplement your diet with fish oil pills, it's best to discuss this with your doctor.

Occasionally, patients with inflammatory arthritis find that a specific food may worsen their symptoms. This is uncommon, but some studies indicate that one patient in 100 may have a food-related flare. Food-related arthritic flares usually occur within 12 to 48 hours after eating the problem food. Food reactions, as well as the offending food, vary from person to person. If you recognize a pattern, it might help to discuss it with your doctor.

Continued on next page

SELF-CARE STEPS FOR CHRONIC ARTHRITIS (CONTINUED)

Other approaches

Exercise is important to maintain good health, especially for the patient with arthritis. Exercise helps preserve joint health and function, even for damaged joints. By improving the function of structures that surround the joint—such as the tendons and the muscles—exercise decreases the joint's workload.

There is no preferred exercise for arthritis. The best advice is to choose an exercise that you like and begin adding it to your regular activities. Exercise duration should be slow at first, and gradually increased. Aerobic exercises are ideal and low-impact activities such as walking, biking, and water exercises are usually most comfortable to do. As long as the activity doesn't increase pain or swelling, it is probably not causing any more joint damage. If pain and/or swelling occurs and lasts for more than 30 minutes after the activity, it is probably the wrong type of exercise or it was done too intensely.

Schedule changes

Sometimes, schedule changes make a big difference to the way joint pain affects your life. People with arthritis are often less mobile and suffer more pain in the morning. Shifting activities until later in the day may help you take advantage of your greatest mobility and make it easier to deal with the pain. This strategy is particularly helpful for patients with inflammatory arthritis.

Reducing stress

Stress—personal, social, and emotional—also takes its toll. Finding better ways to deal with stress may help decrease pain from arthritis and other joint conditions. Some stress reduction options include meditation, biofeedback, and professional counseling. Exercise is also an excellent stress reliever.

Community resources

Most communities have organizations and programs to serve people with arthritis or other disabilities. The Arthritis Foundation has chapters in every state. The organization provides educational materials and co-sponsors support groups, self-help programs, educational seminars, and exercise classes. It also supports research of the causes and cures of arthritis.

Transportation services—for people unable to drive or travel by public transportation—are usually available within larger communities. Social service agencies also may offer help in finding child care services, homemaking help, and meals-on-wheels programs. Additional assistance may be available to help explore financial and health care options. Many health care organizations offer specific programs designed to help people cope with arthritis.

ASTHMA

If you have asthma, you have plenty of company. About 13 million Americans cope with this lung disease, including over 4 million children. Asthma causes more days missed from work and school than any other chronic illness.

Asthma tends to run in families. It happens more often to people whose family members have asthma, hay fever, or eczema, but anyone can develop asthma at any age. About half of all people with asthma get the disease before age 10. Another third or so develop it before age 40.

There is no cure for asthma, but by working with their doctors, patients can learn to control the symptoms of the disease. With proper treatment, most asthma patients can lead normal, active lives.

Asthma can cause shortness of breath, wheezing, coughing, and chest tightness. Symptoms range from mild to life threatening.

Asthma is a common disease affecting 5 percent of the United States population, yet each patient is unique. That's why it is so important for people with asthma to understand the disease and their own symptoms and triggers.

Asthma symptoms fall into two categories: acute and chronic. Symptoms may last just a few minutes, several days, or even weeks. Asthma symptoms come on gradually in some patients, very quickly in others.

What Causes the Problem?

No one knows exactly what causes asthma, but doctors do know that the lining of the bronchial tubes—the air passages in the lungs—is extremely sensitive in people with asthma.

When something triggers an asthma episode, the bronchial tube lining gets inflamed and swollen, and more mucus is produced, leaving less room for air to pass through. Meanwhile, the bands of muscle around the outside of the bronchial tubes tighten, further blocking the flow of air and causing coughing, wheezing, and shortness of breath.

Asthma Triggers

Allergies to pollen (from trees, grasses, and weeds), dust mites, mold spores, and animals cause episodes of asthma.

Infections and irritants are nonallergic triggers for asthma. These include viral infections (such as colds and the flu), cigarette smoke, chemical fumes, smog, poor air quality, aspirin and other anti-inflammatory drugs, cold air, and changes in the weather.

Asthma may also be related to exposure to certain materials at work such as grain dust, flour (commonly known as baker's asthma), or chemicals.

Certain types of exertion or exercises may also trigger asthma episodes.

Note: Intense emotions such as fear and worry can trigger an asthma episode, but they don't cause the condition. Experts believe that emotional problems can result from asthma, but should not be considered a cause of the disease.

Treatment

The goal of asthma treatment is to have complete control, so that a person can do the activities of his or her choosing.

Treatment for an asthma episode involves identifying the specific triggers and eliminating patients' exposure to them. Acute attacks can be treated with medicine.

There is nothing more frightening than watching your child struggle for breath and not knowing how to help. Since Andre was diagnosed with asthma, I've learned to watch for the warning signs of an attack, and learned what to do when they occur. Andre still has difficulty breathing sometimes, but we both stay a lot calmer and just follow our action plan. It's made a world of difference to both of us.

Rachelle

Daily Record and Peak Flow Meters

Doctors and the primary asthma care provider work together with asthma patients first to control acute asthma and then to manage the symptoms by finding out what triggers the episodes. Patients may be asked to keep a daily record of symptoms, possible triggers, and medicine taken. They also may be asked to monitor their lung function with an instrument called a **peak flow meter**. It tells how well the patient is breathing. This information will help the doctor decide when to add the next level of medicine needed to keep the patient's symptoms under control. Through this treatment program, patients learn how triggers affect their asthma and how their lungs respond to medicine.

Action Plan

The patient and doctor or primary asthma care provider develop a written asthma action plan so that patients will be able to recognize warning signs of an asthma episode early and take the right steps to treat it. Each patient should also have an emergency plan to follow if an episode should become severe.

Medicines

There are many different types of asthma drugs. Many people need daily doses of prescription drugs to keep their symptoms under control. Medicines are most often taken by adults through an inhaler or nebulizer (a compressed air device for administering medication to the lungs). But medicine can also come in liquid, capsule, or tablet form. Every medicine has its own set of possible side effects. Be sure to ask the doctor or pharmacist what side effects you might have and what to do about them.

There are two general kinds of asthma drugs. The first ones are called **bronchodilators**. These drugs relax the muscles around the airways, so they can open up and let air in more easily. Bronchodilators come in many different forms.

The second type of medicine prescribed for asthma is called **anti-inflammatory drugs**. They reduce the swelling and mucus that lead to congestion. Anti-inflammatory agents, inhaled steroids, are commonly used to effectively treat people with moderate to severe asthma. The person is able to get the benefit of the medicine without the side effects, because when the medicine is inhaled it goes only to the lungs, not to the rest of the body.

Oral corticosteroids (such as prednisone, prednisolone, and methylprednisolone) are stronger types of anti-inflammatory medicine. Although these drugs can have side effects, they are usually safe when taken according to instructions and are primarily used for short-term control.

Another type of anti-inflammatory drug without steroids is cromolyn or nedocromil. These medicines can be given with an inhaler or nebulizer. They don't help during an asthma episode, but do work to prevent asthma episodes. Both cromolyn and nedocromil have few side effects. Although it doesn't work for everyone and can require as much as a month of usage before any benefit is seen, cromolyn can be especially useful for children with allergies. Both drugs are most effective when taken on a regular, preventive basis. Inhaled steroids are occasionally prescribed along with cromolyn or nedocromil.

Patients usually have questions and concerns about these drugs, and should discuss these issues with their doctor.

Asthma is a serious medical condition. It's not something you can treat by yourself. In partnership with your doctor or health care professional, however, you can use self-care techniques to manage your asthma, reduce the severity and frequency of your symptoms, and cut down on your trips to the clinic and hospital.

Home management recommendations assume the patient has seen a doctor and has an asthma action plan and the right drugs for managing asthma episodes. People with undiagnosed coughing, wheezing, chest tightness, or other possible asthma symptoms should see their doctors to set up a plan of care.

SELF-CARE STEPS FOR ASTHMA

• Become an asthma expert. Find out as much as you can about the disease. Attend patient information sessions and asthma support groups. Read books about asthma. Some good ones are *One Minute Asthma: What You Need to Know*, Thomas F. Plaut, M.D.; *Children with Asthma: A Manual for Parents*, Thomas F. Plaut, M.D.; and *Asthma: The Complete Guide to Self-Management of Asthma and Allergies for Patients and Their Families*, Allan M. Weinstein, M.D. Contact any of the following organizations for more information on asthma: the American Lung Association, the Mothers of Asthmatics, the American Academy of Allergy and Immunology, or the National Heart, Lung, and Blood Institute.

• Follow the asthma action plan established by you and your doctor. Know the warning signs of an asthma episode. Make sure you have written instructions for what to do in an asthma emergency. Keep a record of your episodes, drugs, peak flow readings, and responses to drugs.

• Manage your medicines. Know the kinds of drugs you should take, how much, and how often. Know the possible side effects and what you can do to minimize them. Make sure you know which drugs should be taken first, and follow the instructions carefully. Also learn the correct use of an inhaler with a spacer. Don't run out of your medicines. Ask your doctor or pharmacist to check all new drugs for possible interactions with the asthma drugs you are taking.

• Monitor your condition. Learn how to use a peak flow meter. It can help detect an impending episode early, because lung capacity can drop as much as 24 hours before any symptoms appear. If you keep daily records of your symptoms and peak flow readings, you will be able to begin treatment soon enough to reduce the number and severity of asthma episodes.

• Identify and avoid triggers. Your record keeping will help you determine what triggers your asthma episodes. If inhalants such as dust and animal dander are high on your list, take steps to keep your living areas free of these triggers. Steer clear of irritants, wood smoke, and automobile exhaust fumes.

• Don't smoke and stay away from areas where others are smoking.

• When an episode occurs, follow your asthma action plan: stay calm, stop your activity, take a few relaxed breaths, drink extra fluids, and then use your inhaler. Treat symptoms within minutes of their onset. It takes less medicine to stop an episode in its early phase.

• Stay physically fit. You should be able to control your asthma so you can exercise.

• Keep good records of your drugs and dosages. Make sure someone else in your family knows where to find this information in an emergency.

• See your physician for regular follow-up exams.

When we found out that my cat, Whiskers, made my asthma worse, the doctor said we needed to give him away. Whiskers lives with my grandma now. I've also learned more about my asthma. When I use my nebulizer, I don't cough and wheeze as much.

Emily, age 6

SPECIAL CONCERNS FOR CHILDREN

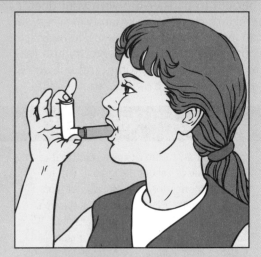

Asthma causes more hospital and emergency room visits than any other chronic childhood disease. Children with well-controlled asthma, however, should be able to do any activity or sport they choose.

Many children "outgrow" their asthma symptoms, although the underlying condition, that extra-sensitive bronchial tube lining, remains throughout life. About half of children with asthma outgrow it by age 15. Asthma can recur in the adult years. Smoking may trigger the return of the problem.

Education of both parent and child is key to treating asthma in children. Understanding the disease and the child's specific triggers and warning signs can help parents follow through with timely, effective treatment.

Children too young to use an inhaler are often treated with a machine called a **nebulizer**. This device uses compressed air to turn a solution of liquid medication into a fine mist that the child breathes in through a mask or mouthpiece.

How to Use an Inhaler

1. Assume a standing position. Shake the container well before using. Remove the cap and hold the container upright.

2. Place a spacer (cardboard or plastic tube) on the end of the inhaler. There are a variety of spacers available. A spacer is a holding chamber that allows you to use inhaled medications more effectively. If no spacer is available, hold the inhaler 1 to 2 inches from your mouth. Without a spacer, too much medication may end up in your mouth rather than in your lungs.

3. Breathe out normally, then position the spacer in your mouth. Place it on top of your tongue and close your lips around it.

4. As you start to breathe in slowly through your mouth, press down on the top of the inhaler container. It will administer a puff of medicine.

5. Continue breathing in slowly for 3 to 5 seconds, until your lungs are full.

6. Hold your breath for 10 seconds to allow the medicine to be deposited in your lungs.

7. In some cases, depending upon the drugs used, you will need to wait 1 to 3 minutes before taking another puff on your inhaler. This allows your lungs to open up, and the second treatment works even better. Check with your doctor for proper instructions.

DECISION GUIDE FOR ASTHMA

SYMPTOMS/SIGNS	ACTION	SYMPTOMS/SIGNS	ACTION
Normal asthma symptoms that can be managed according to asthma action plan	Use self-care	Symptoms during exercise in spite of drugs	Call doctor's office for advice
Minor coughing after exercise	Use self-care	Difficulty breathing, walking, or talking	See doctor
Wheezing when out in cold weather	Use self-care	Lips and/or fingernails turn gray or bluish	Seek help now
A cold or the flu worsens asthma symptoms	Use self-care	Skin of the neck, chest, or rib area is sucked in with each breath; nostrils flare	Seek help now
Severe asthma episode	Use self-care	Peak flow less than 50 percent of your personal best	Seek help now
Unsure about how to take medicines	Call doctor's office for advice	Symptoms worsen despite drugs	Seek help now
Severe reaction to drugs	Call doctor's office for advice	Rapidly getting worse over a few hours	Seek help now
Mucus is yellow, green, or bloody, or is thickening	Call doctor's office for advice	Severe wheezing and/or coughing, gasping for air, sweaty, hunched forward	Emergency, call 911
Temperature of 100° F or greater (101° F rectal) with wheezing or coughing	Call doctor's office for advice	Extremely anxious due to shortness of breath	Emergency, call 911
Peak flow drops into the red danger area	Call doctor's office for advice		
Unable to sleep because of wheezing and/or coughing	Call doctor's office for advice		

Use self-care

Call doctor's office for advice

See doctor

Seek help now

Emergency, call 911

For more about the symbols, see p. 2.

I have smoked since I was a teenager. I've never really had any problems with it, but now that I'm 67, I seem to cough a lot and even simple things like climbing a single flight of stairs or sweeping the floor leave me breathless. My doctor told me I have chronic obstructive pulmonary disease and must quit smoking. It hasn't been easy, but I'm trying, with the help of a nicotine patch and the support and encouragement of my family and doctor. I've also started walking regularly and doing the breathing workouts the nurse showed me. And I plan ahead before I do just about anything, figuring out the easiest way to do it, so I don't get so worn out. If I had known smoking would eventually make me live like this, I never would have started. But I'm making the most of it!

Loren

BRONCHITIS, CHRONIC AND EMPHYSEMA

Chronic obstructive pulmonary disease (COPD) is the fifth leading cause of death in the United States. Although many people think first of emphysema when they hear COPD, chronic bronchitis is actually more common and equally serious because it can lead to emphysema, and eventually cause death if it is not controlled.

Cigarette smoking is the number one cause of COPD, accounting for 82 percent of cases. Other causes include repeated exposure to lots of dust (such as in coal mines, granaries, or metal molding shops), chemical vapors, and possibly air pollution. A small percentage of emphysema cases are inherited.

Like acute bronchitis, **chronic bronchitis** is an inflammation of the lining of the bronchial tubes, which lead to the lungs. This causes the bronchial tubes to produce excess amounts of mucus. As chronic bronchitis progresses, the cilia or tiny hairs that sweep away irritants from the air passages may stop working or die off. Unlike the occasional 1- to 2-week bout with acute bronchitis after a cold or flu in otherwise healthy people, those with chronic bronchitis have inflammation and subsequent coughing, with mucus, for at least 3 months each year.

Emphysema occurs when the tiny air sacks (alveoli) in the lungs become larger and lose their elasticity. When this happens, the lungs become less able to get oxygen into the blood. This leads to shortness of breath, eventually making even the most basic tasks, such as eating or getting dressed, difficult and tiring.

Although neither chronic bronchitis nor emphysema can be cured, with medical treatment the damage they cause to the lungs and heart can be slowed and their symptoms can be eased. Neither disease appears overnight. Chronic bronchitis often begins as repeated cases of acute bronchitis following colds. With chronic bronchitis, however, coughing and mucus production occur more frequently and last longer after each cold, until the bronchitis is finally there whether you've had a cold or not. Likewise, emphysema comes on gradually, often beginning as shortness of breath with exercise or activity.

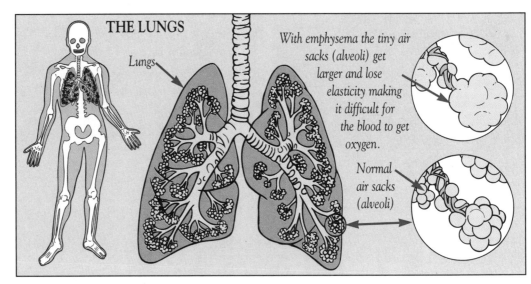

THE LUNGS

Lungs

With emphysema the tiny air sacks (alveoli) get larger and lose elasticity making it difficult for the blood to get oxygen.

Normal air sacks (alveoli)

Because of this gradual onset, you should see a doctor at the first signs of shortness of breath or "smoker's cough." Your doctor may prescribe some combination of bronchodilator drugs (oral or inhaled), which help to relax and open airways; corticosteroids, which help clear away excess mucus; antibiotics; and exercise to help build and support lung function.

In addition to taking drugs prescribed by your doctor, the Self-Care Steps list several things you can do to slow further lung damage and make living with COPD easier.

SELF-CARE STEPS FOR CHRONIC BRONCHITIS AND EMPHYSEMA

• *Quit Smoking!* Read the information in this book on quitting smoking (p. 270) and talk to your doctor. Continuing to smoke will only hasten the progression of emphysema.

• Call your doctor at the first signs of respiratory illness, such as a cold or flu.

• Drink plenty of fluids. Six to eight glasses of clear fluids a day, such as juice or water, will help keep air passages clear of mucus, making it easier to breathe.

• Eat a well-balanced diet. If you have emphysema, spread your meals out. By eating five or six small meals a day, you avoid having a full stomach, which will interfere with your breathing.

• Strengthen your heart with aerobic exercise and build your upper-body strength. Strengthening the muscles in your upper body will make breathing easier. Moderate aerobic exercise, such as 15 minutes of daily walking, will make your heart less susceptible to complications of COPD. Exercise and a healthy diet will also build your resistance to illness and infection.

• Do breathing exercises. If you have emphysema, ask your health care provider about exercises to help you breathe better. Two common exercises are "pursed-lip" breathing (inhaling through your nose and exhaling twice as long through pursed lips) and breathing from the diaphragm (expanding your diaphragm and abdomen, rather than your chest, when you inhale).

• Get a flu shot each fall and a pneumococcal pneumonia vaccination at least once.

DIABETES

Diabetes occurs when the body can't properly use or produce insulin, a hormone made in the pancreas that breaks down carbohydrates in food. Insulin brings glucose from the blood into the cells, where it is used for energy.

When insulin isn't available or the body doesn't use it properly, blood glucose levels rise. Uncontrolled, high blood glucose levels can cause serious health problems, including heart disease, kidney disease, blindness, or nerve damage. Keeping your blood glucose level as close as possible to normal (70 to 115 mg/dl before a meal) is the key to having a more healthy, energetic life.

Although there are different types of diabetes, the cause—the body's inability to use food properly—is the same. The major types of diabetes are Type I (insulin-dependent), Type II (non-insulin-dependent), and gestational diabetes.

Type I (Insulin-Dependent)

This type of diabetes may develop at any age, but most often occurs in children, teenagers, or young adults. Symptoms include being very thirsty, hungry, and tired, and needing to urinate often. Children with Type I diabetes rarely have these symptoms for longer than a few weeks before it is diagnosed.

With Type I diabetes, the pancreas stops producing enough insulin. To make up for this lack of insulin, people with Type I diabetes inject themselves with insulin.

Type II (Non-Insulin-Dependent)

The most common form of diabetes, Type II diabetes usually develops gradually with few, if any, symptoms. The pancreas keeps making insulin; however, the body is not using it effectively. This leads to a buildup of glucose in the blood. Often Type II diabetes is diagnosed by tracking a gradual increase in blood glucose levels.

Gestational Diabetes

This type of diabetes is discovered through a routine blood test for glucose during the course of a woman's pregnancy. Closely monitoring blood glucose levels helps women have safe pregnancies and healthy babies. Gestational diabetes usually disappears at the end of the pregnancy, but mothers may be at increased risk for developing diabetes in the future.

Risk Factors for Developing Diabetes

- Obesity

- Over age 40

- A family history of diabetes

- Race (diabetes is more common among American Indians, Hispanics, and African Americans)

- History of impaired glucose tolerance (IGT)

- High blood pressure or high levels of blood fats (cholesterol, triglycerides)

- Women who have had gestational diabetes

- Women who have had babies that weighed more than 9 pounds

Once you have diabetes, you have it for life. There is no cure. The disease can be successfully managed by controlling blood sugar through proper nutrition and exercise. A healthy lifestyle also can reduce your risk for developing diabetes.

SELF-CARE STEPS FOR DIABETES

Nutrition

A good diet is important for everyone, especially people who have diabetes. Research now shows that sugar, a simple carbohydrate, has the same effect on blood glucose as any other carbohydrate, regardless of the source. (Carbohydrates are the main nutrients in food that affect blood glucose levels.) Watching the total carbohydrates you eat allows you to eat foods with sugar and still keep your blood glucose in control.

Meal planning, such as how much food you need and how to plan meals and snacks accordingly, is key to a blood glucose level that is as normal as possible. A meal plan tells you what to eat and when. It should be suited to your lifestyle and nutritional needs.

Carbohydrate counting is a meal planning method based on total carbohydrates. It allows you to choose from a wide variety of foods for your meals and snacks. Carbohydrate "choices" are servings of food that supply 15 grams of carbohydrate. The carbohydrate may be from a grain, fruit, milk, or small dessert serving. For instance, a small cookie with 15 grams of carbohydrate will have the same effect on your blood glucose as a slice of bread containing the same amount of carbohydrate.

If you are overweight, it is important to reach a reasonable body weight. Often if you lose only 10 or 20 pounds, your blood glucose levels return to normal. For children, it is important to consume enough calories to provide for normal growth and development.

Blood Glucose Monitoring

Whether you have Type I, Type II, or gestational diabetes, checking blood glucose levels and keeping them as close to normal as possible is important. Closely controlling your blood glucose will help you feel better and reduce the risk of problems associated with diabetes.

Glucose levels are monitored by pricking a finger and testing a drop of blood using chemically treated plastic strips that reflect the glucose level in the blood. Color charts or small calculator-sized machines are used to analyze the blood glucose test strips. Your health care provider can teach you how to correctly monitor your blood glucose.

Many people with diabetes monitor their blood glucose up to six times daily, especially those taking insulin to help control Type I or Type II diabetes. Others who have Type II diabetes and are not taking insulin may only need to monitor their blood glucose 2 or 3 days a week if the level remains within or close to normal range.

Exercise

People with diabetes enjoy the same benefits from exercise as everyone else: improved heart and lung efficiency, reduced body fat, increased muscle tone, and improved fitness. But those with diabetes get more benefits: exercise combined with fewer calories will often control Type II diabetes without the need for medication.

Exercise can lower blood glucose levels, making body cells more sensitive to insulin and improving their ability to use and store glucose. Your health care provider can help you determine the benefits of exercise and the type of exercise program that is best for you.

Warning Signs

Call your health care provider if you have any of these symptoms:

- Extreme thirst
- Unusual tiredness
- Excessive appetite
- Frequent urination
- Tingling or numbness in legs or feet
- Cuts or bruises that are slow to heal
- Blurred vision or any change in vision

HEART DISEASE

The most common form of heart disease is known as **atherosclerosis**, or hardening of the arteries. Cholesterol joins with calcium and scar tissue and builds up in the arteries. When cholesterol levels are too high, the circulatory system becomes choked—and the result is a dam of plaque that narrows the channels the blood flows through.

You suffer a **heart attack** when blood can't flow to the heart. This could be caused by narrowing of your arteries or other heart-related problems such as a heart spasm. A **stroke**, on the other hand, occurs when blood can't reach the brain. You may get a warning sign of a heart attack in the form of chest pain that moves to the left arm, jaw, or shoulder blade. This is known as **angina**. Don't ignore it. American Heart Association research shows that hardening of the arteries is responsible for more than 90 percent of all heart attacks.

Another form of heart disease is **congestive heart failure**. The heart is weakened by high blood pressure, previous heart attack, atherosclerosis, rheumatic fever, a congenital heart defect, or a muscle disease known as cardiomyopathy. Just as a weak hand can't squeeze all the water out of a dishcloth, a weak heart can't pump effectively, allowing fluid to collect in the body and lungs. To make matters worse, this fluid contains salt—boosting blood pressure even more.

Risk Factors You Can Control

High Cholesterol

The body tries to flush the excess cholesterol away by "packaging" the cholesterol with a substance known as high-density lipoprotein, or HDL. Low-density lipoprotein, or LDL, on the other hand, carries this cholesterol straight to the artery walls. HDL and LDL are carriers of blood cholesterol.

CLOGGED ARTERIES

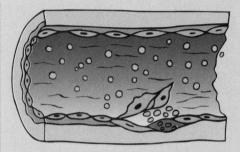

Atherosclerosis begins with a damaged spot in the artery. Cholesterol and other fats from the bloodstream build plaque on artery walls.

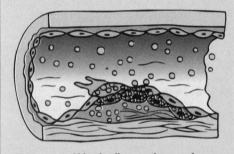

Two types of blood cells contribute to the buildup of plaque: macrophages (large white cells) and platelets (small blood cells that coagulate blood). The macrophages fill up with cholesterol and cholesterol packs in between.

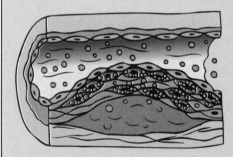

Plaque narrows the arteries. Sometimes a clot can form in an artery narrowed by plaque, causing angina or a heart attack. Blockage in an artery leading to the brain causes a stroke.

Total blood cholesterol is probably the number with which you are most familiar. Guidelines suggest a total cholesterol level of less than 200 is best.

Even if your cholesterol isn't this high, you still need to pay attention to your lifestyle habits. That's why the National Cholesterol Education Program and the National Heart, Lung, and Blood Institute recommend that all adults over the age of 20 have their cholesterol levels measured at least once every 5 years.

Despite many claims to the contrary, there is no single food you can add or subtract from your diet to lower your blood cholesterol level.

Sometimes higher cholesterol levels are hereditary and can't be lowered by diet alone. If your levels do not drop when you change your diet, your doctor may prescribe cholesterol-lowering drugs. Ignore quick fixes and focus instead on eating balanced meals and healthy snacks as in the guidelines discussed under High Blood Cholesterol, p. 219.

High Blood Pressure

The second leading risk factor for heart attacks and the major cause of stroke is high blood pressure, or hypertension. See Hypertension = High Blood Pressure, p. 225.

Below 140 systolic over 90 diastolic is considered normal—120 over 80 is considered an ideal reading. (See the classification table, p. 252, for more information.) Stress, caffeine, exercise, infection, and other factors may temporarily affect blood pressure readings.

Smoking and Secondhand Smoke

Smoking increases your risk of heart attack by lowering your HDL level and raising your blood pressure. According to Dr. W. Virgil Brown, a former president of the American Heart Association and director of the Division of Arteriosclerosis and Lipid Metabolism at Emory University School of Medicine, the HDL cholesterol level of a two-pack-a-day smoker may increase by eight points when that person stops smoking.

In addition, smoke has a glycoprotein that makes your blood clot more easily and weakens the blood vessel walls. The amount of oxygen is reduced, and much of what does make it into the cardiovascular system is replaced with inhaled carbon dioxide. This damages the heart muscle and makes the blood vessel walls even more susceptible to atherosclerosis.

Lack of Exercise

American Heart Association research shows that regular aerobic exercise actually strengthens the heart muscle, boosts HDL levels, lowers blood pressure, slows the progression of diabetes, and helps ward off obesity. About 30 to 40 minutes of moderate exercise, 4 or more days a week, is recommended. It is not necessary to do all of your exercise at once. However, you should increase your heart rate and keep it up for at least 20 minutes.

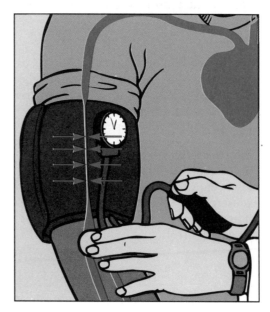

HOW BLOOD PRESSURE IS TAKEN

The blood pressure cuff is inflated tight enough to stop the flow of blood. As the cuff is gradually deflated, the first in a series of sounds that is heard through the stethoscope is recorded as the systolic blood pressure and the last sound heard is recorded as the diastolic pressure.

Obesity

Research shows that obesity should be considered a major risk factor for heart disease, rather than one that just contributes to other risk factors—such as diabetes and hypertension.

Diabetes

People with diabetes are very susceptible to heart disease. People with poorly controlled diabetes often have several health problems, including high cholesterol and other circulatory disorders that lead to atherosclerosis, hemorrhages of the tiny blood vessels in the eyes, and poor circulation to the feet and hands. Smoking makes these problems worse.

Uncontrollable Risk Factors

Age

Heart disease is more common among older people because it reflects the wear-and-tear on the body; however, it doesn't have to be part of aging. For example, atherosclerosis may take 20 to 30 years to get to the point where the arteries are blocked enough to cause trouble—and may be halted in its course if diagnosed in time for the person to make the needed changes.

Gender

Middle-aged men have more heart attacks than women of the same age. This changes after menopause. After the age of 60 the rates are almost equal.

Heredity

Unfortunately, high blood pressure and cholesterol levels run in families. However, don't use your genes as an excuse not to take the necessary steps to offset this risk. Control those risk factors you can control.

Getting More Help

Your family and friends can provide great support and encouragement as you tackle each of your risk factors. Bring one of these people to your next doctor's appointment to help you take notes and ask questions—and to offer emotional support if needed.

Your doctor may refer you to specialists along the way, and surgery may be your only recourse. The two most common surgeries are *angioplasty* and *bypass surgery*. Both are proven techniques. The success rate is 96 percent for the surgeries doctors use to reopen a clogged blood vessel (balloon angioplasty and laser angioplasty). In addition, a new procedure known as *atherectomy* shaves away plaque in a clogged artery. This may be able to cut the reblockage rate in half. In a nonemergency bypass, the risk of a fatal complication is usually less than 1 in 50.

You may need the expertise and help of a nurse or health educator, especially if you have surgery. He or she can give you written materials or information about classes, answer your day-to-day questions, and put you in touch with organizations and support groups that will help you even more.

HIGH BLOOD CHOLESTEROL

High blood cholesterol is one of the biggest risk factors for heart attack, which is the leading cause of death in America. Cholesterol is a waxy substance your body produces to help it function properly. A diet containing too much fat, cholesterol, and calories contributes to high blood cholesterol. Neither fat nor cholesterol dissolves in the bloodstream. Instead, both are carried through the body in packages called *lipoproteins*.

Cholesterol found in low-density lipoproteins (LDL cholesterol) is considered most responsible for plaque formation that clogs the arteries, leading to stroke and heart attack. High-density lipoproteins (HDLs)—known as "good cholesterol"—are thought to be responsible for removing extra cholesterol from the blood and thereby cutting down the risk for coronary heart disease.

Classifying Your Cholesterol

Total blood cholesterol measurements below 200 mg/dl are classified as "desirable," those 200 to 239 mg/dl as "borderline high," and those 240 mg/dl and above as "high." Because cholesterol levels can fluctuate from day to day, an average of two or more measurements should be used for classification. The benefit of "knowing your number" comes from your ability to take action and control your cholesterol—and that means making a long-term commitment to change.

Reducing Your Risk

Your chance of developing heart disease depends on more than just the amount of cholesterol in your blood. To get a better idea of what your cholesterol number means and what action you should take, start by identifying and adding up your other **risk factors for heart disease**. Such factors include:

- Male (45 years and older)
- Female (55 years and older or early menopause without hormone replacement therapy)
- Family history of early heart disease (before the age of 55)
- Cigarette smoking
- High blood pressure (140/90 mmHg or higher)
- Low levels of HDL-cholesterol (less than 35 mg/dl)
- Diabetes or impaired glucose tolerance

Just as these factors combine to increase your risk of heart disease, healthy habits—such as eating a low-fat diet, regular exercise, and not smoking—can reduce your risk. Many people can lower their blood cholesterol simply by increasing their level of physical activity, and changing the way they eat—avoiding foods high in fat, especially saturated fat and cholesterol. The higher your cholesterol level is, the greater the benefits will be if you lower it.

Along with changes in diet, there are drugs that can lower cholesterol in the bloodstream. These drugs, however, can be costly and cause undesirable side effects for some people. For this reason, changes in diet are usually the first step in treatment, unless cholesterol levels are very high.

Dietary Changes

A chart on diet recommendations to reduce blood cholesterol begins on p. 222.

Maintain a Healthy Weight

Taking in more calories than the body needs for energy contributes to a higher cholesterol level for many people. Remember that your calorie needs are based on how many calories your body burns up. People burn calories at different rates depending on many factors—activity, body size, genetics, age, health, and gender. Losing weight and increasing physical activity are important steps toward reducing blood cholesterol and other risks for heart disease.

YOUR CALORIE NEEDS	
Typical Calorie Needs for Maintaining Weight	
	Calories/Day
Women.	1,800–2,100
Men.	2,100–2,400
Recommended Calorie Ranges for Losing Weight	
	Calories/Day
Women	1,200–1,500
Men	1,500–1,800

Eat Less Fat

Fat is the most concentrated calorie source. By reducing fat, you can also reduce your calorie intake. If you're currently at a healthy weight, you'll need to replace these calories to maintain your weight. There are two major types of fat: saturated and unsaturated. All fat sources contain a mixture of these types of fat, although certain sources contain more of one kind or the other. Cutting down on total fat will help you reduce the amount of saturated fat in your diet.

Keeping your calories from fat under 30 percent of your total daily calories doesn't require any complicated calculations. Use the chart above to calculate your fat limits.

YOUR FAT LIMITS	
If your planned daily calorie intake is:	Your daily fat intake should be less than:
1,200 calories	40 grams
1,500 calories	50 grams
1,800 calories	60 grams
2,400 calories	80 grams

Eat Less Saturated Fat

Since animal products are a major source of saturated fat—and the only source of dietary cholesterol—as you limit high-fat meat and dairy choices, you'll also cut down on saturated fat and dietary cholesterol. A few vegetable fats, such as palm and coconut oil, are also high in saturated fat. These fat sources are mainly found in commercially prepared foods. Less than one-third of the total fat you eat should come from saturated fat. Use labeling information to help you limit your saturated fat intake.

Eat Fewer High-Cholesterol Foods

Cholesterol in food can also raise your blood cholesterol level, but its effect is not as significant as that of saturated fat. This waxy, fatlike substance is essential for several important body functions, including hormone production and fat digestion. Your body makes cholesterol in the liver to meet your needs in response to a number of factors.

It's important to understand the difference between cholesterol found in blood and cholesterol found in food. The cholesterol you eat does not automatically add to the cholesterol in your blood. Cholesterol is not the same as fat and does not supply any calories. Cholesterol-free foods, therefore, can be full of fat and calories. Usually when you limit high-fat and high-saturated fat choices, you automatically limit high-cholesterol foods. Liver and egg yolks are notable exceptions because, although they are not extremely high in fat, they are high in dietary cholesterol and should therefore be limited. Shrimp is somewhat higher in dietary cholesterol than some other choices, but because it's very low in fat, it is an acceptable choice for occasional use.

Eat More Carbohydrate-Rich, High-Fiber Foods

Reducing calories from fat means you'll need to increase your carbohydrate-rich choices: legumes, breads, grains, pasta, rice, fruits, and vegetables. Carbohydrate sources include simple sugars and complex carbohydrates (starches and fibers). Most foods contain a combination of these carbohydrate sources. Eating more complex carbohydrates ensures a better balance of vitamins, minerals, and fiber.

Dietary fiber is found in all plant foods and is usually divided into two types: soluble and insoluble. These two types of fiber provide different benefits. By adding a variety of fiber-rich foods, you'll be sure to meet your needs for both types.

Soluble fiber is found in certain fruits and vegetables; dried peas, beans, and other legumes; oats; and barley. Studies show that by eating more soluble fiber, you may lower your blood cholesterol level and reduce your risk of heart disease.

Insoluble fiber is found mainly in wheat bran and other whole grains, such as wheat, corn, and rye. This type of fiber is also found in many fruits and vegetables. Insoluble fiber may help reduce the risk of certain cancers and digestive diseases by shortening the amount of time it takes food to pass through the intestine. Insoluble fiber also helps relieve constipation.

Foods to choose and those to limit are based on typical items in each category. Adjust the size and number of your servings to meet your calorie needs in order to reach or maintain a desirable weight.

Making Realistic Changes

Once you recognize the health threat posed by high blood cholesterol levels, it may seem like an emergency. However, the heart disease caused by high blood cholesterol is a chronic condition that develops over many years. And, just as it takes time to build up plaque in the arteries, it takes time to start healthy eating and exercise plans. The diet recommended for cholesterol reduction should usually be introduced gradually over 4 to 6 months. The changes in eating and exercise habits you make are likely to result in cholesterol changes that are also gradual and progressive. If the response is not enough to meet your treatment goals, further reductions in fat, saturated fat, and cholesterol can help you progress. However, keep in mind that fat is necessary in small amounts for good health. Fat is needed to carry fat-soluble vitamins and to provide essential fatty acids. These functions require as little as 8 to 10 grams of fat per day.

DIET RECOMMENDATIONS TO REDUCE BLOOD CHOLESTEROL

The following chart summarizes the current National Cholesterol Education Program Step I and Step II diet recommendations. The Step I diet emphasizes reducing total fat intake, especially major saturated fat and excess calories. The Step II diet calls for even less saturated fat and cholesterol, depending on the response to the initial changes. The following pages will translate these recommendations into changes in lifestyle and eating patterns.

Nutrient	Recommended Intake	
	Step I Diet	Step II Diet
Total fat	Less than 30% of total calories	Less than 30% of total calories
Saturated fat	Less than 10% of total calories	Less than 7% of total calories
Polyunsaturated fat	Up to 10% of total calories	Up to 10% of total calories
Monounsaturated fat	10–15% of total calories	10–15% of total calories
Carbohydrates	50–60% of total calories	50–60% of total calories
Protein	10–20% of total calories	10–20% of total calories
Cholesterol	Less than 300mg/day	Less than 200mg/day
Total calories	To achieve and maintain healthy weight	To achieve and maintain healthy weight

FOOD CHOICES GUIDE

Meats

Limit intake of lean meat, chicken, turkey, and fish to 6 ounces or less each day (cooked weight).
3 ounces cooked meat = 4 ounces raw meat.
Hint: A 3-ounce portion of cooked meat is the size of a deck of cards.

Choose Lean Meats (with no more than 3 grams of fat per ounce) such as:

• Chicken, turkey, fish and shellfish (without skin or added oil)

• Lean, trimmed cuts of beef, pork, and lamb such as: beef or veal tenderloin, sirloin tip, round steak, rump roast, flank steak; pork-loin chops, tenderloin, center-cut ham, Canadian bacon; Lamb-loin or leg roasts, chops

Limit High-Fat, High-Cholesterol Meats

• High-fat, processed meats such as: bacon, bologna, salami, sausage, hot dogs

• High-fat cuts of beef, pork, and lamb such as: prime-grade steaks, roasts, ribs, veal cutlets

• High-cholesterol meats such as: liver, sweetbreads, brains, kidneys

Eggs

Limit egg yolks (including those used in baked goods and cooking) to no more than three per week.
One egg yolk has 5 grams of fat.

Dairy

Use at least two servings of nonfat or low-fat dairy products per day.

A serving size equals:

• One 8-ounce glass of milk

• 1 ounce of cheese

• $1^1/2$ cups cottage cheese or dairy dessert

Choose Nonfat (Skim) or Low-Fat Dairy Products

• Skim or 1% milk and milk products such as: skim or 1% evaporated milk or yogurt

• Nonfat or low-fat dairy desserts such as: sherbet, sorbet, frozen yogurt, in moderation

• Nonfat or low-fat cheese (any cheese with no more than 5 grams of fat per ounce) such as: low-fat cream cheese, low- or nonfat cottage or cream cheese, part skim mozzarella, farmer cheese, or string cheese

Limit High-Fat Dairy Products

• Regular and 2% milk and milk products such as: regular evaporated milk or yogurt

• Whole milk; processed and natural cheeses such as: Cheddar, Swiss, brick, Brie, Monterey Jack, Colby, American, cream cheese

• Rich dairy desserts such as, or containing: ice cream, whipped toppings, sour cream, half-and-half

Continued on next page

FOOD CHOICES GUIDE (CONTINUED)

Fats and Oils

Limit all added fats, especially sources of saturated fat, to no more than three to eight servings per day. One serving contains 4 to 5 grams of fat. Added fat also includes fat used in cooking or baking, and fat contained in convenience foods. Limit fat carefully to avoid extra calories.

One serving of fat equals:

- 1 teaspoon butter, margarine, or oil
- 2 teaspoons salad dressing or 2 tablespoons light salad dressing
- 1/8 medium avocado

- 1 tablespoon nuts and seeds
- 5 large olives (black or green)
- 2 teaspoons peanut butter

Choose Unsaturated Fats (in limited quantities—as above)

- Unsaturated oils such as: olive, canola, corn, safflower, sesame, soybean, sunflower
- Peanut butter, nuts, seeds, olives, avocados

Limit Saturated Fats

- Saturated fats and oils such as: butter, lard, bacon fat, coconut oil, palm oil, and cocoa butter
- Hydrogenated oil found in shortening, some margarines, and salad dressings
- Coconut

Fruits and Vegetables

Eat two to four servings of fruit and three to five servings of vegetables per day.

One serving equals:

- 1/2 cup cooked or 1 cup of raw vegetables
- 1/2 cup or 1 small piece of fresh fruit

Starches, Grains, and Legumes

Eat six to eleven servings per day, especially whole-grain products. The type of fiber found in oat, rice, and barley bran, along with beans, peas, and some fruits and vegetables has been shown to lower blood cholesterol.

Choose Low-Fat Starches (containing no more than 2 grams of fat per serving)

- Angel food cake, low-fat cookies and crackers, bagels, english muffins, yeast breads
- Cereals, rice, pasta, corn, potatoes, peas, beans, lentils, pretzels, bread sticks

Limit High-Fat Baked Goods and Snacks

- Pies, cakes, doughnuts, pastries, croissants, muffins, quick breads, high-fat cookies and crackers
- Granola, potato chips, tortilla chips, french fries

HYPERTENSION = HIGH BLOOD PRESSURE

Hypertension is the most prevalent chronic adult illness in America today. Treating high blood pressure is a lifelong process requiring a team approach. As part of the team, *you can prevent future problems* by understanding your condition, making lifestyle changes now, taking drugs if needed, and having your blood pressure checked as recommended.

Hypertension does not mean you are overly tense, although anxiety can raise blood pressure. As blood pressure increases, so does the strain on your heart to push blood through your circulatory system. High blood pressure usually has no immediate symptoms, therefore your blood pressure needs to be measured at least every 2 years.

What Is Blood Pressure?

Each time the heart beats, blood is pumped to all parts of the body. For blood to circulate, it needs a certain amount of force or pressure. Blood pressure is the force the flow of blood exerts on your arteries.

Two numbers are used to measure your blood pressure:

132 (systolic)/ 84 (diastolic)

The higher number, the **systolic pressure**, refers to the pressure inside the artery when the heart squeezes to pump blood through the body. The lower number, the **diastolic pressure**, refers to the pressure inside the artery when the heart is relaxed and filling with blood. The numbers are recorded as "mmHg" (millimeters of mercury)—meaning how high the column of mercury is raised by the pressure of your blood.

You are considered to have high blood pressure when your readings are consistently 140 mmHg or greater systolic and/or 90 mmHg or greater diastolic.

The term **borderline** is sometimes used to describe hypertension in which the blood pressure only occasionally rises above 140/90 mmHg.

High blood pressure is referred to as the "silent killer." Since most people with high blood pressure don't have noticeable symptoms, and since it's not clear who will get it or when, it is important to have your blood pressure checked regularly. (See the classification table on p. 252 to determine your blood pressure classification.) To confirm the diagnosis of hypertension, readings from two or more visits are needed.

High Blood Pressure and Overall Health

The strength of your heart, the condition of your blood vessels and how well your kidneys work all affect your blood pressure. If your heart is more efficient because you exercise regularly, it will push more blood with each stroke—and it will not need to beat as often to sustain normal blood pressure.

The hardening and narrowing of arteries that can result from a high-fat diet or aging can make it harder for blood to flow and cause blood pressure to rise. And if the arteries begin to clog, your heart has to work even harder. Your kidneys maintain the volume of water and salt in your body. If they retain too much, blood pressure will also increase. In effect, the river banks overflow.

Long-term uncontrolled hypertension can damage your body by increasing the workload on your heart and arteries. Controlling high blood pressure will reduce your risk of stroke, coronary artery disease, enlarged heart, aneurysm, heart attack, eye problems, and kidney disease. Risk relates to not only how high, but how long the blood pressure has been raised.

Having other risk factors for heart and blood vessel (cardiovascular) disease adds to your overall risk. The three major risk factors for **cardiovascular disease** that you can control are high blood pressure, high blood cholesterol, and smoking. Any one of these increases your risk by about 30 percent. If you have two of these risk factors, your risk for cardiovascular disease is three times as great. If you have all three risk factors, you have seven times the risk.

Other major risk factors for cardiovascular disease include age, gender, diabetes, family history, and your individual health history.

Standardized Measurement
The Importance of Standardized Measurement

Measuring blood pressure is not as quick and easy as it may seem. In addition to the normal minute-by-minute fluctuations in blood pressure, several biological factors, such as anxiety, eating, and pain, can also influence a blood pressure reading. If the people taking the readings don't use the same technique to measure blood pressure, the results may vary as well. Since blood pressure readings are an important test for diagnosing and treating high blood pressure, a standardized measurement technique is recommended to reduce as many of these variables as possible.

You should expect your doctor to follow the American Heart Association standards when measuring your blood pressure:

- Measure your arm for proper blood pressure cuff size
- Support your arm at the level of your heart
- Get an estimate of your systolic blood pressure by feeling the pulse at your wrist and inflating the cuff
- Inflate the cuff quickly and deflate it slowly
- Tell you your blood pressure numbers

To guard against incorrectly diagnosing high blood pressure on one elevated reading, readings from two or more separate visits should be used. In a study of Park Nicollet patients being screened for high blood pressure, 275 patients with

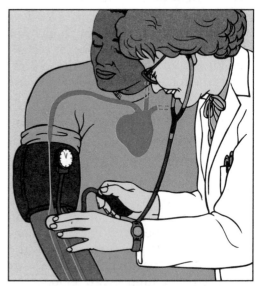

HOW BLOOD PRESSURE IS TAKEN

The blood pressure cuff is inflated tight enough to stop the flow of blood. As the cuff is gradually deflated, the first in a series of sounds that is heard through the stethoscope is recorded as the systolic blood pressure and the last sound heard is recorded as the diastolic pressure.

high blood pressure on one reading were referred for three more blood pressure screening visits. Normal blood pressure was recorded for 215 (78 percent) of these patients after these visits.

Your Contribution to Accuracy

Worry, poor eating habits, tobacco, air temperature changes, exertion, and pain can create results that are not your usual blood pressure. **To maximize the accuracy of your blood pressure measurement:**

- Do not eat, smoke, drink caffeine, or exercise for at least 30 minutes before you have your blood pressure measured.

- Wear short sleeves or loose sleeves that can be easily pushed up when you have your blood pressure taken. For consistency, use the same arm for each reading.

- Sit quietly with your legs uncrossed for a period before having your blood pressure measured.

- Bring along your blood pressure records and a list of any drugs you are currently taking.

- If using home blood pressure equipment, follow the standard measurement technique and bring equipment in yearly for comparison.

High Blood Pressure Exam

If your blood pressure has been classified as higher than normal, an exam by your doctor is needed. He or she will check for any known causes for the elevated blood pressure and find out if there is any damage to your heart, kidneys, brain, or eyes. This involves a detailed history, physical exam, and specific laboratory tests. Your doctor will also check for cardiovascular risk factors, such as smoking, diabetes, or high blood cholesterol. About 90 to 95 percent of patients have "primary" or "essential" hypertension, in which the cause is unknown. Only about 5 to 10 percent of patients have "secondary" hypertension (high blood pressure from a known cause such as organ problems or diseases).

During your exam, your physician will ask you questions about your health and medication history and your family's health history. A physical exam and some lab tests will be done to look for possible causes of high blood pressure and to determine your risk of heart disease. Other lab tests will provide a baseline for comparison after treatment.

Treatment

Treatment decisions are based on your blood pressure stage, presence or absence of organ damage, and presence of other risk factors. Your doctor may give you drugs right away or may try a period of lifestyle changes (such as regular exercise or a change in your diet) for 3 to 6 months. Depending on your treatment plan and drugs prescribed, your doctor will tell you how often to have your blood pressure checked.

Lifestyle Changes

Lifestyle and hereditary factors affect your risk of developing high blood pressure and cardiovascular disease. Changing health habits may reduce health risks and help control blood pressure. Lifestyle changes to prevent and manage high blood pressure include weight control, limiting salt, limiting alcohol, and regular exercise. See High Blood Pressure, p. 251, for detailed recommendations on lifestyle changes for prevention and control of high blood pressure.

Medicine

Drugs have proven very effective in controlling high blood pressure. Your doctor can help you determine if you will need drugs, in addition to lifestyle changes. The goal of drug treatment is to achieve and maintain regular blood pressure readings of less than 140/90 mmHg with few or no side effects. Your doctor will advise you if your treatment goals are different. Because it is still unclear why one type of drug works for a particular person while another is less effective or creates side effects, your medicine may need to be changed several times before the most effective one is found.

Continuing Care

The goal of treatment is to lower and control your blood pressure to reduce your risk of stroke, heart attack, and kidney disease. The risk is related to how high and how long your blood pressure has been raised. Therefore, the sooner your blood pressure is controlled, the less you risk future problems.

After your blood pressure is controlled, you should continue to have your blood pressure checked regularly by a health care professional or by home monitoring. You should be seen at least once a year by your doctor to see if your blood pressure is under control.

LOW BACK PAIN

Pain in the lower back is very common. It can be caused by inflammation of structures in the back—such as the joints, muscles, or discs. Most often it is made worse by certain activities. It can also be affected by physical or psychological stresses.

Uncommonly, back pain can be caused by serious problems like infection or other conditions that your doctor can distinguish from the more common types of back pain described here.

Fortunately, over 90 percent of people with low back pain completely recover within 4 to 6 weeks. When pain or weakness last longer than 6 weeks, however, more specialized treatments may be needed. For this reason, it is important to keep your doctor informed of your progress.

Acute Low Back Pain

Acute low back pain is also called lumbar muscle strain or backache. It is described as low back pain that you've had for 6 weeks or less that does not go past the knees. Although quite painful, it usually improves after a few days of simple treatment.

Acute Sciatica

Acute sciatica—also known as "disc pain" or "radiating leg pain"—usually resolves more slowly over time than acute low back pain. Acute sciatica is described as low back pain that you've had for 6 weeks or less where the pain extends below the knee. Sciatica pain is often caused by nerve irritation from discs in the lower back.

Chronic Back Pain and Sciatica

If your back pain and sciatica persist longer than 6 weeks, your condition is considered chronic and other evaluation will be needed. You may be asked to return to the doctor after 6 weeks for X-rays or other tests. Some type of back education class or instruction should be considered if you have chronic back pain and sciatica to help you learn to handle your back problems.

If there has been no significant improvement, you may need to consult with experts in the problems that can cause chronic back pain. Most often, these are doctors who work in departments of rehabilitation medicine, orthopedics, and neurosurgery. In certain cases, other medical specialists in neurology, occupational medicine, and rheumatology, among others, may be consulted.

Although each patient is a special case, the procedures described follow a typical pattern of care for back pain. Your doctor may follow procedures similar to these or make other arrangements for your treatment. Either way, it is important to understand how back problems get better and what to expect if they don't.

Warning Symptoms

Tell your doctor right away if you have any of these symptoms or conditions:

- Unexplained weight loss
- Constant night pain
- Fever
- Trouble urinating
- Leg weakness

Tests

X-rays are usually considered unnecessary in the early stages of treatment because they do not show inflamed muscles and discs. X-rays are rarely needed except for severe trauma (like a fall or motor vehicle accident), in older patients, or in patients who have other medical problems.

If you have back pain that is not improving after 6 weeks (chronic low back pain), back X-rays will probably be ordered if they have not already been done. If you have sciatica pain longer than 6 weeks (chronic sciatica) and surgery is being considered, then CT scans or other procedures may be done.

EXERCISES TO KEEP YOUR BACK FIT

It is important to keep your back flexible and strong. Back exercises can help prevent back problems and improve posture. Aerobic exercise also is very effective for patients with lower back pain. You should plan regular, daily walks as soon as you can, along with other exercise as tolerated. Swimming or biking are also good activities for the lower back.

The back exercises shown below should be started at home or with the help of a physical therapist, and should be started as soon as the pain improves. Do not do any exercises that make the pain or stiffness much worse.

Knee Raise

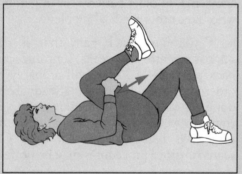

Lie flat on your back, knees bent, feet flat on floor. Do a pelvic tilt (see above) and raise your knee slowly to your chest one at a time as shown. Hug knee gently, let go, then lower your bent leg slowly. Do not straighten your knees.

The Pelvic Tilt

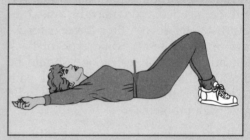

Lie flat on your back (or stand with your back to a wall), knees bent, feet flat on floor, body relaxed. Tighten abdominal muscles and tilt pelvis so that the curve of the small of the back is flat on the floor (or wall). Tighten the buttocks muscles. Hold 10 seconds and then relax.

Partial Press-up

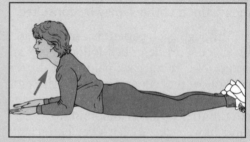

First, lie face down on a soft, firm surface. Rest for a few minutes, relaxing completely. Second, staying in the same basic position, raise your upper body enough to lean on your elbows. Let your lower back and your legs relax as much as you can. Hold this position for 30 seconds at first. Slowly work up to 2 minutes.

SELF-CARE STEPS FOR LOW BACK PAIN

• Medical studies show that prolonged bed rest is not necessary for most back problems. In fact, staying in bed for more than 2 days may increase the pain and stiffness. Moderate activity is more helpful, avoiding anything that makes the pain much worse.

• Ice or cold packs can reduce the pain and swelling of a muscle strain or spasm. Use them for 20 minutes three or four times a day during the first few days. After that, a hot bath or heating pad may be used to reduce pain and stiffness, but ice may still be helpful.

• Anti-inflammatory medicines like ibuprofen (Motrin or a generic) or aspirin can help ease the pain and swelling in the lower back. If they cause stomach upset, then acetaminophen (Tylenol or a generic) can be used instead. Muscle relaxers can also be used during the first few days to ease muscle spasms, but they often cause drowsiness. Narcotic painkillers are rarely prescribed because they may become addictive.

• Good posture keeps the body's weight aligned and reduces stress on the back muscles. Often, the most comfortable positions for sleeping are lying on the back with a pillow under the knees or lying on the side with a pillow between the lower legs. Being overweight increases stress on the lower back, and weight loss is important to prevent future problems.

• Returning to work or usual daily activity in a few days or less is an important part of the recovery process, either with lighter duties or limited hours. Some discomfort will occur, but this prevents the back from becoming weak and stiff.

• To manage lower back problems, back pain experts suggest avoiding lifting heavy objects, and repeated bending and twisting. It is also important to change positions frequently and use a chair with good lower back support.

• Financial worries, family problems, or work pressures can affect back pain. Learning to accept and deal with everyday stress can help your recovery from back pain. If you have concerns about these areas, please discuss them with your doctor.

• Physical therapists work to restore normal mobility, strength, and function through special exercise, manual therapy technique, pain relief techniques (like ultrasound, heat, cold), and patient education. Your doctor will consider physical therapy if you have: severe incapacitating pain for more than 1 week, no improvement after 2 weeks of home therapy, or you are unable to return to work (limited activity) within 1 week.

• Fortunately, surgery is rarely needed for either back pain or sciatica. Many studies show that nonsurgical treatments and exercise are often as effective at relieving pain and preventing relapse. Surgery is usually only considered after months of nonsurgical treatment have failed to ease the pain or improve the function of the back. In these cases, an orthopedic surgeon or neurosurgeon can help decide. Only 5 to 10 percent of patients with sciatica ever need surgery.

OBESITY

Despite many claims, there is no "perfect or ideal" weight. Good health comes in a variety of sizes and shapes. A combination of many factors adds up to a healthy weight, including how much weight is fat, where the fat is stored, and any medical problems that would benefit from more or less weight. Obesity or having extra body fat increases the risk of developing non-insulin-dependent diabetes, high blood pressure, high blood cholesterol and triglycerides, and some cancers, as well as other health problems. Consider the following questions and chart to help determine your healthy weight range.

- Are you within the suggested weight range? The higher weights in the ranges generally apply to men, who tend to have more muscle and bone. The lower weights more often apply to women.

- Where is your fat stored? Extra fat stored below the waist seems especially difficult to shed. However, on the plus side, it's also less likely to pose a health risk. Studies show that fat stored above the waist, in the upper abdominal area, is linked with an increased risk of diabetes and heart disease. One easy way to identify the level of health risk your weight is causing is to find your waist/hip ratio. This ratio is a quick, easy way to determine your risk. Here's the formula: Waist measurement divided by hip measurement equals risk ratio. A ratio of more than 1.0 for men and more than 0.8 for women may mean a higher health risk.

Higher weights generally apply to men and lower weights to women in each height category.

* Without shoes   † Without clothes
Source: National Research Council, 1989.

Example:

Waist (38 inches) / Hip (42 inches) = Risk ratio (0.9)

- Do you have a weight-related medical problem or a family history of one? If you—or a relative—have had elevated blood pressure, cholesterol, or blood sugar levels, a weight in the lower end of the range could be best for your health.

SUGGESTED WEIGHTS FOR ADULTS

Height*	Weight in Pounds†	
	19–34 yrs	35+ yrs
5' 0"	97–128	108–138
5' 1"	101–132	111–143
5' 2"	104–137	115–148
5' 3"	107–141	119–152
5' 4"	111–146	122–157
5' 5"	114–150	126–162
5' 6"	118–155	130–167
5' 7"	121–160	134–172
5' 8"	125–164	138–178
5' 9"	129–169	142–183
5' 10"	132–174	146–188
5' 11"	136–179	151–194
6' 0"	140–184	155–199
6' 1"	144–189	159–205
6' 2"	148–195	164–210
6' 3"	152–200	168–216
6' 4"	156–205	173–222
6' 5"	160–211	177–228
6' 6"	164–216	183–234

Causes of Obesity

There are many complex risk factors for obesity, including environment, genetics, physical inactivity, and eating too many calories and fats. Just as there are no simple explanations for how weight problems start, there are no simple solutions. Weight loss requires a combination of fewer calories taken in, more calories used up, and behavior changes.

Dangers of Fad Diets

If there were a simple solution to take off extra pounds, no one would have a weight problem. And although most people recognize that fad diets aren't the answer, the short-term reward of rapid weight loss is hard to resist. These quick weight-loss plans cost consumers up to $5 billion annually.

Most people, however, don't know how risky these diets may be. Very low-calorie diets or diets that restrict certain foods can be dangerous and should never be used without medical supervision.

There is growing concern that long-term use of very low-calorie diets may actually make lasting success more difficult to maintain. When the body is threatened by a drastic reduction in calories, it responds by conserving energy output—slowing down the rate at which calories are burned. Increasing calories back to a normal level results in a rapid weight gain. A repeated pattern of quick loss followed by rapid gain (often called "yo-yo dieting") may even sabotage future weight loss attempts by actually altering body composition. The loss usually reflects a loss of "metabolically active" muscle tissue which is then replaced by "metabolically inactive" fat when normal eating is resumed.

Changes in body composition after cycles of losses/gains can be dramatic enough that, even when a stable weight is achieved, the body is "fatter" and has a lower metabolic rate. Instead of enduring a "diet" you can hardly wait to go off, focus on developing better eating and exercise habits.

Your Calorie Needs

Remember that eating and exercise aren't the only factors that affect your weight, but they are the ones you can control. Studies have shown that people who are overweight don't necessarily eat any more than their thin counterparts. Often they are more efficient energy users and, thus, are more likely to build up fat. Metabolism and body composition help determine the number of calories your body burns at rest, and these tendencies are often inherited.

The number of calories you need depends on how many calories your body burns up. People burn calories at different rates, depending on many factors, including activity, body size, genetics, age, health, and gender. Calories also describe how much energy a food supplies. People need over 50 nutrients from foods, including those that supply calories—such as carbohydrates, proteins, and fat—and those that help with other body functions, such as vitamins, minerals, and water. Quality calorie choices meet nutrient needs without adding extra, unneeded, calories.

YOUR CALORIE NEEDS

Typical Calorie Needs for Maintaining Weight

	Calories/Day
Women	1,800–2,100
Men	2,100–2,400

Recommended Calorie Ranges for Losing Weight

	Calories/Day
Women	1,200–1,500
Men	1,500–1,800

CALCULATING YOUR FAT LIMITS

To limit your fat calories to less than 30 percent:

If your planned daily calorie intake is:	Your daily fat intake should be less than:
1,200 calories	40 grams
1,500 calories	50 grams
1,800 calories	60 grams

Or use the following formula:

(Calorie intake x 0.3) / 9 = your maximum grams of fat per day

Example:

1,800 calories x 0.3 = 540 / 9 = 60 grams of fat per day

Controlling Portions

As important as it is to choose quality calories over empty ones, it's also important to eat a reasonable amount. Even the most nutritious and low-calorie foods can add to a weight problem if eaten in large enough quantities. Practicing portion control can help ensure that you're not getting too much of a good thing.

Calculating Your Fat Limits

Since fat is the most concentrated source of calories in a diet, it is a good target for extra calorie-cutting. It is encouraging to note that a lower-fat diet, combined with exercise, has shown effective results in studies with calorie reductions of only 150 to 200 calories per day.

Losing at a Healthy Rate

To lose weight you need to burn an extra 3,500 calories for each pound you would like to lose; this is the approximate number of calories in 1 pound of body fat. To lose 1 pound per week, you need 500 fewer calories per day than the calories required to maintain your weight. It's best to get the 500 fewer calories from cutting your usual calories and increasing your activity level. Try eating 250 calories less per day and adding 250 calories in activity to lose that pound of fat.

Eating habits are developed throughout life in response to family and social patterns. That's why it's important to remember that the habits of a lifetime are not changed overnight. Fortunately, changes in these eating habits don't need to be dramatic to work. A good starting point is to identify and include healthy foods you enjoy.

There isn't a single ideal meal plan that works for everyone. The sample plans in this chapter are examples of just one way to meet basic nutrient needs at different calorie levels. You can use these samples as a starting point, and add or subtract servings to reach your desired calorie level.

YOUR DAILY FOOD PLAN

Food Group/ Nutrients Supplied	Serving Size*	Range of Recommended Servings/Day*	Calories per Serving	Grams of Fat per Serving	Planned Servings & Calories
Starch/bread *Thiamin, iron, niacin, fiber, carbohydrate*	• 1 slice bread; 1/2 c. pasta, rice, or potato; 1 oz. cereal; 4–5 crackers; 1/2 English muffin or bagel; 1 dinner roll	6 or more	80	1–2	
Meat *Protein, niacin, iron, thiamin*	• 1 oz. cooked, lean meat (poultry, fish, lean beef, pork); 1/4 c. cottage cheese; 1/4 c. chopped meat	4–6 oz.	55	3	
	• 1 oz. cooked, medium-fat meat (beef or pork roast, steak, ground beef); 1 oz. low-fat cheese	4–6 oz.	75	5	
	• 1 oz. cooked high-fat meat (luncheon meats, hot dogs, fried meats, prime meats); 1 oz. cheese	4–6 oz.	100	8	
Vegetables *Vitamins A and C, fiber, carbohydrate*	• 1/2 c. cooked or 1 c. raw	3 or more	25	0–1	
Fruits *Vitamins A and C, fiber, carbohydrate*	• 1/2 c. unsweetened (canned or frozen) or 1 small piece fresh	2 or more	90	0–1	

Continued on next page

YOUR DAILY FOOD PLAN (CONTINUED)

Food Group/ Nutrients Supplied	Serving Size*	Range of Recommended Servings/Day*	Calories per Serving	Grams of Fat per Serving	Planned Servings & Calories
Milk *Calcium, riboflavin, protein, vitamin D*	• 8 oz. skim milk or yogurt; 1/2 c. frozen yogurt	2 or more	90	1/2–3	
Fat *Essential fatty acids; and vitamins A, D, and K*	• 1 tsp. butter, oil, margarine, shortening; 2 tsp. salad dressing or peanut butter	3–5	45	5	

* These are averages. Check product labels for more precise information.

Free foods: Noncaloric beverages, and one or two servings per day of condiments or snacks that add less than 20 calories per serving.

SAMPLE MEAL PLAN

	1,200 Calories	1,500 Calories	1,800 Calories
	SERVINGS PER DAY		
Starch, Bread	6	7	9
Meat, lean	4 oz.	5 oz.	6 oz.
Vegetables	3	3	4
Fruits	2	4	4
Milk, skim	2	2	2
Fat	3	4	5

There isn't a single ideal meal plan that works for everyone. The plan to the left is an example of how to meet basic nutrient needs at different calorie levels. You can use these samples as a starting point and add or subtract servings to reach your desired calorie level.

SECTION FOUR
PREVENTING HEALTH PROBLEMS

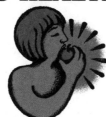

No one likes unpleasant surprises, especially when they concern one's health. The sooner you learn about your health risks, the better. Preventing health problems helps increase your chances of living a longer, healthier life.

Many people assume that an "annual physical" is the best way to prevent problems. Today, most doctors agree that an annual physical is a worn-out tradition. There is simply no scientific evidence that a yearly pilgrimage to your doctor will prevent health problems. The U.S. Preventive Services Task Force has stated that the emphasis of preventive exams should be on health counseling and health behavior rather than on the traditional physical exam.

Experts question the value of many routine tests such as blood tests and urinalysis and are increasingly recommending tests based on personal health risks. This section offers guidelines on how often you need preventive exams. You may be surprised to learn that many tests are not needed as often as were previously recommended.

For some health tests, the recommendations of different expert groups conflict. When this is the case, this section offers a balanced presentation of the options and suggests that you need to consider your personal preferences, values, and beliefs about health care risks and benefits before making a decision.

Your doctor can help you weigh the pros and cons of having certain exams. If it is unclear to you if a screening test would help you, ask yourself these questions: Is it likely that many other tests and exams will be done if the results of a screening test are inconclusive? What are the odds of detecting a disease through this test? Could any harm come from having this test? Given my age and health history, how effective is the treatment for the disease that may be detected through this test? If you ask these questions and pay careful attention to the answers, you can be a partner with your health care provider in deciding whether the test is appropriate for you.

Sharing in Decisions about Preventive Exams

Some preventive health services—like immunizations—can help you avoid certain health problems. Also, doctors use screening tests to detect diseases before symptoms actually appear. Such early detection can help stop the disease or keep it from getting worse. Despite this, many health experts question the effectiveness of screening tests in detecting disease soon enough to prevent health problems. Even for those tests that experts agree are effective, there is still debate on how often the tests should be done. This disagreement means you need to play an active role in your health care.

How can you help prevent future health problems? By learning more about health care prevention, and finding out what screening tests can and cannot do for you. With your health care provider you can discuss your personal health habits and set behavior change goals—the primary focus of any prevention discussion.

There are guidelines in this section for exams that are recommended by the Institute for Clinical Systems Integration based on scientific evidence from sources such as the U.S. Centers for Infectious Disease Control, the U.S. Preventive Services Task Force, the American Academy of Family Physicians, and the American Academy of Pediatrics. Read these guidelines; better yet, *study* them. Then, together with your physician, plan a preventive exam schedule appropriate for you. You may notice that many tests considered part of a "complete physical exam" are not listed in our recommendations. There is not enough evidence to justify routinely doing tests such as urinalysis, blood glucose, prostate specific to antigen, or resting EKGs. To put it another way, preventing disease does not outweigh the possible harm of doing these tests. Still, you may find such tests recommended elsewhere. Ask your doctor which tests tend to be traditional and which have clear scientific merit. By asking the right questions, you will be able to make more informed decisions about avoiding illness, while cutting the costs and inconvenience of unnecessary tests.

WEIGHING HEALTH RISKS

Medical experts believe that the counseling and education about your health risks from your health care provider are likely to have more impact on your health than physical exams and laboratory testing. And, in the long run, your health decisions and your lifestyle have more impact on your health than anything the doctor can accomplish during preventive exams.

The following questions will remind you of health choices that you make every day that can dramatically affect your well-being now and in the future. Share the results with your health care provider during a preventive medical visit as a way to talk about the preventive health issues that concern you the most.

PREVENTIVE STEPS

You can do more to protect your health than all the doctors, hospitals, new medical equipment, and medical scientists put together. That's because the decisions you make about exercise, diet, and substance use are clearly the best predictors of your long-term health.

If you are ready to make positive changes in your lifestyle, consider your personal priorities and readiness for change before starting a preventive self-care program. For example, if you smoke, this habit represents the single most preventable cause of future health problems that you have to address. But if you are sure that this is not the best time for you to quit, you may be better off working on a different health habit for now. Use the recommendations in this section to ensure that you are basing your decisions on the best available examples of effective behavior change.

Reading across each row, mark the one box in each row that is closest to your current situation.

HEALTH ASSESSMENT ONE: LIFESTYLE CHOICES

COLUMN 1 (1 POINT)	COLUMN 2 (2 POINTS)	COLUMN 3 (3 POINTS)
☐ I am a nonsmoker, or I quit smoking over 12 months ago.	☐ I smoke one to nine cigarettes per day or quit less than 12 months ago.	☐ I smoke 10 or more cigarettes per day.
☐ I regularly eat a well-balanced diet that includes bread/cereal/rice/pasta, fruit, vegetables, meat/poultry/fish/beans/eggs, and milk/yogurt or cheese.	☐ I sometimes eat a well-balanced diet, but do not consistently eat foods from all the food groups.	☐ I rarely or never eat a variety of foods in a well-balanced diet.
☐ I do aerobic exercise, like brisk walking, swimming, biking, jogging and/or aerobics, three or more times a week.	☐ I do aerobic exercise one or two times a week.	☐ I seldom or never do aerobic exercise.
☐ I am within 10 pounds of my healthy weight.	☐ I am 10 to 20 pounds over or under my healthy weight.	☐ I am more than 20 pounds over or under my healthy weight.
☐ I seldom or never drink more than two alcoholic beverages per occasion. I am not concerned, nor are people close to me, about how much alcohol I drink.	☐ I sometimes drink more than two alcoholic beverages per occasion and/or sometimes I am concerned, or people close to me are concerned, about how much alcohol I drink.	☐ I often drink more than two alcoholic beverages per occasion and/or I am often concerned, and people close to me are concerned, about how much alcohol I drink.
Column 1 total: _____	Column 2 total: _____	Column 3 total: _____

Add your points from columns 1, 2, and 3 together to arrive at your "Lifestyle Choices" total and enter it here. **Total Points:**_____
Key: 6 or less: Healthy choices   7–11: Somewhat risky choices   12 or more: Risky choices

HEALTH ASSESSMENT TWO: PERSONAL SAFETY

☐ I always wear my seat belt when driving or riding in a car.	☐ I sometimes wear my seat belt.	☐ I rarely or never wear my seat belt.
☐ I always wear a helmet when riding a bicycle.	☐ I sometimes wear a helmet when riding a bicycle.	☐ I rarely or never wear a helmet when riding a bicycle.
☐ I never ride in a car with a driver who has been using alcohol or other drugs.	☐ I sometimes ride in a car with a driver who has been using alcohol or other drugs.	☐ I often ride in a car with a driver who has been using alcohol or other drugs.
☐ I always follow "safer sex" practices or don't have intercourse.	☐ I sometimes follow "safer sex" practices.	☐ I rarely or never follow "safer sex" practices.
☐ I always or almost always use sun block to protect my skin from the sun.	☐ I sometimes use sun block to protect my skin from the sun.	☐ I rarely or never use sun block to protect my skin from the sun.
Column 1 total: _____	Column 2 total: _____	Column 3 total: _____

Add your points from columns 1, 2, and 3 together to arrive at your "Personal Safety" total and enter it here. **Total Points:**_____
Key: 6 or less: Healthy choices   7–11: Somewhat risky choices   12 or more: Risky choices

PREVENTING HEALTH PROBLEMS

Reading across each row, mark the one box in each row that most closely reflects your current situation.

HEALTH ASSESSMENT THREE: HOME SAFETY

COLUMN 1 (1 POINT)	COLUMN 2 (2 POINTS)	COLUMN 3 (3 POINTS)
☐ I have a working smoke detector in my home that I check regularly.	☐ I have a smoke detector in the home but rarely check to see if it's working.	☐ I do not have and/or do not check on a home smoke detector.
☐ I keep all possibly poisonous items in my home locked and stored away from children.	☐ I have some or most poisonous items in my home locked and stored away from children.	☐ I do not keep poisonous items locked or stored away from children.
☐ My water heater is set to a maximum of 120° F to prevent burns.	☐ I do not know the temperature setting of my water heater.	☐ My water heater is set above 120° F.
☐ I do not have firearms or weapons at home, or I keep them locked, stored, and unloaded where children can't get them.	☐ I keep firearms or weapons stored and locked most of the time.	☐ I do not keep firearms and weapons stored away from children.
☐ I always keep electrical cords or carpets secured to prevent slips and falls.	☐ I sometimes check to be sure cords or carpets will not cause slips and falls.	☐ I rarely or never check cords or carpets to prevent slips and falls.
Column 1 total: _____	Column 2 total: _____	Column 3 total: _____

Add your points from columns 1, 2, and 3 together to arrive at your "Home Safety" total and enter it here. **Total Points:**_____
Key: 6 or less: Healthy choices   7–11: Somewhat risky choices   12 or more: Risky choices

HEALTH ASSESSMENT FOUR: PERSONAL HEALTH DECISIONS

☐ I rarely or never feel overwhelmed with problems.	☐ I sometimes feel overwhelmed with problems.	☐ I often feel overwhelmed with problems.
☐ I rarely or never feel afraid in my relationships.	☐ I sometimes feel afraid in my relationships.	☐ I often feel afraid in my relationships.
☐ I am not presently concerned about an unwanted pregnancy.	☐ I am concerned about an unwanted pregnancy and always take steps to prevent pregnancy.	☐ I am concerned about an unwanted pregnancy and sometimes take measures to prevent pregnancy.
☐ I have a complete and current living will that states my wishes for care if I should become unable to make my own decisions.	☐ I have a living will that needs updating.	☐ I do not have a living will.
☐ I have many social contacts and do not feel isolated from others.	☐ I have some social contacts but sometimes feel isolated from others.	☐ I have few social contacts and often feel isolated from others.
Column 1 total: _____	Column 2 total: _____	Column 3 total: _____

Add your points from columns 1, 2, and 3 together to arrive at your "Personal Health Decisions" total and enter it here. **Total Points:**_____
Key: 6 or less: Healthy choices   7–11: Somewhat risky choices   12 or more: Risky choices

AGE GUIDE TO WEIGHING AND PREVENTING HEALTH RISKS

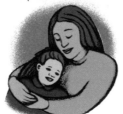

CHILDREN AND TEENAGERS

The growth and development of children is one of life's wonders. Keeping children safe and healthy is a main concern as we watch them cut new teeth, hit growth spurts, and struggle through adolescence into adulthood. The health risks children and teenagers face are as varied as the many interests and skills they learn as they grow up. From infections as infants to falling out of trees to experimenting with sex, some health issues facing children and teenagers will always stay the same, while other health threats are new and unnerving.

Many factors need to be weighed when deciding how often to bring in children and teens for a routine prevention visit. The schedules here are based on the Institute for Clinical Systems Integration's recommendations. There is no scientific evidence to support any particular schedule of well-child visits. Therefore, visits to cover needed immunizations are recommended. Other visits can be scheduled to fit the needs of individual patients and providers. A child's developmental stages or behavior, a family history of health risks, or significant changes in a child's environment or behavior are all reasons that could prompt additional visits. As your child enters adolescence, your doctor may ask to see the child alone so that he or she can discuss sensitive issues openly.

It is likely that you will continue to see greater involvement in preventive care from the entire health care team. As the health care system continues to seek greater efficiency, along with personalized care, you will see primary care doctors joined by nurse practitioners, physician assistants, and other health professionals trained to give your family preventive services. This makes prevention a priority, and involves the patient and health care team more in improving general health care.

Childhood Immunizations

Among the greatest achievements in modern medicine, vaccines protect children from serious diseases including mumps, measles, diphtheria, and polio. Some immunizations work by giving a very weak dose of the disease—strong enough to prompt the body's immune system to develop antibodies against the disease but not strong enough to cause it. Others offer immunity but do not cause the disease itself. The following section describes each of the major vaccines and how they are used.

Diphtheria/Pertussis/Tetanus (DPT)

The DPT shot combines all three vaccines to protect against these life-threatening diseases. Most children should have five DPT shots before they enter kindergarten. Babies should have three shots by the time they reach 6 months of age—at 2, 4, and 6 months—plus one at about 15 months of age.

Oral Polio Vaccine (OPV)

Since becoming available in the 1950s, this vaccine has nearly wiped out polio. Experts warn, however, that without continued vaccination, the risk of contracting this crippling, potentially fatal disease could return. Children should receive four doses of oral polio vaccine by age 6. This, in most cases, provides protection for life.

Haemophilus Influenzae Type B (HIB)

HIB is a dangerous bacterium that can cause meningitis, pneumonia, and infections of other body systems. The HIB vaccine protects almost all children who receive the full four doses. It is given by injection three times before a child is 7 months old, followed by a booster at 12 to 15 months.

Measles/Mumps/Rubella (MMR)

The MMR vaccine is given by injection once at 15 months of age and again at age 12 to guard against these common childhood infections. In most people, these two doses provide protection for life.

Hepatitis B Vaccine

Hepatitis B is an inflammation of the liver that can cause a range of problems—from simple flulike symptoms to severe reactions requiring hospitalization. Hepatitis B is considered the most serious form of hepatitis. The hepatitis B vaccine is given three times before age 1.

Chicken Pox (Varicella) Vaccine

The American Academy of Pediatrics recommends chicken pox (varicella) vaccine for children over 12 months of age who have not had chicken pox (see Chicken Pox, p. 152). A single dose should be given between 12 and 18 months of age. Older children can be immunized at the earliest convenient opportunity, also with a single dose. Healthy adolescents past their 13th birthday who have not been immunized previously and have not had chicken pox should be immunized with two doses of vaccine 4 to 8 weeks apart.

The following tables summarize the preventive health care schedules for children and teenagers. They are mainly for children without symptoms of health problems and who do not have special health risks. If you have a family history of certain illnesses, your doctor should recommend a schedule of preventive visits that is more appropriate to your child's needs.

Use this chart to keep track of your child's immunizations.

Child's Name _____ Date of Birth _____	Date Dose 1	Date Dose 2	Date Dose 3	Date Dose 4	Date Dose 5
DPT (Diphtheria/pertussis/tetanus)					
OPV (Oral polio vaccine)					
HIB (*Haemophilus influenzae* type B)					
MMR (Measles/mumps/rubella)					
Hepatitis B vaccine					
Chicken pox (Varicella) vaccine					

PREVENTIVE SERVICES RECOMMENDATIONS

PREVENTION STEP	SCREENING RECOMMENDATIONS
Birth to Age 23 Months	
Lab Tests	
Hemoglobin or hematocrit	Once during infancy
Cholesterol	Not recommended for healthy children
Urinalysis	Not recommended for healthy children
Tuberculin skin test	Not recommended for healthy children[1]
Lead screening	Recommended for children at high risk[4]
Immunizations	
HIB	2, 4, 6, and 12 to 15 months
Oral polio vaccine (OPV)	2, 4, and 6 to 15 months
Diphtheria/pertussis/tetanus (DPT)	2, 4, 6, and 15 months
Measles/mumps/rubella (MMR)	15 months
Hepatitis B	Birth, 1 and 6 months *or* 2, 4, and 10 months
Exams	
Hearing exams	Special hearing tests given by primary caregiver if child is at risk[2]
Ages 2 to 6	
Lab Tests	
Cholesterol	Recommended for children at high risk[3]
Urinalysis	Not recommended for healthy children
Tuberculin skin test	Not recommended for healthy children[1]
Lead screening	Recommended for children at high risk[4]
Immunizations	
Oral polio vaccine (OPV)	4 to 6 years old
Diphtheria/pertussis/tetanus (DPT)	4 to 6 years old
Exams	
Blood pressure	Every 2 years
Eye exam	Once by age 5
Hearing exam	Only if hearing ability is questioned[2]

Risk Factors

(1) Children suspected of having tuberculosis, children who live in households with cases of tuberculosis, or children who are new immigrants from areas known to have tuberculosis should be tested.

(2) Vision and hearing tests given at school do not need to be repeated by the health care provider. Special hearing tests should be given to children with infections at birth, family history of hearing problems, low birth weight, low Apgar scores, or malformation of the head or neck.

(Additional risk factors follow on p. 244.)

(Continued on next page)

Risk Factors

(3) Children over age 2 who have a family history of heart disease before the age of 55 or who have a parent with cholesterol readings of over 300 may need to be tested for high cholesterol.

(4) Children at high risk include those who live in—or often visit—housing built before 1950 that is run down or undergoing renovation; who come into close contact with other children who have high lead exposure; whose parents work in lead-related occupations; or who live near hazardous waste sites, busy highways, or lead processing plants.

(5) More frequent tetanus boosters are recommended if the child has ever had a serious open wound.

PREVENTIVE SERVICES RECOMMENDATIONS (CONTINUED)

PREVENTION STEP	SCREENING RECOMMENDATIONS
Ages 7 to 12	
Lab Tests	
Cholesterol	Recommended for children at high risk[3]
Urinalysis	Not recommended for healthy children
Tuberculin skin test	Not recommended for healthy children[1]
Immunizations	
Measles/mumps/rubella (MMR)	12 years old
Exams	
Blood pressure	Every 2 years
Vision and hearing exams	If problems are suspected[2]
Scoliosis screening	Not recommended for healthy children
Ages 13 to 18	
Lab Tests	
Urinalysis	Not recommended for healthy teens
Immunization	
Tetanus/diphtheria	Once at 14 to 16 years old[5]
History/Counseling	
Sexual practices	Weigh risks and provide appropriate information/advice
Tobacco/alcohol/drug use	Weigh risks and provide appropriate information/advice
Exams	
Blood pressure	At all visits
Pap smear (women)	At age 18 or after first sexual activity

THE BEST PREVENTION YEARS: AGES 19 TO 39

At a time when you are building a career, starting a family, establishing a home, or all the above, paying attention to your health habits may not be a high priority. After all, the odds are in your favor. Your chances of falling victim to a major illness, such as heart disease or cancer, are very remote before the age of 40.

But the lifestyle habits you establish now can affect how you feel and what health problems you may have in the future. For example, during early adulthood, you tend to gain weight faster than at any other time in your adult life. And although the combined effects of smoking, extra calories, or lack of exercise may be reversible, habits of 10 or 20 years are tough to change. Now is the time to invest in a healthy future by making positive health choices—like regular exercise and a low-fat, low-salt diet.

Besides forming your personal health habits, you should also begin to develop a schedule of preventive health exams that fits your health history and build a good relationship with your health care provider.

Leading Health Threats

Although it may seem that physical ailments are for "old" people, you're certainly not invincible before age 40. You face the major risk of death for your age group every day when you get into your car. Wearing your seat belt, never drinking and driving, staying within the speed limit, and using a helmet when you ride a bicycle are the main ways to ensure you'll reach age 40.

This stage in your life is also the time to identify your risks for diseases you may get later in life and adjust your health habits to lower those risks. Regular blood pressure checks and cholesterol screenings are important for everyone. For women, regular Pap smears and pelvic exams are important to detect cervical cancer early.

The following table highlights recommendations for preventive services you should discuss with your doctor. Men should note that although you need to schedule an exam only every 5 years, getting blood pressure measured every 2 years is vital. Women need to schedule a checkup only every 3 years as long as you schedule other visits for blood pressure checks, clinical breast exams, and mammography.

Risk Factors

(1) High blood pressure, elevated cholesterol, smoking, fat stored above or near waist.

(2) Residents of chronic care facilities such as nursing homes; people with diabetes or chronic lung or kidney disease; health care workers with patients at high risk.

(3) Chronic heart, kidney, or lung disease; diabetes; alcoholism; Hodgkin's disease; cirrhosis; sickle cell disease.

(4) Male, smoking, high blood pressure, African American, family history of heart disease, diabetes, obesity, sedentary lifestyle.

(5) Regularly scheduled visits are recommended for those with a history of ulcerative colitis, severe dysplasia (abnormal changes in cells), or Crohn's disease; mother, father, sister, or brother with colon cancer; obstruction in flow of urine.

(6) Yearly if at risk due to history of sexually transmitted disease, first intercourse before age 18, had several sexual partners, smoker, sexual partner who had several other partners.

(7) More frequent tetanus boosters are recommended if the person has ever had a serious open wound.

(8) Mother, sister, or daughter with breast cancer, previous breast biopsy, or personal history of cancer.

PREVENTIVE SERVICES RECOMMENDATIONS

PREVENTION STEP	SCREENING RECOMMENDATIONS
Ages 19 to 39	
Lab Tests	
Cholesterol and HDL	Every 5 years (test more often if risk factors are present[1] or if total cholesterol is higher than 240)
Blood pressure	Every 2 years (test more often if risk factors are present[4] or if blood pressure is higher than 130/85)
Chest X-ray	Not recommended for healthy adults
Urinalysis	Not recommended for healthy adults
Rubella titer	Women lacking evidence of immunity
Immunizations	
Diphtheria/tetanus	Every 10 years [7]
Influenza	Yearly if at risk[2]
Pneumonia vaccination	At least once if at risk[3]
Hepatitis B	If at risk[3]
For Women	
Breast exam	Professional exam—every 3 years, beginning at age 20 (test more often if risk factors are present[8])
	Self-exam—monthly
Mammography	Age 35 if at risk[8]; otherwise, age 40
Pelvic exam/Pap smear	Annually beginning at age 18 (or at age of first intercourse); then every 3 years after three normal exams in a row[6]

THE EARLY DETECTION YEARS: AGES 40 TO 64

After you turn 40, your body will sometimes remind you that middle age brings physical changes. But this does not have to be the age for physical decline. Studies show that those who stay active can slow the usual decreases in stamina or strength that come with aging. For many, the middle years are a time of self-renewal. You may be more ready to attend to some personal health goals you postponed during your 20s and 30s. If you smoke, now is the time to quit before cancer, heart disease, or shortness of breath begins. And if you've been putting off improving your eating habits, it's time to get on track.

If it's been years since you exercised regularly, start soon but start slow. Exercise is very important for many health conditions—such as hypertension or diabetes—that begin to show up during middle age. Slowly changing your routine is safest, and you will be more likely to stay with new habits if they can be built into your lifestyle.

Major Health Threats

This is a critical time for detecting the start of health conditions that—if left unchecked—can be life threatening. **Heart disease** is the major cause of death for adults in midlife. The best exams for detecting problems of the circulatory system are blood pressure and cholesterol tests. **High blood pressure** is the most common cardiovascular disease in the United States, and controlling blood pressure is the best way to decrease the death rate from heart attack and stroke.

Most people know that **high cholesterol** increases the risk for heart disease and stroke, but fewer than 20 percent know their own cholesterol number. For both high cholesterol and high blood pressure, obesity is a major risk factor.

Lung cancer remains the most common cause of cancer-related death for men, and the incidence of lung cancer among women is increasing at an alarming rate—more than doubling in the last two decades. Cigarette smoking accounts for at least 75 percent of these deaths. Although breast cancer is the most probable cancer for nonsmokers, lung cancer is by far the leading cause of cancer for women who smoke. In fact, lung cancer is now the most frequent cancer for women in general.

The following table highlights recommendations for preventive services you should discuss with your doctor. Even though a routine exam for preventive services is needed only every 3 years, blood pressure checks every 2 years are recommended for everyone, and breast exams and mammography are recommended more frequently than before for women.

PREVENTING HEALTH PROBLEMS

Risk Factors

(1) High blood pressure, elevated cholesterol, smoking, fat stored above or near waist.

(2) Residents of chronic care facilities such as nursing homes; people with diabetes or chronic lung or kidney disease; health care workers with patients at high risk.

(3) Chronic heart, kidney, or lung disease; diabetes; alcoholism; Hodgkin's disease; cirrhosis; sickle cell disease.

(4) Male, smoking, high blood pressure, African American, family history of heart disease, diabetes, obesity, sedentary lifestyle.

(5) Regularly scheduled visits are recommended for those with a history of ulcerative colitis, severe dysplasia (abnormal changes in cells), or Crohn's disease; mother, father, sister, or brother with colon cancer; obstruction in flow of urine.

(6) Yearly if at risk due to history of sexually transmitted disease, first intercourse before age 18, had several sexual partners, smoker, sexual partner who had several other partners.

(7) More frequent tetanus boosters are recommended if the person has ever had a serious open wound.

(8) Mother, sister, or daughter with breast cancer, previous breast biopsy, or personal history of cancer.

PREVENTIVE SERVICES RECOMMENDATIONS

PREVENTION STEP	SCREENING RECOMMENDATIONS
Ages 40 to 64	
Lab Tests	
Cholesterol and HDL	Every 5 years (test more often if risk factors are present[1] or if total cholesterol is higher than 240)
Rubella titer	Women lacking evidence of immunity
Urinalysis	Not recommended for healthy adults
Chest X-ray	Not recommended for healthy adults
Immunizations	
Influenza	Yearly if at risk[2]
Pneumonia vaccination	At least once if at risk[3]
Diphtheria/tetanus	Every 10 years[7]
Exams	
Health counseling	Every 3 years for women, every 5 years for men
Blood pressure	Every 2 years (test more often if risk factors are present[4] or if blood pressure is higher than 130/85mmHg)
Hemoccult test (for "hidden" blood in stool)	Beginning at age 50, optional[5]
Sigmoidoscopy	Every 5 years beginning at age 50[5]
For Men	
Prostate specific antigen	Not recommended for healthy males
For Women	
Breast exam	Professional exam—yearly
	Self-exam—monthly
Mammography	Every 2 years beginning at age 40, and yearly if at risk[8]; yearly for all women beginning at age 50
Pelvic exam/Pap smear	Every 3 years after three normal exams[6] (yearly if risk factors present)

THE HEALTH MAINTENANCE YEARS: AGE 65 AND OLDER

Some people believe disease prevention is for younger people and that by age 65 chronic illnesses have already developed. Although it's true that four out of five persons aged 65 and older have one or more chronic conditions—such as arthritis, heart disease, or diabetes—preventive health care is still important.

Advice you followed—or ignored—about diet, exercise, and use of alcohol and tobacco are as important now as ever. For example, exercise—even in the frail elderly—remains one of the most effective ways to become or stay vital. Aging should bring a renewed focus on keeping existing health problems from getting worse. Here are some tips to help you make the most of your health care:

• If you see more than one doctor, make sure each one knows what drugs the others have prescribed for you; this will help prevent drug interactions.

• Tell your doctor about your physical ailments. Not all aches, pains, discomforts, or functional declines are "normal" parts of aging—yours may be treatable.

• If you become ill and can no longer live independently, remember that nowadays a nursing home isn't the only option. Hospital social workers and area agencies may be able to help you find support services so you can remain at home.

Major Health Threats

Although the main threats to your physical health at this age are complications of chronic illnesses you already may have, simple cases of influenza or pneumonia can also become life-threatening illnesses. Likewise, preventing falls is more important than ever—particularly for women, who are more likely than men to have osteoporosis, making them more likely to break bones.

The "golden" years are not always happy for everyone. Depression is common among older adults because of the many losses they often experience—including the death of friends and loved ones and loss of health or independence. Depression can lower your immunity and put you at risk for suicide. Fortunately, depression can be treated with drugs, counseling, or both.

The following table highlights recommendations for preventive services you should discuss with your doctor. The evidence for the effectiveness of several screening tests after the age of 75 or 80 is incomplete. Your doctor can help you decide whether you will benefit from having certain exams that may have been routine for you in the past.

Risk Factors

(1) High blood pressure, elevated cholesterol, smoking, waist measure greater than hip measure.

(2) Routine urinalysis is only recommended for male smokers over age 65.

(3) Male, smoker, high blood pressure, African American, diabetes, obesity, sedentary lifestyle, or family history of heart disease.

(4) Pelvic exams are not effective for detecting ovarian cancer. Patients may consider discontinuing Pap smears after age 65 if there are no high risk factors. Risk factors include history of sexually transmitted disease, first intercourse before age 18, had several sexual partners, smoker, sexual partner who had several other partners.

(5) More frequent tetanus boosters are recommended if the person has ever had a serious open wound.

PREVENTIVE SERVICES RECOMMENDATIONS

PREVENTION STEP	SCREENING RECOMMENDATIONS
Age 65 and Older	
Lab Tests	
Cholesterol	Every 5 years (test more often if risk and HDL factors are present[1] or if cholesterol is higher than 240)
Urinalysis	Not recommended for healthy adults[2]
Chest X-ray	Not recommended for healthy adults
Immunizations	
Influenza	Yearly
Pneumonia vaccination	Once, at age 65
Diphtheria/tetanus	Every 10 years[5]
Exams	
Blood pressure	Every 2 years (test more often if risk factors are present[3] or if blood pressure is higher than 130/85)
Hemoccult test (for "hidden blood" in stool)	Periodically, optional
Sigmoidoscopy	Every 5 years until age 80
Vision/hearing exams	Starting at age 65
For Women	
Breast exam	Professional exam—yearly
	Self-exam—monthly
Mammography	Yearly
Pelvic exam/Pap smear	Every 3 years (optional if low risk)[4]

PREVENTION AND EARLY DETECTION OF COMMON PROBLEMS

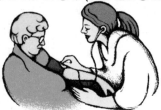

HIGH BLOOD PRESSURE

High blood pressure, or hypertension, affects one in every four adults. As a main risk factor for two of the top three leading causes of death in America—heart disease and stroke—high blood pressure is perhaps the number one killer in this country. Left unmanaged, high blood pressure can also damage the kidneys.

Although hypertension cannot be cured, it can usually be controlled. Advances over the last 30 years in detecting and treating it have contributed to a 50 percent reduction in deaths from heart disease, and a 57 percent reduction in deaths from stroke since 1972. (See Hypertension = High Blood Pressure, p. 225, for a full description of what blood pressure is, how it is taken, and what happens during and after a blood pressure exam.)

The risks for developing high blood pressure are greater for certain groups of people. **People at particular risk include:**

- African Americans
- People whose parents have high blood pressure
- People with high-normal blood pressure
- Young adult and early-middle-age men

Scheduling Readings

Blood pressure can vary widely from time to time, so several readings need to be averaged from two or more visits before you can be classified as having high blood pressure. The Joint National Committee on High Blood Pressure (JNC) has developed new classifications that now identify different stages of hypertension. These stages need to be considered, in addition to your health history and risk factors for heart disease, to decide how to manage and follow up hypertension. The JNC recommends routine blood pressure checks at least once every 2 years for people with normal blood pressure (below 130/85mmHg).

Many doctors routinely check blood pressure every time a patient is seen at the office. The following blood pressure classification table has more guidelines on how often you should have your blood pressure checked.

*If you are not taking antihypertensive drugs and are not acutely ill.

†When systolic and diastolic pressures fall into different categories, the higher category should be used to classify your blood pressure status.

CLASSIFICATION OF BLOOD PRESSURE FOR ADULTS AGE 18 YEARS AND OLDER*

Category	Systolic† (top number)	Diastolic† (bottom number)	What to do
Normal	Less than 130	Less than 85	Recheck in 2 years
High-normal	130–139	85–89	Recheck in 1 year
Hypertension			
Stage 1	140–159	90–99	Confirm within 2 months
Stage 2	160–179	100–109	See provider within 1 month
Stage 3	180–209	110–119	See provider within 1 week
Stage 4	210 or higher	120 or higher	See provider immediately

Source: 1993 Joint Committee on Detection, Evaluation, and Treatment of High Blood Pressure

SELF-CARE STEPS FOR HIGH BLOOD PRESSURE

Reduce high blood pressure and cardiovascular risks by:

• **Losing weight.** Being overweight increases your risk of developing high blood pressure. Weight loss in even modest amounts can lower and help control blood pressure. Weight loss can also decrease blood cholesterol, triglyceride, and blood sugar levels. Of all the nondrug methods of hypertension control, weight loss is by far the most effective.

• **Exercising regularly.** Regular, aerobic exercise—such as walking, running, bicycling, or swimming laps—can prevent and reduce high blood pressure. More activity can also help reduce weight and stress. Many experts recommend 30 to 45 minutes of aerobic exercise three to five times a week.

• **Controlling salt in your diet.** Not everyone is sensitive to the blood pressure-raising effects of too much sodium, but there is no simple way to find out such sensitivity. Since the amount of salt in the average American diet raises blood pressure for about half of those with high blood pressure and interferes with some blood pressure-lowering drugs, cutting down on salt is recommended for anyone with high blood pressure. Limit salt to less than 2,300 milligrams per day by not adding it to your food and by limiting processed, convenience, and fast foods, which are traditionally high in sodium.

• **Limiting alcohol.** Drinking too much alcohol can raise blood pressure, add weight, and make high blood pressure control harder. Avoid alcohol or do not have more than two drinks a day. A drink is defined as 12 ounces of beer, 4 ounces of wine, or 1.5 ounces of 80-proof liquor.

• **Quitting smoking.** Smoking cigarettes does not cause high blood pressure, but smoking is a major risk factor for cardiovascular disease. That is why everyone, especially people with high blood pressure, needs to quit smoking—better yet, never start.

• **Eating less fat.** Some evidence shows that a low-fat diet may reduce blood pressure and lower blood cholesterol. Eating less fat will also aid in weight loss.

CANCER PREVENTION AND MANAGEMENT

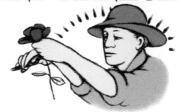

On your way to work you notice the American Cancer Society billboard, and one of the seven warning signals of cancer leaps out at you: a nagging cough or hoarseness. You've been thinking your dry morning cough was allergies or too many cigarettes or not enough humidity—but now you fear the worst. Should you?

Only your doctor and other medical specialists can find out for sure. So, **see your doctor if you have any of these symptoms:**

- A change in bowel or bladder habits
- A sore that does not heal
- Unusual bleeding or discharge, especially from the rectum or vagina
- A thickening or lump in a breast or elsewhere
- Indigestion or difficulty in swallowing
- An obvious change in a wart or mole
- A nagging cough or hoarseness

Other signs of possible cancer include a constant, low-grade fever, fatigue, unusual and persistent headaches with changes in vision or behavior, nagging and unexplained pain in the bones or elsewhere, easy bruising, loss of appetite, and sudden, unexpected weight loss. For more on breast cancer, see p. 260; cervical cancer, p. 264; colon cancer, p. 255; prostate cancer, p. 257; and testicular cancer, p. 259.

PREVENTION: RISK FACTORS YOU CAN CONTROL

Smoking and Secondhand Smoke

Smoking causes two-thirds of all lung cancer deaths, and also increases the risk of cancers of the mouth, pharynx, larynx, esophagus, pancreas, uterus, cervix, kidney, and bladder. Research also shows that the smoke blown your way from others' cigarettes may even be worse than smoke directly inhaled because its tar content has not been reduced by going through the cigarette's filter. When you quit smoking, your lungs begin healing themselves, and some smoking-induced precancerous changes can be totally reversed.

Alcohol

Heavy drinkers may have a twofold to six-fold risk of developing throat or mouth cancer. The chances of developing cancer of the pancreas, liver, breast, stomach, and rectum also are greater if you drink alcohol. The news is even worse for drinkers who smoke. The risks of throat and mouth cancers escalate 15-fold, and the risks of esophageal cancer may increase by as much as 25-fold. Heavy drinking may keep the liver from detoxifying potentially cancer-causing substances from smoking. It also may irritate and make tissues of the mouth, throat, and esophagus more prone to cancer.

Eat Less Fat

Scientists are finding that a high-fat diet can increase the risk of breast and colon cancer. It also is a suspect in prostate and ovarian cancer. Fat may cause the body to make some bile acids that promote cancer, and definitely increases production of hormones. This tends to trigger the growth of some tumors in overweight people. Several suspected cancer-causing chemicals are first stored in animal fat and then in the body fat of humans who eat the animals.

Eat More Fiber

Research from the National Cancer Institute shows that if most people had 20 to 30 grams of fiber daily, their risk of getting colon cancer would be cut in half. The insoluble fiber found in wheat bran, whole-grain cereals and breads, vegetables and fruits, and the soluble fiber in such foods as oat bran and beans flushes possible cancer-promoting waste through the intestines and colon. It also flushes out fats and bile acids.

Protect Your Skin from the Sun

Most skin cancers are caused by too much exposure to the sun's ultraviolet rays and the high-energy bulbs in tanning parlors. It's easy to protect yourself from this threat: try to avoid direct sunlight between 10:00 a.m. and 2:00 p.m., wear protective clothing when you are out in the sun, and use sunscreen with a sun protection factor of at least 15.

Maintain a Healthy Weight

Overweight women have higher death rates from cancer of the uterus, gallbladder, cervix, ovaries, and breast. More overweight men die from colon, rectal, and prostate cancers. Eating healthy foods in moderation and exercising regularly will help you tone up and lose weight. Researchers are trying to find out exactly how exercise protects the body. Not only does 30 minutes of exercise at least three times each week combat obesity, it also helps reduce stress and regulate bowel movements.

Avoid Environmental Hazards

Workplaces are now regulated so that hazardous materials are not routinely released into the air, but if you work around chemicals or dust, let your doctor know this during your next physical examination. Whenever you use paint, varnish, or any other chemical indoors, leave windows open. Have your house checked for radon leakage. Use pesticides and herbicides carefully, and wash fruits and vegetables before eating them.

When the Diagnosis Is Cancer

After cancer is detected and confirmed, several treatment options or combined options may be available. Surgery, radiation, and chemotherapy are the most common treatments. Antihormone therapy, immunotherapy, and regional perfusion are less common.

Surgery

The oldest form of cancer treatment, surgery involves removing a tumor or cancerous growth.

Radiation Therapy

Radiation works by killing the cancer cells by exposing them to high doses of X-rays.

Chemotherapy

Drugs that kill cancer cells by interfering with how they reproduce are taken orally or injected into the body.

Antihormone Therapy

These drugs have been successful in treating breast and prostate cancers. The antihormone medication most commonly used to treat breast cancer, tamoxifen, has some side effects, including hot flashes.

Immunotherapy

Drugs are used to boost the body's own ability to fight cancer in the same way it wards off infections. The best known of these, Interferon, has been successful in treating a rare form of leukemia but less successful against other cancers.

Regional Perfusion

Drugs are introduced to only the part of the body that has cancerous tissue. Damage to healthy tissue is minimal, the drugs may be more effective, and there are fewer side effects.

Support Is Available

Discovering you have cancer and looking ahead to an uncertain future can be frightening. Many cancer patients and their families find it helpful and reassuring to talk with others who also are dealing with cancer. Emotional support is available for those who wish to join a cancer support group. For more information on how to locate a support group, ask your health care provider or contact the American Cancer Society.

COLON CANCER

Colon cancer is a common cancer that can be detected and prevented in many people if simple steps are followed. The rate of colon cancer among men and women is about the same, with 6 percent of women and 5 percent of men getting this disease during their lifetime.

Colon cancer ranks second only to lung cancer, with more than 152,000 new cases reported each year. The earlier the cancer—or any changes in the colon that might lead to cancer—is found, the better the chance for cure. Indeed, early detection increases the cure rate to 91

percent. The death rate, however, among people with late stages of colon cancer at the time of diagnosis is high—about 60 percent—and the statistics are not improving.

Understanding Your Risk

No one knows for sure what causes colon cancer, but we do know some of the risk factors. Your chances of developing colon cancer are higher if you have a history of ulcerative colitis, severe dysplasia (precancerous changes), or Crohn's disease or if your mother, father, sister, or brother has had colon cancer.

Age plays a role, too. Most cases occur in people over age 65. Fewer than 2 percent of cases occur in those under age 40.

Screening Tests

The three tests most commonly used for colon cancer screening are the digital (finger) rectal exam, testing the stool for blood, and sigmoidoscopy. Screening exams can be mildly uncomfortable, but generally these tests are easy and safe to do. Experts still disagree about how often the colon should be examined and how effectively tests detect cancer in people who have no symptoms. Your doctor can help you decide if you need any of these tests:

Sigmoidoscopy

A slender lighted tube called a flexible sigmoidoscope is inserted into your rectum after you have had an enema. With this device, the physician can see about 27 inches into your colon. About 80 percent of cancers and polyps (growths) that might become cancer can be found this way, because they tend to build up at the lower end of your bowel.

Stool Test for Blood

Because polyps and cancers produce small unnoticeable amounts of blood, which are carried away in the stools, tests such as "Hemoccult" or "guaiac" are used to detect bleeding. By carefully following the directions for the test, you will make the results more reliable. Some medical guidelines suggest this test is unnecessary for average risk patients.

Digital Rectal Exam

Using his or her finger, the doctor feels for lumps (polyps) in your colon that could be cancer. The effectiveness of this screening method is limited because less than 13 percent of colon cancers are within a finger's reach.

If the results of any of these tests are abnormal, your doctor will probably order more studies. Sometimes these tests are not accurate, creating either a false promise of good health or a false alarm about the frightening possibility of cancer.

The recommendations for colon exams vary. The Institute for Clinical Systems Integration recommends annual digital rectal exams beginning at age 50, and sigmoidoscopy every five years between ages 50 and 80. The U.S. Task Force on Preventive Services is now revising its recommendations. The American Cancer Society and national medical societies recommend annual digital rectal exams for adults over 40, annual stool blood testing starting at age 50, and sigmoidoscopy every 3 to 5 years beginning at age 50.

Given the cost, inconvenience, and uncertainty about the effectiveness of colon cancer screening, you and your doctor may decide it is unnecessary for you. On the other hand, if you are at high risk for colon cancer—particularly if you have a close family member who has had the disease—your doctor may recommend more extensive testing.

Those with a history of cancer are clearly candidates for regular screening. Remember, these are only screening tests and if you have symptoms that persist you should see your doctor no matter what your last screening test showed.

SELF-CARE STEPS FOR COLON CANCER

• Since cure by early detection is the goal of colon cancer screening, your quick response to warning signs is critical. If you have a change in your bowel habits (black stools, thin stools, blood in your stools, or intermittent or persistent diarrhea or constipation) an exam of your colon to find the cause may be done, regardless of your age. Cancer, however, is just one of the many possible causes of these symptoms.

• Several dietary factors are thought to play a role in colorectal cancer. Obesity, total calorie intake, and high-fat diets have been implicated in causing cancer in both animal and human research. A diet high in fiber may be helpful in preventing colon cancer. Foods high in fiber include whole-grain cereals and breads, beans, potatoes, brown rice, fruits and vegetables.

HEALTH RISKS FOR MEN AND WOMEN

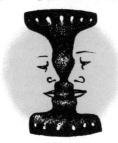

HEALTH RISKS FOR MEN

Many people believe that women have more health risks than men. Whether this is true or not, men too have special health issues they need to know about, like smoking, violence, and alcohol-related problems.

Reproductive and sexual health for men includes the potential for cancer of the testicles and the prostate. During a routine examination your doctor will probably check for signs of these cancers, and for hernias.

At some point in their lives, most men struggle with impotency. In the past, impotency was passed off as a psychological condition. But today it's known that somewhere between 50 percent and 75 percent of all cases have a physical cause. When impotency does not go away on its own within a short period of time, it's important to seek treatment or at least to find out the cause. Left untreated or undiagnosed, impotency can lead to loss of self-confidence, problems in intimate relationships, and other psychological concerns.

Men also face a higher risk for heart disease. This makes regular blood pressure checks, cholesterol screening, a low-fat diet, and regular exercise particularly important.

Another area of high risk for men is that of work and sports injuries. Insurance companies report that young men who exercise vigorously tend to have higher health care claims than those who don't. Of course it's not suggested that you avoid exercise to prevent injury, but you should know limits for safe exercise, and avoid too much exertion and strain. Other precautions like warm-up and cool-down periods, and stretching before and after your workout routine, can help prevent injuries.

Work-related back injuries are also common among men. If you do a lot of lifting on your job—or elsewhere—remember to lift from your legs instead of your back. Keeping your abdominal muscles in good shape can also help prevent injury to your back.

Smoking is also a major health issue for men. See Smoking, p. 270, for more information on this topic.

Prostate Cancer

The prostate is an organ that surrounds the bladder opening and urethra of males. Enlargement of the prostate is a common disorder among men over 60 years of age. Cancer of the prostate is as common as lung cancer among males. However, less than 1 percent of men under age 50 have detectable prostate cancer. Past the age of 80, more than 50 percent of males have been shown to have some stage of prostate cancer.

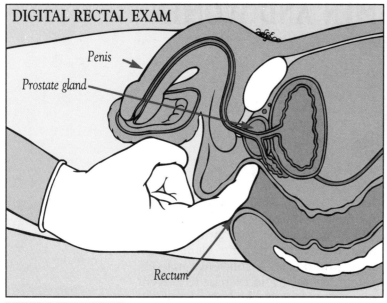

DIGITAL RECTAL EXAM

Penis

Prostate gland

Rectum

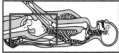

The digital (finger) rectal exam is the most commonly used method for early detection of prostate cancer. The doctor uses his or her finger to feel through the wall of the rectum for abnormal growth in the prostate.

Although prostate cancer is serious, only a small percentage of men who get the disease die of it.

If you have a relative (father or brother) who has had prostate cancer, you may be at higher risk for getting this cancer.

Symptoms

You should consider any block to your normal flow of urine a warning sign, even though such symptoms rarely mean you have cancer. Other more common problems such as **prostatitis** (infection of the prostate), stones, or a noncancerous growth of the prostate are the main causes of urinary problems.

What You Can Do

Several studies suggest that diets high in fat may contribute to prostate cancer. Countries with the highest fat consumption also have the highest prostate cancer rates. Other than growing older, there is little evidence that prostate cancer has early, easily identified symptoms. (Also see Cancer Prevention and Management, p. 253.)

Screening

There is no clear evidence that screenings are of value.

Prostate cancers are being diagnosed more often in younger and middle-aged men. The most commonly used method for early detection of prostate cancer is a digital rectal exam in which the doctor uses his or her finger to feel through the wall of the rectum for abnormal growth in the prostate (see illustration). However, because only part of the prostate can be felt, many prostate cancers are likely to be missed by such an exam. Studies also show that as often as 60 percent of the time an abnormal finding proves to be a false alarm after further tests.

Your doctor may also consider some of the new approaches for detecting prostate cancer, including transrectal ultrasound or a prostate-specific antigen blood test—especially if you are at high risk or if your rectal exam was abnormal. These tests, however, haven't been proved effective when used alone for screening. But when a digital rectal exam is abnormal, these screening studies greatly increase the rate of cancer detection.

Prostate Screening Recommendations

The National Cancer Institute and the American Cancer Society recommend a digital rectal exam every year for men over age 40. Recently, the U.S. Preventive Services Task Force recommendations differed. That Task Force concluded that for men without symptoms or special risk factors there is not enough evidence to recommend either for or against routine digital rectal exams. Other, more extensive prostate screening methods—such as transrectal ultrasound or prostate specific antigen testing—are not recommended for routine screening.

Testicular Cancer

Although cancer of the testes is pretty rare, it is the most common form of cancer in men between the ages of 20 and 35. It accounts for 12 percent of all cancer deaths in young men. It is four times more common among Caucasian men than African American men. Testicular cancer usually responds well to treatment, particularly when it is detected early. In most cases, it affects just one testicle, and the other remains perfectly healthy.

Understanding Your Risk

Testicular cancer can develop any time after puberty starts but is most common in men between the ages of 29 and 35. Men whose testes have not descended into the scrotum or did not descend until after age 6 are at a much higher risk for this type of cancer.

Screening Recommendations

Not all experts agree on how effectively testicular self-examination detects cancer. Nor do they agree on the need for men who have no special risk factors to have routine testicular examinations by a professional. If you have a history of undescended testes, however, you should be examined periodically by your doctor. If symptoms such as pain, swelling or heaviness in your testicles last as long as 2 weeks, you should see your doctor as soon as possible.

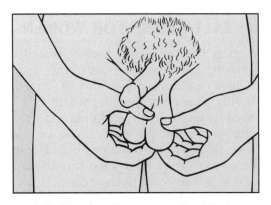

How to do a testicular self-exam—Begin by standing in front of a mirror. Look for signs of swelling in the scrotum. Next, examine each testicle with both hands. With your index and middle fingers underneath and your thumbs on top, gently roll each testicle, feeling for lumps.

SELF-CARE STEPS FOR TESTICULAR CANCER

While there is no way to prevent testicular cancer, organizations such as the National Cancer Institute and the American Cancer Society recommend that men do a monthly self-exam to check for possible lumps or nodules in the testes.

Testicular self-examination (TSE) is easy and takes only a few minutes. Testing is best done after a warm shower or bath, when the scrotal skin is relaxed. **You should see your doctor if you notice any of these symptoms:**

• Pain, swelling, or a feeling of heaviness in your scrotum or testicles

• A dull ache in your lower abdomen or groin

• A lump or a change in the way a testicle feels when examined

These symptoms may be signs of other illnesses, such as infections or other nonmalignant disorders, but you should let your doctor make the diagnosis. (Also see Cancer Prevention and Management, p. 253.)

HEALTH RISKS FOR WOMEN

Gender creates unique health issues for women. For the most part, these are related to reproductive and sexual health. The most obvious, perhaps, is the need for obstetrical care during and right after pregnancy. But even if you are not sexually active, or have never had children, you still need to take care of your sexual and reproductive systems.

Breast cancer and cervical cancer are perhaps the most easily detected diseases you may have as a woman. In addition to having a Pap smear and a breast exam, a routine gynecological examination gives your doctor a chance to check for other problems related to your reproductive system. For example, an internal pelvic exam can detect ovarian cysts, malignancy, or signs of infection. If you are using birth control pills or an intrauterine device (IUD), regular gynecological exams are very important.

If you are a smoker, you should be aware that 18 percent of cases of low birth weight, premature delivery, respiratory distress syndrome, and sudden infant death syndrome are caused by smoking during pregnancy. Regardless of pregnancy, smoking is bad for your health, and the benefits of quitting are tremendous.

Menopause is another time when routine exams can be very helpful for maintaining good health. For some women, hormone-replacement therapy can help relieve uncomfortable symptoms of menopause. Symptoms include unusual vaginal bleeding, which you may think is just a normal part of menopause but may actually be a sign of other more serious conditions, such as uterine or ovarian cancer. These problems may not be detected with a Pap smear, so it's important to mention your symptoms to your doctor.

Female hormones also play a role in osteoporosis. Lower estrogen levels after menopause can contribute to the bone loss of osteoporosis. Even though osteoporosis usually affects only postmenopausal women, it's important that women of all ages exercise regularly and get enough calcium in their daily diets to prevent osteoporosis later in life.

Back pain is also common among women. Practicing proper lifting and keeping abdominal muscles strong should protect you from sprains and strains.

Breast Cancer

Breast cancer is the most common type of cancer in American women. Each year in the United States, more than 182,000 women learn they have this disease. Although breast cancer may not be prevented, it often can be survived. Early detection increases the breast cancer survival rate. Women with small, localized breast cancers (where the cancer has not spread beyond the breast) have a 90 percent chance of living more than 10 years after cancer treatment.

Understanding the Risk

The average woman has a one-in-eight chance of having breast cancer during her lifetime. Several factors, however, can increase your risk:

Family history. Your risk doubles if your mother or sister has had breast cancer. It is even higher if they developed breast cancer before menopause.

Premalignant cells on biopsy. Women who have had a previous breast biopsy that was benign but showed certain suspicious cells are at increased risk.

Age. Two-thirds of all breast cancers occur in women over 50. As you grow older, your risk increases.

Childbirth and menstruation. Never having children, or giving birth to your first child after age 30, increases your risk of breast cancer. Having your period begin before the age of 12 or starting menopause after the age of 50 may also add to your risk.

Other factors. Other factors linked to breast cancer include obesity and a history of ovarian or endometrial cancer. Even so, the most important risk factors are growing older and a personal or family history of breast cancer. You'll want to be very careful if you are at a higher risk. (Also see Cancer Prevention and Management, p. 253.)

Screening Tests

Mammograms. The most effective early detection method available today is mammography—a low-dose X-ray of the breast. Mammograms can detect breast cancers while they are very small, sometimes 2 years earlier than they can be felt by a woman or her doctor.

In the past 25 years, mammograms have improved considerably. The X-rays are much more sensitive, and far less radiation is used. Today we use 1/40 the amount of radiation required just 20 years ago. The risk of 10 mammograms causing breast cancer is one in 25,000—much less than many of the normal risks of daily life.

Mammography, however, is not perfect. In some cases, a lump that you can feel during a breast exam may not appear on a mammogram. The lump would still need to be checked, even if the mammogram is normal. Mammography, like most other tests, can also show abnormal results where there is no cancer. This occurs in about one out of every 100 mammograms.

Professional breast exam. Many doctors do routine breast exams for women of all ages during general physicals or pelvic exams. The doctor will check each breast using fingertips to feel for lumps, and look for other suspicious changes—such as dimpled, scaling, or puckered skin or fluid leaking from the nipple. When combined with a mammogram, a breast exam by a doctor is the best way to detect cancer in its early stages.

Breast self-exam. Many women are afraid to examine their breasts because of what they might find. Most breast lumps are not cancerous. Even if a breast lump is cancerous, your best defense is early detection. Breast self-examination (BSE), described on p. 263, is easy and takes only about 5 minutes a month. Among women with breast cancer, 34 percent said they first discovered their breast cancer through BSE. BSE is a way to discover any change from what is "normal" for you. Your doctor can review this technique with you.

Scheduling Breast Screening Exams

Mammograms. The Institute for Clinical Systems Integration recommends a baseline mammogram between ages 35 and 40 only for women with any high-risk factors (p. 260). Between the ages of 40 and 49, all women should have a mammogram at least once every 2 years. A yearly mammogram is recommended for women over the age of 50.

Other experts, such as the panel of the U. S. Preventive Services Task Force, say women who are not at special risk for breast cancer do not need breast exams by their doctor until they are age 40 and that regular mammograms are not needed until age 50. There is little debate, however, that women with special risk factors should begin routine mammograms and breast exams at about age 35.

They also suggest that women who have not had breast cancer detected may stop mammography screening at age 75.

The American Cancer Society recommends that women start having mammograms every 1 to 2 years at age 40. After age 50, the ACS recommends women have a mammogram once each year.

After looking at research from around the world on the potential benefits and harms of mammography for women younger than age 50, the National Cancer Institute concluded that there is no clear overall benefit and also no clear overall harm to using this screening test for women under the age of 50.

However, many people in the medical community still disagree on this issue. Now that you know more about these issues, you may want to discuss your options with your doctor or nurse practitioner. Whether or not you decide to have a mammogram at this time, it's important to remember that regular breast self-exams and clinical breast exams by your doctor are wise practices to follow for early detection of breast cancer.

Breast self-exam (BSE). There is some disagreement in the medical community about the effectiveness of BSE. Some believe BSE is not very accurate and can create needless anxiety and expense. This is especially true for younger women who have no special risk factors. However, those who say there is not enough evidence in favor of monthly BSE do not advise women who already do a self-exam to stop.

Performing a Breast Self-Exam

Despite the disagreement about breast self-exams, many health professionals strongly recommend that women perform monthly breast self-examinations (BSE) to increase their chances for early detection if they develop breast cancer. In fact, the American Cancer Society recommends monthly BSE for all women age 19 and older. The procedure is actually quite simple and takes only about 5 minutes a month.

The best time to do BSE is 1 week after the start of your period. If you have already passed through menopause, do BSE on the first day of each month. If you've had a hysterectomy, ask your doctor to advise you on the best time for you to perform BSE.

What to Look For

It's normal for women's breasts to feel lumpy, to swell, or to become tender, especially around the time of menstruation. By performing BSE each month, you will become familiar with the feel, shape, and size of your breasts, making it easier for you to notice changes should they occur. **Here are some things to look for while examining your breasts:**

- New lumps or changes in the size or shape of existing lumps

- Change in the shape or contour of your breasts or unusual swelling

- Changes in skin color or texture

- Dimpling, puckering, crusting, or rash in the skin, especially around the nipple

- Any fluid leaking from the nipple

Remember that even if you have some of these signs, it doesn't necessarily mean you have breast cancer. Most breast lumps are not cancerous. You should call your doctor if you notice any lumps or changes that concern you. He or she can tell you if you should schedule an appointment.

HOW TO DO A BREAST SELF-EXAM

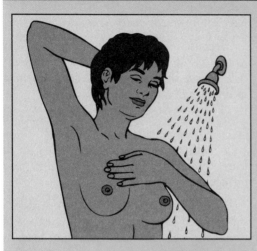

1. While in the shower, raise your right arm, placing your hand on the back of your head. Starting at the outer edge of the right breast, use the pads of the fingertips of your left hand. Feel for lumps or changes as you firmly move your fingers in small circles, working in a spiral toward the nipple. Check the other side in the same way, then gently squeeze each nipple to check for any discharge.

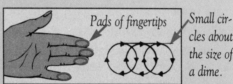

Pads of fingertips   Small circles about the size of a dime.

2. After your shower, clasp your hands together and raise your arms above your head with elbows bent. In a mirror, look for changes in shape or contour, as well as any skin changes, such as dimpling or rashes.

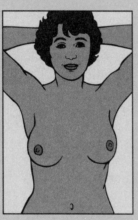

3. Still standing before the mirror, lower your arms. Place your hands on your hips, pull your shoulders and elbows forward, and lean slightly toward the mirror. Look again for any changes in shape or contour, and for skin changes.

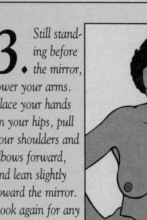

4. Finally, lying down, place a rolled towel or pillow under one shoulder and place the hand on that same side over your head. Examine your breast again as you did in the shower, this time checking your armpit as well. Repeat this on the other breast.

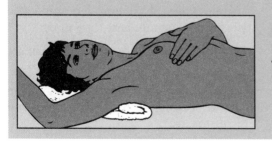

5. Call your doctor if you find anything that concerns you. After age 50, the Institute for Clinical Systems Integration recommends annual mammograms for all women.

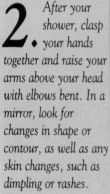

I know that a woman has a 1-in-8 chance of developing breast cancer during her lifetime. And I understand that premenopausal breast cancer is a more aggressive disease than breast cancer that develops later in life. I'm very concerned for myself, and so I'll be having a mammogram every other year until I'm 50. Then I'll have yearly mammograms.

Aritha, age 42

I've read the statistics on breast cancer, and most—75 percent—of the women who get it are over age 50. We don't have a family history of the disease, and I don't have any of the other risk factors. I practice breast self-exams and have exams done by my doctor regularly. I won't be having mammograms until I'm 50.

Eloise, age 46

Several of my friends have had breast cancer and my co-worker died from it. But I know that there's a chance that even if I have a mammogram—and it's negative—I could still have breast cancer. I think I will talk this over with my doctor and then decide on the best plan for future mammograms.

Christine, age 39

I hadn't been in to see my doctor for a Pap smear in years. But my daughter kept reminding me about the importance of having this screening test, so I started going for a Pap test again.

Betty, age 62

My doctor recommends I see her every year for a breast exam. I plan to continue regular yearly visits, even though I need a Pap smear only every 2 or 3 years.

Linda, age 41

My friends always tell me how much they dread having Pap smears done. But when one of my co-workers was diagnosed with cervical cancer, I decided it would be smart for me to start having Pap tests. After my first one, I found it wasn't as bad as my friends told me it would be!

Kathy, age 19

Cervical Cancer

The most effective early cervical cancer detection method available today is the Pap test, or Pap smear. It is a simple procedure that involves swabbing a small sample of cells from a woman's cervix and transferring them to a slide. The cells are then examined and evaluated by a certified laboratory.

Women should begin having regular Pap smears at age 18 or earlier if they are sexually active. There is some disagreement about when women should stop having Pap smears. Some say there is no upper age limit; others suggest having your last Pap smear at age 65 if there is no history of problems. Talk with your doctor about your situation.

Done regularly, Pap smears make it possible for doctors to find early evidence of cervical cancer. This can be done before any visible symptoms are present, when the disease is easier to cure. Also see Cancer Prevention and Management, p. 253.

Cervical cancer is one of the most common female cancers in the United States. It is diagnosed in an estimated 13,500 women yearly. About 4,400 women die each year from the disease. For those women diagnosed early, the survival rate is 89 percent. If the disease hasn't spread, the survival rate is virtually 100 percent.

Scheduling Pap Smears

Most women consider the Pap smear and pelvic exam to be the major part of an annual checkup. The tradition has been to have a "yearly Pap and pelvic."

However, a panel of experts analyzed the most recent scientific and medical research about Pap smears and concluded:

While it is extremely important to have Pap smears on a regular basis, it is no longer considered necessary for most women to have a Pap smear every year.

Because most cervical cancers grow very slowly, a Pap smear done every 2 to 3 years will provide the same early detection benefit as an annual Pap smear.

You may be able to extend the interval between Pap smears to 2 to 3 years if you have had annual normal Pap smears for at least 3 years in a row (documented in your medical records).

More frequent Pap smears are still recommended for women with a history of abnormal cell changes that may lead to cancer in the next 5 years and for women who are HIV positive (or otherwise immunosuppressed).

You and your doctor can decide together on a Pap smear schedule that is most appropriate for you. Remember that he or she may recommend more frequent visits for other reasons—such as a breast exam—depending on your age and health status.

For Best Results

Try to schedule your periodic health exam (that may include a Pap smear) to take place about 1 week before the start of your period. If this isn't possible, at least try to avoid the days when your menstrual flow is heaviest.

Don't use a vaginal douche or any type of vaginal medication or lubricant for 24 hours before having a Pap smear.

Help your physician determine the Pap smear schedule best for you by:

- Telling him or her the approximate dates of your previous Pap smears.

- Discussing any concerns you may have about waiting 2 to 3 years between Pap smears.

LIFESTYLE CHOICES

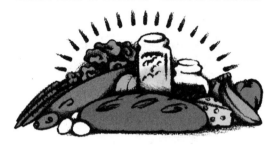

DIET

A "balanced diet" means eating a variety of foods that supply calories and nutrients you need without excess fat, salt, sugar, or alcohol.

Daily, each person needs more than 50 nutrients from food, including those that supply calories (carbohydrates, protein, and fat) and those that help with various body functions (vitamins, minerals, and water). Despite claims to the contrary, there are no known advantages to consuming large quantities of a specific nutrient or food.

The amount of food you need depends on your age, gender, physical condition, and activity level. Almost everyone should have at least the minimum number of servings from each food group daily. Many men, women, older children, and most teenagers need more. When grocery shopping, and planning and preparing meals for yourself and others, use this guide to maintain a healthy weight.

- Choose foods daily from each of the five major groups shown in the Food Guide Pyramid. (See illustration, page 266.)

- Include a variety of different foods from each group to balance calorie and nutrient needs.

- Choose, most often, foods that are low in fat.

- Go easy on sweets, salt, and alcoholic beverages.

Eat Less Fat

The U.S. Department of Agriculture 1990 *Dietary Guidelines for Americans* notes the health benefits of low-fat, fiber-rich food choices. Eating the typical high-fat American diet can increase your risk of heart disease, certain cancers, and obesity. It's recommended that adults and children over the age of two get no more than 30 percent of their calories from fat.

Fat is the most concentrated calorie source. By reducing the amount of fat, you can also reduce your calorie intake. Cutting down on total fat will help you reduce the amount of saturated (cholesterol-raising) fat in your diet (see Obesity, p. 232).

Eat More High-Fiber Foods

Getting fewer calories from fat means you'll need to increase your carbohydrate-rich choices: legumes, breads, grains, pasta, rice, fruits, and vegetables. Carbohydrates include simple sugars and complex carbohydrates (starches and fibers). Most foods contain a combination of these carbohydrate sources. Although there's no major health risk associated with simple sugars (other than tooth decay and excess calories), getting more complex carbohydrates will give you a better balance of vitamins, minerals, and fiber.

Fiber is found in all plant foods. Studies have shown that eating foods high in fiber may help lower blood

THE FOOD GUIDE PYRAMID

Build your diet from the bottom up. *Grains, fruits, and vegetables should make up the bulk of your diet. These foods supply energizing carbohydrates, help replace those unwanted fat calories, and supply fiber.*

Don't count on one food group to do it all. *You need more than 50 different nutrients, and no one food group has them all. Have at least the minimum number of servings from each group.*

Eat regularly to keep energy flowing. *Don't go longer than 5 hours without food. Develop an eye for portion size. The number of servings from each food group may sound like a lot, but it's really not. For example, a cup of pasta is two bread servings. One serving of meat is the size of a deck of cards.*

Don't feel guilty about an occasional treat. *But remember, occasional doesn't mean daily, either.*

Fats, Oils, & Sweets
Use sparingly

Milk, Yogurt, & Cheese
2–3 servings

Meat, Poultry, Fish, Beans, Nuts, & Eggs
2–3 servings

Vegetables
3–5 servings

Fruits
2–4 servings

Breads & Grains 6–11 servings

cholesterol, reduce the risk of heart disease, and protect against certain cancers and digestive diseases.

Dietary guidelines encourage eating a variety of foods, decreasing fats, and increasing carbohydrates. The Food Guide Pyramid (above) was developed by the U.S. Department of Agriculture to show the ideal proportions of the foods we eat each day. Study the Pyramid and think of your present eating patterns, so you can make goals that bring you closer to eating the amounts of foods suggested.

EXERCISE

Exercise is very good for you. It would be difficult to find any other health habit with so many good side effects. Exercise increases longevity and reduces the risk of heart disease, diabetes, hypertension, and osteoporosis. And increasing your activity level will help you resist stress, and may help lower your blood pressure and cholesterol. While there is a predictable decline in health and stamina during the middle years, those who stay physically active have nearly twice as much endurance as those who are not active.

How much exercise is enough? Two recent studies may have the answer. A review of the 25-year exercise history of almost 17,000 Harvard alumni revealed that those who were more active lived longer—up to 2 years longer—than their sedentary counterparts. Health improvements resulted from burning as little as 500 calories per week through exercise. However, burning 2,000 calories provided the best health benefits.

In another study, 13,000 men and women were divided into five fitness groups. The least-fit group had, by far, the highest number of deaths. But surprisingly, the most dramatic drop in death rate occurred in the second-least-fit group. This group exercised moderately—the equivalent of 30 to 60 minutes of walking per day—for a weekly total of 1,000 to 2,000 calories burned.

These studies dispel the idea that activity has to be aerobic to produce a health benefit. There is convincing evidence that lower intensity activities like walking, gardening, or golfing have very favorable health benefits. Ultimately, doing any activities that use up to 2,000 calories per week is a healthy goal. Use the chart on page 268 to estimate how your various calorie-burning activities are adding up to better health.

Fitness and Weight Control

Exercise is closely linked to success in weight control. Indeed, doctors and dietitians now believe that trying to control weight without exercise is counterproductive. Since using your muscles is what burns calories, balancing your calorie needs in the future depends on keeping your muscles in shape. If you are not active, your muscles weaken and you need fewer calories to fuel your body.

Unfortunately, if you are like most people, you continue to eat the same amount of calories you did years ago when you may have been more active, thereby replacing muscle with fat. Also, if you lose weight and you are not exercising, you are likely to lose even more muscle. This starts a cycle that leads to a body composed of increasingly more fat and less muscle and, ultimately, needing fewer and fewer calories. That is why many dieters report that it becomes harder to lose weight every time they try. Making time for exercise is the most effective way to avoid middle-age spread.

What You Can Do

The risks of not exercising far outweigh the risks of exercise. Still, for those with existing chronic illness—such as diabetes, heart disease, or high blood pressure—an exercise test would be a good idea before you start an exercise program. Competitive athletes often suffer sports injuries, but moderate activity rarely leads to injury. In fact, the intense type of exercise—the kind that leads to injuries related to wear and tear on the joints—is simply not necessary to achieve long-term health benefits.

EXERCISE AND CALORIES	
EXERCISE ACTIVITIES	**CALORIES BURNED***
Biking (5 1/2 mph)	210
Walking (2 1/2 mph)	210
Gardening	220
Golf	250
Swimming	300
Walking (4 mph)	300
Tennis, doubles	300
Biking (10 mph)	415
Tennis, singles	420
Aerobics	445
Jogging	585
Running (8 1/2 mph)	700
Cross-country skiing	900

Average calories burned for a 150-pound person in an hour of activity.

From **Lifetime Fitness and Wellness 4th Edition** by *Werner W. K. Hoeger and Sharon A. Hoeger. Copyright 1995 Morton Publishing Co., Engelwood, CO. Reprinted with permission.*

How to Get Started

- Get off to a slow start! If you are just beginning, 30 minutes of walking three times a week is plenty. Move slowly toward a daily routine of 30 minutes of activities you enjoy. But only increase your activities when you feel your present level is getting too easy.

- Keep a diary of your activity. As your entries build so will your commitment.

- Avoid high-impact activities. Try low-impact activities like walking, swimming, or biking, especially if your joints are sore.

- Try a variety of activities to keep exercise fresh and interesting.

- Exercise at the same time every day. If you can't lock into a regular time, then schedule your exercise in advance—as an appointment to keep with yourself. There is some evidence that people are more successful at sticking with a morning routine.

- Join a club or start a regular routine with friends to add a social element to your activity.

The Activity Pyramid

There is no secret formula for deciding how much exercise is enough or which types of activities are best. The Activity Pyramid was developed to show the relative value of different types of exercise. In general, when it comes to activity, the more, the better. Examine the Activity Pyramid on p. 269 to help think about your current activities and make goals for the future.

THE ACTIVITY PYRAMID

Each week, try to increase your physical activity using this guide. Here's how to start...

If you are inactive
(Rarely active)

Increase daily activities at the *base* of the Activity Pyramid by:

- Taking the stairs instead of the elevator
- Hiding the TV remote control
- Making extra trips around the house or yard
- Stretching while standing in line
- Walking whenever you can

If you are somewhat active
(Active some of the time, but not regularly)

Increase activity in the *middle* of the pyramid by:

- Finding activities you enjoy
- Planning activities in your day
- Setting realistic goals

If you are often active
(Active most of the time, or at least 4 days each week)

Include activities from the *whole* pyramid by:

- Changing your routine if you start to get bored
- Exploring new activities

**Above all...
Have fun
and good luck!**

CUT DOWN ON
- *Watching TV*
- *Computer games*
- *Sitting for more than 30 minutes at a time*

2–3 TIMES A WEEK

LEISURE ACTIVITIES
- *Golf*
- *Bowling*
- *Softball*
- *Yardwork*

FLEXIBILITY & STRENGTH
- *Stretching and yoga*
- *Push-ups/curl-ups*
- *Weight lifting*

3–5 TIMES A WEEK

AEROBIC EXERCISE
(20+ minutes)
- *Brisk walking*
- *Cross-country skiing*
- *Bicycling*
- *Swimming*

RECREATIONAL
(30+ minutes)
- *Soccer*
- *Basketball*
- *Martial arts*
- *Hiking*
- *Tennis*
- *Dancing*

EVERY DAY
OR AS MUCH AS POSSIBLE

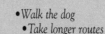

- *Walk the dog*
- *Take longer routes*
- *Take the stairs instead of the elevator*

BE CREATIVE IN FINDING A VARIETY OF WAYS TO STAY ACTIVE

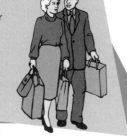

- *Walk to the store or the mailbox*
- *Park your car farther away*
- *Add extra steps to your day*

Adapted from **Activity Pyramid**. Copyright 1995 Park Nicollet Medical Foundation. Reprinted with permission.

SMOKING

Years ago, smokers were left alone to enjoy their habit. Those days are gone. It's getting to be more and more of a hassle to be a smoker. And given the overwhelming evidence that tobacco use is very hazardous to health, most smokers want to quit. In fact, estimates are that 80 percent of smokers want to quit and most have tried several times. The good news is that each failed attempt puts you one try closer to reaching your goal of becoming a nonsmoker.

And the reasons to keep trying to quit are more compelling than ever. According to the Centers for Infectious Disease Control, one out of every six deaths in America is related to smoking. Smoking is responsible for large numbers of deaths from cancer, heart attacks, stroke, and lung disease. About 18 percent of cases of low birth weight, premature deliveries, respiratory distress syndrome (SIDS), and sudden infant death syndrome are linked to smoking during pregnancy. And, 25 percent of all deaths from home fires are from fires that were started by smoking materials.

Lung cancer isn't the only cancer caused by smoking; others include cancer of the larynx, esophagus, kidneys, pancreas, and stomach. Although many people may believe smokeless (chewing) tobacco poses fewer health hazards than do cigarettes and other smoking tobacco, it can cause cancer of the mouth. Tobacco of all kinds is one of the most potent cancer-causing agents for humans.

More than 50 million Americans—slightly less than one-quarter of the population—smoke, and another 10 million use smokeless tobacco. Because tobacco is both physically and psychologically addictive, quitting is often hard—but it's not impossible. Some smokers must make several attempts before they actually quit smoking for life.

The health benefits of quitting are tremendous. After 5 to 15 years of non-smoking, ex-smokers' risks of developing heart and lung diseases, cancer, and lung problems drop to the same—or nearly the same—levels as if they had never smoked.

Obviously, if you don't smoke, don't start. But if you do smoke, here are some tips to help you quit.

Steps to Quitting

- Set your goal. Pick a date on which to stop smoking and plan to quit completely and for good. Switching to a lower-tar brand or cutting back just doesn't work.

- Take it one day at a time. Focus on making it through today without a cigarette, rather than on how you will go without one for the next week. If you do falter and light up, don't give up. Forgive yourself and work on resisting the next one.

- Find support. Tell as many as 10 friends that you are quitting, then take advantage of as much encouragement and prodding as they can give you. Check in with your doctor for support, as well. He or she may be able to prescribe a nicotine substitute to help you. Organizations such as the American Lung Association and the American Cancer Society offer classes and support groups for people trying to quit smoking. Many employers and health care providers also offer such help.

- Find a substitute. Avoid the temptation to smoke by finding other things to keep your mouth and hands busy. Try sugarless gum, hard candy, or flavored toothpicks. Try woodworking, needlework, snapping a rubber band on your wrist, or playing with fidget toys.

- Exercise to avoid weight gain. If you're afraid of gaining weight, keep in mind that the average weight gain after quitting smoking is only 5 pounds. Only 3 percent of those who quit smoking gain 20 pounds or more. While you are quitting, eat a well-balanced diet and avoid excess calories in sugary or fatty foods, drink six to eight glasses of water a day, and exercise. By walking just 30 minutes a day or doing some other activity, you will ward off excess pounds and ease some of the tension of tobacco withdrawal.

- Avoid smoking situations. Go places where smoking isn't allowed, such as the nonsmoking section of a restaurant or a movie theater. Take your work breaks with nonsmoking co-workers. After eating, take a walk or do the dishes instead of lighting up a cigarette. When you can't avoid a smoking situation, plan in advance for ways to curb the desire to smoke, such as having sugarless gum or a healthy snack close by.

YOUR PERSONAL HEALTH RECORD

Test — Age:	20	22	24	26	28	30	32	34	36	38	40	42	44	46	48	50	52	54	56	58	60	62	64	66 or over
Blood Pressure Every 2 years, more often if at risk																								
Cholesterol Every 5 years, more often if at risk																								
Diptheria/Tetanus Every 10 years																								
Influenza Yearly from age 65																								
Pneumococcal Vaccine Once, at age 65																								
Hearing Every 2 yrs. from age 65																								
Vision/Glaucoma Every 3 yrs. from age 65																								
Hemoglobin, Urinalysis, Rubella Titer																								
Rectal Exam and Hemoccult																								
Sigmoidoscopy																								
WOMEN																								
Pap Smear and Pelvic Exam																								
Professional Breast Exam Every year from age 40																								
Mammography Every 2 yrs. from age 40; yearly from age 50																								

This table provides a way to chart your screening tests and immunizations. Use the following letters to record what happened during your last visit. Enter (A) if you met with your doctor but took no tests; (B) if a test was completed and passed with no problems; or (C) if tests indicated health problems.

SECTION FIVE: HEALTH CARE CONSUMERS AND SHARED DECISIONS

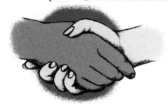

As in any other industry, professionals in health care should be expected to offer the best service at the most reasonable price if they expect to keep you as a customer. But how do you know if you are getting the best results for your money? And why is it that health care has grown to such a large American industry? The government, insurance plans, doctors, nurses, technicians, hospitals, and employers are all concerned about the rising cost of health care. Yet, they all seem to be looking in different places for the solution to this troubling national problem. Where does that leave you, the health care consumer?

If you answered, "Confused," you're not alone.

Few people understand the full complexities of the changing American health care system. But one thing is certain: Individuals play one of the most important roles in the battle against rising health care costs. Each consumer decides when to get health care and what type of service to use. These decisions have a very big impact on the cost of health care.

Becoming an active, prudent consumer requires some effort and some new ways of thinking and behaving. But it's clearly the best route to ensuring your good health and your financial well-being.

This section explains some of the reasons why health care costs are off the scale and what you can do about it.

SEEKING QUALITY HEALTH CARE

Because so much is riding on your decisions, consumers need to make wise choices about health care. You need information and skills to make those decisions. And you need to become an active partner with your doctors in dealing with your own health and well-being.

You can start by building a relationship with a primary care doctor such as a family practitioner or internist. Since there are no industry standards for health care quality, a primary care doctor can ensure that diagnostic tests and treatment recommendations from other doctors are appropriate, based on your history and health problems. A long-term relationship with your primary care doctor results in consistent treatment that meets your needs. Such coordinated care improves the quality of your care and lowers costs.

Finding Good Health Care

Concerned consumers of any products need accurate, up-to-date information to judge the quality of their purchases. The same is true for health care consumers. Most of us hold onto old ideas from the days when we followed the doctor's orders without question. Times have changed, and so should our attitudes about medical care.

When it comes to your health, there are basically four health care providers that have the best chance to offer you successful treatment and prevent problems. Understanding how each of these contributors can influence your choices is the first step in finding quality care.

You

Many people believe that the doctor's role is to manage their health care. But when it comes down to it, you are the one who does the real managing. You decide when to seek care and whether or not to follow your doctor's advice. You also decide how to live your life— whether you will exercise, what foods you will eat, and what risks you will take with your health.

Your Doctor

Doctors can guide you to better health. But they can't cure everything. Our doctors are our link to medical science, but they might not always have the answers. A good doctor will admit uncertainty and seek help and advice from other health care professionals when needed. Keep in mind that more treatment, testing, or medication doesn't necessarily mean better care. And no matter how good your doctor is, all medical care involves some risk.

The Pharmacy

Whether it's self-care, over-the-counter remedies, or a prescription drug, your drugstore is often the place to find the tools you need to control or relieve illness. Pharmacists can guide you through the maze of over-the-counter drugs. They can also give you clear directions on how to care for minor problems yourself or how to follow your doctor's advice on prescription drugs.

The Hospital

In the past, most medical tests and surgery were performed in the hospital and often required an overnight stay. Advances in technology, changes in philosophy, and findings that people tend to recover more quickly at home have led the way for many forms of minor surgery and lab tests to be performed on an outpatient basis. When hospitalization is needed, recovery often comes more quickly if you return home as soon as you are medically ready, rather than staying in the hospital an extra day or two.

Choosing Necessary, Appropriate Care

Wise health care consumers choose only needed and appropriate health care services. But just what is needed and appropriate when it comes to health care?

Needed care is medical care required to improve or preserve your health. Getting childhood vaccinations, setting broken bones, and treating serious infections are all examples of necessary care.

Appropriate care means weighing your options and choosing procedures best suited to your circumstances. Appropriate care is different for everyone. If you have severe headaches, appropriate care might be as simple as pain relievers and relaxation exercises. If your headaches and other symptoms make your doctor suspect a serious problem, such as a brain tumor, expensive tests and procedures such as CT scans, MRIs, and surgery may be considered appropriate care. Appropriate care doesn't mean you can't have expensive tests when you need them. It means not having an MRI when an aspirin will do the trick.

Unfortunately, our health care system hasn't worked this way. All too often, patients have expensive, inappropriate, or repeated procedures. They usually don't object because they are just following doctors' orders. Besides, the insurance companies pay for it all. Right? Wrong. In the end, we all end up paying for inappropriate care through higher medical costs and insurance rates. In fact, that kind of wastefulness is a major reason why our medical costs are skyrocketing.

We're not paying more for health care because we're getting better, faster, or more effective medical services. Too often, we're paying more because new technologies and procedures are overused.

What You Can Do

The best way to track down high-quality, reasonably priced medical care is by becoming an active, prudent consumer. This means:

- Staying healthy through lifestyle choices, exercise, nutrition, and preventive health care that can reduce the risk of needing treatment.

- Asking questions and gathering information so that you can actively participate in decisions about your health.

A New Direction

Your role as an active consumer is to seek a doctor group that is continually improving the quality of health care. Such a group will focus on weighing the results of patient care, using a single medical record that contains your complete medical history, and developing medical practice guidelines. The successful health practitioners of the future will not only follow standard procedures for care, they will be able to show why their approach is more effective than other approaches. Staying informed as new options in health care arise is one of the best ways to keep your own health care headed in the right direction—toward higher quality and lower cost.

It is important to find a doctor who matches your needs and values. Finding a doctor with whom you feel comfortable and building an ongoing relationship helps you get the best possible care.

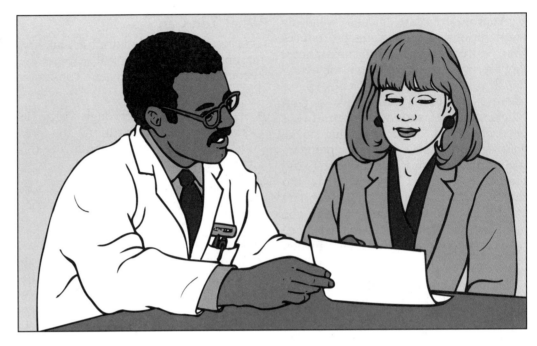

CHOOSING A DOCTOR

Having a good talk with your doctor may be the best medicine around. Studies show that patients who are satisfied with how comfortably they can discuss problems with their doctors tend to recover from illnesses more easily. Still, for many people a trip to the doctor is stressful. And unless you are prepared to play an active role during your visit, you are apt to forget much of what the doctor tells you, and you will be less likely to follow his or her advice.

Finding a Good Match

Finding a doctor with whom you feel comfortable can make a big difference in the quality of your health care. Doctors, like everyone else, vary widely in their communication skills and the value they place on the personal aspects of your relationship. It is very important, then, that you establish a relationship with a doctor who matches your needs and values.

Use your first meeting with your doctor as a time to explore your expectations of one another. In fact, your first meeting doesn't have to be for an examination. Many doctors are willing to meet with prospective patients for informational interviews. In addition to increasing the doctor's knowledge of your medical history, the interview will help him or her understand how much of the medical decision-making you wish to participate in and how much information you want about your health condition. One study showed that doctors often underestimate how much information patients want, but they overestimate their patients' desire to be in on personal health decisions.

For some people, a good relationship with a doctor is a very important part of their health care. For others, the doctor's personality and communication skills can be overlooked so long as he or she is highly skilled and knowledgeable. If you fall in the first group and are seeing a doctor who, although highly skilled, has a poor bedside manner, you may be better off changing doctors. If you are in the second group, however, you may well think this type of doctor is highly professional.

No matter what it is you look for in a doctor, it's important that you find one with whom you feel comfortable and confident—even if that means changing doctors. But remember that an ongoing relationship with a doctor increases your chances of getting the best possible health care.

Your Doctor as Educator

The average adult visits the doctor more than four times a year, and the most common reason for a visit is for preventive services such as physical exams or health screening. Many find the doctor's advice about preventing health problems to be very motivating, so judge a doctor on how interested he or she is in your personal health habits. Will the doctor advise you on habits such as drinking and smoking? Is the doctor concerned about your diet or exercise practices? Finally, keep in mind that most of the health problems you will face are chronic conditions such as high blood pressure or diabetes—conditions that require long-term care involving many health professionals. So find out if your doctor works well with other health care team members such as dietitians, physical therapists, counselors, and health educators. When it comes to handling long-term health problems, a team approach is considered the most effective. Keep in mind that an effective team approach is one where you are at the center of the team, involved and communicating your needs clearly and consistently. Choose a doctor you want on your team, working as an expert, concerned partner.

PREPARING FOR AN OFFICE VISIT

Of the many barriers to effective communication during a typical visit to a health care provider, the most common is time. A typical visit lasts 15 to 20 minutes, during which evaluation, diagnosis, treatment planning, and teaching occur. Accordingly, you need to present your most pressing problem to the doctor and avoid bringing a laundry list of other unrelated complaints. To avoid communication problems:

- Write down your most important concerns. Before your visit, review all of your symptoms, including when they started; the history of the problem, including whether you've had the problem before; and any treatments you have tried. List these things in order of importance to you so you will be sure to get your most pressing concerns answered.

- Bring related records. If you have information about drugs you use, allergies, or other health problems, bring these records along if you are seeing a doctor for the first time. If your appointment is with a doctor you've been with for a while, be sure to let him or her know what over-the-counter remedies you are using and whether you are taking medicine prescribed by another doctor.

- Be brief and clear. As you describe your symptoms to your doctor, avoid vague statements like "I've been feeling sick lately." Be specific: "I've had a headache and nausea for the past week, and I don't know what's causing it."

Making the Most of Your Visit

Researchers have interviewed patients after office visits and learned that over half of the doctors' instructions are routinely forgotten within minutes of the visit. It is difficult for you to benefit from the doctor's good advice if you can't remember the details. Here are three ways to increase your recollection of the visit:

- Take notes. Even if you can't write down everything you hear, an outline of the discussion will dramatically increase your memory of the information. Take some time immediately after the visit to fill in other details you remember about the discussion. It may also help to talk your visit over with a friend or family member soon afterward.

- Ask for information that is organized. Studies on communication show that understanding improves a lot when information is well organized. Ask the doctor to put information into categories such as what is wrong, information about tests, treatment approaches, and, finally, advice about what you must do.

- Ask for explanations. When in doubt about a term your doctor uses—ask. A good way to ensure that you understand is to restate what you believe the doctor has told you. Then if you've misunderstood something, your doctor can explain it again.

FAMILY AND PERSONAL MEDICAL HISTORY

Keeping good medical records is an important part of being an active health care consumer.

Many health problems run in families. Other health problems are easier to anticipate when you and your doctor have a complete picture of your personal medical history. That's why it's important to keep up-to-date records of your family and personal medical history. Make copies of the Family Medical History worksheet on p. 279 and Your Medical History worksheet on p. 280, and complete one for yourself and for each member of your family. Keep them with your medical records and update them as necessary.

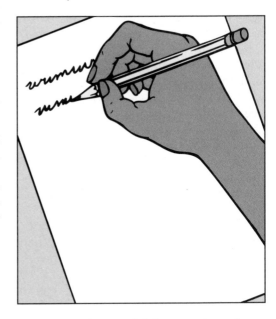

Keeping up-to-date records helps you and your doctor have a complete picture of your medical history.

FAMILY MEDICAL HISTORY

Blood Relative:	Significant Health Problem	If Deceased: Cause of Death/Age at Death
Mother	_____	_____
Father	_____	_____
Brothers & Sisters	_____	_____
	_____	_____
	_____	_____

Mother's Side:		
Grandfather	_____	_____
Grandmother	_____	_____
Aunts & Uncles	_____	_____
	_____	_____

Father's Side:		
Grandfather	_____	_____
Grandmother	_____	_____
Aunts & Uncles	_____	_____
	_____	_____

Have any of your blood relatives (mother, father, brothers, sisters, grandparents, aunts, uncles) had any of the following diseases or conditions?

Condition	Name/Relationship	Condition	Name/Relationship
❑ Allergies	_____	❑ Glaucoma	_____
❑ Anemia or other blood disorder	_____	❑ Heart disease	_____
❑ Arthritis	_____	❑ High blood pressure	_____
❑ Asthma	_____	❑ High blood cholesterol	_____
❑ Bowel disorder	_____	❑ Liver disease	_____
❑ Cancer	_____	❑ Lung disease	_____
❑ Cataracts	_____	❑ Nervous system disorder	_____
❑ Diabetes	_____	❑ Stroke	_____
❑ Eczema	_____	❑ Thyroid disorder (type:_____)	_____
❑ Emphysema	_____	❑ Ulcer	_____
❑ Epilepsy	_____	❑ Other	_____

YOUR MEDICAL HISTORY

Name _____

Date of birth _____

Blood type _____

Acute Diseases

Disease	Date of Illness
❑ Chicken pox	_____
❑ Ear infection	_____
❑ German measles (rubella)	_____
❑ Hepatitis	_____
❑ HIV	_____
❑ Mononucleosis	_____
❑ Measles	_____
❑ Mumps	_____
❑ Polio	_____
❑ Scarlet fever	_____
❑ Sexually transmitted disease	_____
❑ Sinus infection	_____
❑ Strep throat	_____
❑ Whooping cough	_____
❑ Other	_____

Chronic Disorders

Disorder	Date Diagnosed	Treatment
❑ Arthritis	_____	_____
❑ Asthma	_____	_____
❑ Blood disorder	_____	_____
❑ Cataracts	_____	_____
❑ Diabetes	_____	_____
❑ Epilepsy	_____	_____
❑ Gastrointestinal disorder	_____	_____
❑ Glaucoma	_____	_____
❑ Heart disease	_____	_____
❑ High blood pressure	_____	_____
❑ High blood cholesterol	_____	_____
❑ Kidney disease	_____	_____
❑ Ulcers	_____	_____
❑ Other	_____	_____

MEDICAL RESOURCES

Doctor _____

Clinic _____

     Telephone _____

Doctor _____

Clinic _____

     Telephone _____

Hospital _____

     Telephone _____

After-hours medical care center _____

     Telephone _____

Pharmacist _____

     Telephone _____

Poison control center _____

     Telephone _____

MANAGING YOUR MEDICINE

Today's prescription and over-the-counter drugs control chronic disease, relieve pain, and cure infections. They can help us feel better, but they can't do the job unless they are taken correctly.

Take an Active Role

You can make sure your medicines work for you—instead of against you—by following a few simple steps when you talk with your doctor or pharmacist.

Tell your doctor and pharmacist about all drugs you are taking. Whenever you visit your doctor, be ready with a complete list of any prescription or over-the-counter drugs you are taking. Over-the-counter medications include aspirin, acetaminophen (Tylenol or a generic), antacids, laxatives, cough and cold medicines, and vitamin supplements, to name a few. Most drugstores have a computer program that checks for drug interaction and drug allergies. If you see more than one doctor, be sure each knows what the others have prescribed.

Tell your doctor and pharmacist about any past reactions to specific drugs. If you are allergic to a certain drug, such as penicillin, your doctor needs to know this.

Ask about generic drugs. Many brand-name drugs have less-expensive generic equivalents. To save money, ask your doctor or pharmacist if a generic drug is available. In some cases, however, your doctor may advise using a specific brand.

Ask about nondrug options. For many conditions, drugs aren't the only solutions. When talking with your doctor, ask about alternative ways of treating your condition. For example, losing weight and increasing your physical activity can help lower high blood pressure.

Keep Complete Records

Keeping records of the drugs you take gives you easy reference to important medical information. Use the Personal Medication Record worksheet on p. 286 to list current drugs and past reactions. Refer to this record when discussing a new prescription with your doctor or pharmacist.

Update your records whenever you receive a new prescription. You'll be more likely to take your medicine as directed—and you may avoid a bad reaction.

Choosing a Drugstore

There are many drugstores to choose from in any community—but each one handles things a little differently. Whether it's near your home or in your clinic, you should select one drugstore that suits your needs and use it consistently. That way, the pharmacist can check your records for possible drug interactions and allergies whenever a new prescription is filled. Your file will be complete if you always use the same drugstore.

Your pharmacist is a good source of information about the drugs you take. For your regular drugstore, look for one where pharmacists will take the time to thoroughly answer all your questions, either in person or over the phone.

Cost is another consideration when choosing a drugstore. Call around and comparison shop, especially if you take certain drugs regularly. If your health plan covers prescriptions, find out whether you can only use certain drugstores.

Some drugstores offer special conveniences such as 24-hour emergency service, computerized records of the drugs you purchase, senior citizen discounts, and delivery service. Consider cost, helpful service, and convenience when deciding which drugstore to use.

Prescription Drug Worksheet

On the following page are some questions to ask your doctor or pharmacist whenever you receive a new prescription for medicine. Make copies of this form and keep them on hand for your entire family to bring along to the doctor's office or your drugstore.

PRESCRIPTION DRUG WORKSHEET

Name of Drug and Date
What was prescribed and when? _____

_____

What type (class) of drug is this? _____

_____

Purpose
Why am I taking it? _____

_____

What does it do? _____

_____

How does it work? _____

_____

How long does it take to work? _____

_____

Dosage
How much should be taken? _____

When and how often should it be taken? _____

_____

What should I do if a dose is missed? _____

_____

How Long?
How long should it be taken? _____

Is it all right to quit when symptoms stop? _____

Special Instructions
Take with food or on an empty stomach? _____

_____

Any other precautions? _____

_____

Side Effects/Reactions
What are the most common side effects or allergic reactions?

_____

What should I do if I have an allergic reaction?

_____

_____

Will side effects decrease after routine use?

_____

_____

Drug/Food/Alcohol Interaction
What other drugs, foods, or activities should be avoided while taking this medication? _____

_____

Follow-Up
When should I report back to the doctor?

_____

Are lab tests necessary to monitor changes?

_____

Refills
How many and when? _____

Storage
What's the expiration date? _____

How should it be stored? _____

_____

Does my household require childproof or easy-to-open caps?

_____

Cost
How much does it cost? _____

Is there a less expensive generic form? _____

_____

Making Your Medicine Work for You

When packing a suitcase, you try to make the most of every inch of space. To get the most out of your medicine, follow these steps.

Understand what you're taking.

Know what the drug does, the correct dosage, when and how to take it, and how long to take it. Some drugs aren't effective unless you take the entire prescription. Others, such as pain relievers, can be stopped when symptoms disappear.

Ask about side effects and report reactions promptly.

Some side effects are common and are not dangerous. Others can signal that a drug isn't right for you. If you don't feel right, call the doctor or pharmacist. Report the name of the drug you're taking and the reaction(s) you're having.

Bad reactions to drugs are more common as we age. Be wary of such symptoms as dizziness or drowsiness. They could interfere with driving or cause falls. Regardless of your age, such symptoms may mean a change in dosage or drug is in order.

Be sure to tell your doctor or pharmacist if you have a reaction to a particular drug or if you have a condition that may affect or be affected by the prescribed drug. For example, pregnant and nursing mothers should avoid many drugs.

Follow instructions.

Read labels carefully and ask your pharmacist about other special precautions. Some drugs must be taken with food, and others work best on an empty stomach. You may also need to avoid alcohol or stay out of the sun while on certain drugs. Even instructions like "shake first" or "refrigerate" can make a big difference in the drug's effectiveness.

Be consistent.

Remember to take your medication regularly—and on time. If you miss a dose, check with your doctor or pharmacist. Sometimes you might be told to double the next dose. Other times that could be harmful. Don't make the decision on your own.

Remember to take your medication.

Remembering to take your prescription can sometimes be hard. Try to link taking medicine with other activities that are part of your daily routine, such as meals or bedtime. Here are some examples:

- **Once a day.** Watching the evening news.

- **Twice a day.** Brushing your teeth. (Turn the bottle upside down in the morning and right side up in the evening.)

- **Four times a day.** At three meals and at bedtime. (If the medicine should be taken on an empty stomach, take 1 hour before meals.)

Over-the-Counter Care

Many people underestimate the health consequences of nonprescription drugs. But over-the-counter drugs can cause overdoses, allergic reactions, and dangerous interactions with other drugs just as prescription drugs can.

Over-the-counter drugs can also interfere with your prescription drugs. For example, a seemingly innocent antacid can destroy the effectiveness of certain antibiotics. The side effects of cough or cold medicines can be serious if you're taking medicine for high blood pressure, diabetes, or glaucoma.

Not all over-the-counter drugs are the same. Those called "cough or cold medicines" have a variety of ingredients to treat different symptoms of colds and flu. Read the label to make sure you're taking medicine that will treat the symptoms you have. Or ask your pharmacist for a recommendation.

Many drugs that once required a prescription are now sold over the counter. Check with your pharmacist about whether a drug is available over the counter. To help you make the right decision, use the following Nonprescription Drug Worksheet as a reminder of what to consider when choosing an over-the-counter drug.

List Nonprescription Drugs

You may want to list a summary of options and compare the uses, dose, costs, and side effects of medicine you commonly use. For example, the Pain Medication Chart on p. 287 can be kept in a convenient place for times when you need to decide about using these common medicines.

NONPRESCRIPTION DRUG WORKSHEET

Keep copies of this worksheet readily available so family members can use it whenever they consider taking a nonprescription drug.

Evaluate

What symptoms do you want the medication to relieve?

Can home remedies do the job?

Are you supposed to avoid certain drugs for any reason (pregnancy, breastfeeding, drug interactions, allergies)?

Consult

Ask your pharmacist or doctor or check a reference book for help in choosing the proper product.

Investigate

Read the label thoroughly. What are the ingredients?

Do they conflict with any other drugs you are taking?

Are you allergic to any of the ingredients?

What does the drug do?

What is the recommended dosage for you?

Do any warnings or cautions apply to you?

Confirm

Ask your pharmacist about possible interactions with food, alcohol, or your other medicines.

Decide

What is your motive for buying this drug?

Are you being influenced by recommendations, price, or advertising?

PERSONAL MEDICATION RECORD

Make copies of this record as needed.

Prescription Drugs

List any prescription drugs you've taken in the last 2 to 4 weeks, as well as any you have on hand to use as needed, but that you haven't taken recently. Add new drugs as they are prescribed.

Drug
(brand or generic name) _____

Purpose _____

Dose _____

Instructions_____

Date started _____

Nonprescription Drugs
(Make a similar list for nonprescription drugs.)

Drug _____

Purpose _____

Dose _____

Instructions_____

Date started _____

Drug Allergies and Past Reactions

List any drugs you know you are allergic to and those to which you have had a bad reaction in the past. You may also include the names of prescription drugs that haven't worked for you.

Drug _____

Purpose _____

Drug _____

Purpose _____

Drug _____

Purpose _____

What happened to make you think you are allergic to this drug?

PAIN MEDICATION CHART			
	Acetaminophen Tylenol Tempra to	**Ibuprofen** Advil, Nuprin, Motrin IB	**Aspirin** All brands are equal [Ecotrin is coated,
Use	First choice for: fever, headache, mild burns, stings	Sports injuries, acute trauma, menstrual cramps, headache, "—itis"(tendon/joint inflammations)	Stroke/heart attack prevention; fever in adults
Dose	Children: by weight Adults: two 325 mg tablets	Take with food Adults: one or two 200 mg tablets	DON'T USE FOR CHILDREN Adults: one or two 325 mg tablets
Use for pain	Yes	Yes Increasing dose will increase relief; take up to 3,200 mg/day	Yes Increasing dose will not increase relief
Use for fever	Yes	Yes, small doses	Yes
Use for muscle/joint pain	No	Yes, higher doses of 2,400–3,200 mg/day	Yes
Use for blood thinning	No	Some	Yes
Side Effects	Safe for short-term use (large overdose can be dangerous)	Can irritate stomach	Ulcers, gastro- intestinal bleeding; easy to overdose

This table will help you decide which type of pain reliever is the right choice for your condition.

Be careful of combination products; some may have caffeine and some mix these drugs.
Do not use more than one pain reliever at a time.
Do not take with cold medicines.

DECIDING ABOUT SURGERY

When the doctor recommends surgery, patients need to play an active role in decision making. Your values and beliefs are often a key part of choosing surgery as a road to better health versus exploring other types of treatment. Surgery can be risky and difficult, but sometimes it's clearly the only way to go. Other times, alternatives to surgery are the wisest choice.

Learning to ask the right questions to get the information you need is vital to helping you decide whether or not surgery is right for you. Being a responsible health care consumer starts with taking an active role in decisions about your health. That way, you're more likely to feel calm and confident about whatever course of treatment you choose.

Deciding Which Option Is Best

The very thought of having a problem that could be serious enough to warrant surgery scares many people. That's why only 10 to 40 percent of elective surgical procedures—those a person can choose to have or not have—are performed to relieve basically harmless conditions or ones that are causing only minor symptoms.

So how do you decide about surgery? The first step is to find out whether the surgery your doctor is recommending is nonelective or elective.

Nonelective Surgery

When surgery is needed to save a person's life (such as to remove a ruptured appendix) or must be done immediately to prevent permanent disability (such as to surgically repair a badly broken bone), it is considered nonelective. That means you have little or no choice but to have the operation. And you probably do not have time to explore other options. Fortunately, few surgical procedures are truly nonelective.

Elective Surgery

Most surgical procedures involve some degree of choice for the patient. In some cases, alternatives to surgery exist, such as drugs or other ways of dealing with the problem. In other cases, surgery may be the only option for correcting a particular problem, but the symptoms don't merit the risk of surgery. For example, many people who have gallstones have no pain, discomfort, or other symptoms and do not need treatment.

Surgery is appropriate if it is needed to:

- Relieve or prevent pain
- Restore or preserve normal function
- Correct a deformity
- Save or prolong your life

Even if surgery is appropriate, it may not be the only choice of treatment. It's always best to investigate all other options before choosing surgery.

Make an appointment with your doctor to discuss the Questions to Ask before Surgery worksheet on p. 289. Write down or tape-record the answers. If you feel anxious or nervous, take a friend or relative along for moral support. Then, assess the information and decide what you want to do.

Make sure it's your own decision. Don't let yourself be pressured into having surgery you don't need or want.

Asking for a Second Opinion

Getting more information can help when you're deciding about surgery. One way to do this is to get a second opinion (also called a "review of treatment"). Some health plans require second opinions before they will cover certain procedures. But a second opinion can also give you more facts for and reassurance of making an informed decision.

Although a second opinion isn't needed in every instance, you would be wise to seek one if:

- The procedure is experimental or high-risk, such as an organ transplant

- Your symptoms aren't severe and the outcome of surgery isn't clear

- The procedure has a reputation for being performed when not absolutely needed

QUESTIONS TO ASK BEFORE SURGERY

Name and Procedure
What's the operation called? _____

_____

What will be done?_____

_____

How is it performed? _____

_____

How long will it take?_____

_____

How serious is it? _____

_____

Reason
Why is this surgery recommended? _____

_____

Results
How will this procedure help my condition?

_____

What are the benefits? _____

_____

Alternatives
What other treatment options are available?

_____

Is outpatient surgery an option? _____

_____

What will happen if I don't have the surgery?

_____

Is nontreatment an option? _____

_____

Timing
How soon should I have the surgery?_____

_____

How soon must I make a decision?_____

_____

What will happen if I postpone the operation?

_____

Risks
What are the risks involved? _____

_____

What percentage of patients die from this procedure?_____

_____

Complications
What complications may occur?_____

_____

Which complications are common for my age and state of health? _____

Postoperative information
Are there any side effects of anesthesia? _____

_____

Will I have tubes, catheters, or dressings after surgery? _____

Recovery
What's the typical recovery period?_____

_____

How long will I be unable to care for myself?

_____

When can I return to work and my normal activities? _____

Experience
How frequently do you perform this procedure?

_____

How frequently is this surgery done at your hospital? _____

Cost
How much is this surgery likely to cost? _____
What are your fees? _____
What's the average hospital charge? _____
What will be covered by my health plan? ____

_____

AVOIDING UNNECESSARY SURGERY

Getting a second opinion is a good idea if your doctor recommends any of the surgeries listed below. These procedures tend to be performed more often than is medically necessary.

- Tonsillectomy (removal of tonsils)

- Hysterectomy (removal of uterus and sometimes ovaries)

- Coronary bypass

- Radical mastectomy (removal of the breast)

- Orthopedic surgery (back, bones, or joints)

- Cholecystectomy (removal of gallbladder)

Learning more about the pros and cons of any recommended procedure is the best way to decide whether the risk outweighs the benefits, given your personal preferences. Other controversial procedures that warrant special study and discussion include:

- Fixing a fracture of the femur (internally or externally)

- Transurethral resection of the prostate (TURP)

- Delivering a baby with a vacuum instrument or instrument for a baby low in the vagina (vacuum extraction or low forceps delivery with episiotomy)

- Balloon angioplasty

- Unilateral thyroid lobectomy

- Total knee or hip replacement

Don't Be Timid

You might feel uncomfortable asking for a second opinion, but most doctors today are used to this and are very cooperative. A doctor who responds with anger or refuses to cooperate with such a request may not have your best interests at heart.

To find a second surgeon, ask your primary doctor, your health plan, or your local hospital for a recommendation. If you ask the first surgeon for a referral, you are less likely to get a truly objective second opinion.

Avoid the expense of repeating tests and procedures by bringing your medical records and X-rays, if any, along with you. If this is not possible, you can have them sent to the second surgeon before your appointment by signing a records release form.

If the second surgeon disagrees with the first, find out why. You may find that one surgeon's philosophy and reasoning fit with your own more than the other's.

IF YOUR DOCTOR RECOMMENDS HOSPITALIZATION

Many procedures that used to require hospitalization are taken care of at clinics today. What's more, surgeries and rehabilitation that used to require days and weeks in the hospital now are often taken care of in a matter of hours. Because procedures that required lengthy hospitalization in the past have changed so much over the past few years, it is vital that you understand all the reasons that justify the need for you to be treated at the hospital instead of at home or in a clinic. Besides, going to the hospital is a major disruption of life for most people, so being sure you understand why it is necessary will help you cope with the stress of hospitalization.

Because doctors are so busy, they try to be brief. But you need to know exactly why your doctor recommends hospitalization. To get your questions answered efficiently, take a copy of the Questions to Ask before Hospitalization worksheet (below) with you when you visit your doctor and jot down or tape-record the answers. For some people, it helps to bring a friend or relative along who can help remember the details of the discussion with the doctor.

QUESTIONS TO ASK BEFORE HOSPITALIZATION

Reason
Why is hospitalization necessary? _____

_____

Procedure
What tests and/or procedures will be done? _____

_____

Must the tests and/or procedures be done at the hospital? _____

Alternatives
What other choices do I have? _____

_____

How much will I be involved in deciding about my treatment? _____

_____

_____

Risks
Are there any risks involved with any of the tests or procedures? _____

_____

What are they? _____

_____

Results
What will the tests tell us? _____

_____

Timing
How long will I be in the hospital? _____

_____

Recovery
How soon can I return to normal activities? __

_____

How long will I be away from work? _____

REVIEWING MEDICAL FEES AND BILLS

Wise consumers of goods such as cars or groceries routinely check prices before making decisions. Knowing what to expect in the way of cost is a smart idea when planning for surgery or hospitalization, too. The first step is to find out what your insurance covers and whether there is anything special you need to do to qualify for coverage, such as getting preauthorization from the health plan or getting a second opinion. For care provided by a specialist, many plans also require a referral from a primary care doctor for the highest level of benefits. Most of all, find out what copayments or what percentage of the bill you will have to pay.

The next step is to find out what the total bill—for you and your health plan—is likely to be. Medical fees can vary greatly from doctor to doctor and hospital to hospital. If you have a choice of hospitals, call each to find out what a stay for your type of surgery usually costs or at least what the daily room rate is.

Feel free to also discuss financial questions with your surgeon or the office staff. Find out if the doctor's office will fill out and submit insurance forms or if that's your responsibility. Also ask if the doctor accepts the insurance payment as the full fee (called "accepting assignment"), or if you must make up the difference between the doctor's fee and insurance payment.

Reviewing Your Hospital Bill

After your surgery or hospital stay is over, you can avoid financial unpleasantness by reviewing your hospital bills carefully. Hospitals try hard to provide accurate bills, but errors do occur.

Ask the hospital billing office to explain unclear charges, terms, or tests. You can also ask for a copy of your bedside log or other medical records to use when checking your bill. If you need further help, your doctor's office might be able to help.

Just like reading the labels on the foods you buy or checking the sticker to see what options come with a car you may buy, checking your hospital bills requires some time and attention on your part to be sure you are getting value for your dollar. Don't hesitate to look at the fine print and ask for more information about the bill if you think things are not adding up the way you anticipated. The following questions should help you identify any special problems with a hospital bill:

• Ask for an itemized bill instead of the summary most hospitals send.

- Were you billed for a semiprivate or a private room? Which did you have?

- Does the room rate multiplied by the number of days you stayed come to the same total as on the bill? (Most hospitals do not charge for the day of discharge.)

- Did you have each of the tests and procedures listed? You may be charged for something you didn't have simply because of a clerical error or because your doctor cancelled the orders, but the billing records weren't changed.

- Do any charges seem unusually high to you? For example, $3 for a dose of acetaminophen (Tylenol)?

If you find an error, call the hospital's billing department and ask that it be corrected. If necessary, ask to speak with the department supervisor. Once the hospital agrees to correct the mistake, ask for a revised bill, and then send a copy to your health plan. If you run into problems, call your health plan for help.

Before paying your portion of the bill, make sure your questions have been answered, errors are corrected, and your health plan has already paid its portion.

NOTES

INDEX

F

CREDITS

 Park Nicollet
Medical Foundation

Editor-in-chief
Paul E. Terry, Ph.D., Park Nicollet Medical Foundation

Medical Editors
David Abelson, M.D., Park Nicollet Medical Center; Allan Kind, M.D., Park Nicollet Medical Foundation

Section Editors
Joseph Alfano, M.D., George Halvorson, HealthPartners Health Plans; Spencer Holmes, M.D., Park Nicollet Medical Center; Thomas Kottke, M.D., Mayo Clinic; Gordon Mosser, M.D., Institute for Clinical Systems Integration; Linda Peitzman, M.D., Park Nicollet Medical Center; James L. Reinertsen, M.D., HealthSystem Minnesota; Leif Solberg, M.D., Group Health Foundation; Steve Wetzell, Business Health Care Action Group

Writers/Contributing Editors
Paul E. Terry, Ph.D.; Lisa Bartels-Rabb, M.S.J.; Tom Brandes, M.A.; Scott Glickstein, M.D.; Robert Gorman, M.D.; Kathy Tingelstad

Contributors
Suzanne Bennett, M.P.H.; Joan Bissen, R.D.; Debra Boal, R.N.; Mark DePaolis, M.D.; Marion Franz, R.D.; Lisa Graham-Peterson; Susan Hanson, R.D.; Mary Kruse, M.A.; Judy Monn; Jane Norstrom, M.A.; Joan Nyberg; Linda Pietz, R.N.; Marta Simpson, R.N.; Susan Sullivan, Ph.D.

Medical Reviewers
Internal Medicine: Avis Baumann, R.N.; Jane Oh, M.D.; Jennifer Olson, M.D.; Barbara Steigauf, R.N.

Pulmonary Medicine: Kevin Komadina, M.D.; A. Stuart Hanson, M.D.; Kathleen Hornsby, R.N.; Richard Woellner, M.D.

Infectious Diseases: Pat Dahlman, R.N.; Paul Carson, M.D.

Family Practice: Donald Abrams, M.D.; Joseph Alfano, M.D.; Barbara Benjamin, M.D.; Alan Carter, M.D.; Susan Carter, M.D.; Michael Dukinfield, M.D.; Janet Frost, R.N.; John Haugen, M.D.; Mark Hench, M.D.; Jeanne Hesse, M.D.; Bonita Hill, M.D.; Julie Hudson, R.N.; John Kaintz, M.D.; Michael Lano, M.D.; Douglas Lowin, M.D.; Joseph Lukaska, M.D.; Alston Lundgren, M.D.; Jean Lundgren, M.D.; Donald Lynch, M.D.; Rosa Marroquin, M.D.; Charles McCoy, M.D.; Kenneth Olson, M.D.; Carolyn Torkelson, M.D.; David VonWeiss, M.D.

OB/GYN: Janet Claxton, N.P.; Barbara Davenport, N.P.; Deborah Meade, R.N.; Leslie Pratt, M.D.; Lois Satterberg, N.P.; Deborah Thorp, M.D.

Pediatrics: Renner Anderson, M.D.; Jayne Boche, M.D.; David Griffin, M.D.; Thomas Helm, M.D.; Robert Karasov, M.D.; Kristi Klett, M.D.; Beth Leaneagh, R.N.; Douglas Martin, M.D.; John Meurer, M.D.; Michael Pryor, M.D.; Theresa Ryan, M.D.

CREDITS

Urgent Care: Shelly Barton, R.N.; Paul Bearmon, M.D.; Carol Manning, M.D.; Linda Peitzman, M.D.; Mary Ratz, M.D.; Suzanne Schaefer, M.D.; Omri Shochatovitz, M.D.; Susan Vitalis, M.D.

Allergy: David Graft, M.D.; William Schoenwetter, M.D.; Richard Sveum, M.D.

Cardiology: Steve Benton, M.D.; J. Mark Haugland, M.D.

Gastroenterology: Matthew Bagamery, M.D.; Michael Levy, M.D.

Dermatology: Spencer Holmes, M.D.; Michael McCormick, M.D.; Louis Rusin, M.D.; Victoria Vanroy, M.D.

Oncology: Steven Duane, M.D.; Charles Murray, M.D.

Neurology: Daniel Freking, M.D.; Sandra Hanson, M.D.; Debra Heros, M.D.; Eric Schenk, M.D.

ENT: David Buran, M.D.

Orthopedics: Matthew Putnam, M.D.; Gregg Strathy, M.D.; Thomas Youngren, M.D.

Ophthalmology: Robert Campbell, M.D.; Timothy Diegel, M.D.; Rodney Dueck, M.D.; Richard Freeman, M.D.; Anne Towey, M.D.; Anton Willerscheidt, M.D.

Rheumatology: Eric Schned, M.D.

Urology: Steven Bernstein, M.D.; Clyde Blackard, M.D.; William Borkon, M.D.; Sharon Reiter, R.N.; William Sharer, M.D.; Erol Uke, M.D.; Gang Zhang, M.D.

Senior Health: Sharon Marx, M.D.

Rehabilitation Medicine: Ann Brutlag, M.D.; Robert Gorman, M.D.; George Kramer, M.D.; Daniel Kurtti, M.D.

Occupational Medicine: David Parker, M.D.

Pharmacy: Richard Bleck R.Ph., Scott Bryngelson R.Ph., Roger Mickelson R.Ph.

Specialty Reviewers: Gail Amundson, M.D.; Dale Anderson, M.D.; Debra Boal, R.N.; Stephen Bonfilio, Ph.D.; Hyacinth Campbell-Roberts; Timothy Culbert, M.D.; Stacie Emberley; Mary Figueroa, M.D.; Jinnet Fowles, Ph.D.; Stanley Greenwald, M.D.; Carmen Gutterman, Ph.D.; Carol Hersman, R.N., M.A.; Rebecca Kajander, C.P.N.P., M.P.H.; Judy Kelloway, Ph.D.; James Li, M.D.; Janet Lima; Sheila McCormick, R.N.; Jeanne Nelson, M.D.; Joseph Nelson, L.P.; Stephen Olsen, Ph.D.; Anthony Pojman, M.D.; Stephen Powless, M.D.; Ira Rabinowitz, D.M.D.; Judson Reaney, M.D.; Michael Rethwill, M.D.; Peter Smars, M.D.; Paul Spilseth, M.D.; Linda Strohmayer, R.N.; Andrew Wood, R.P.T.

Production Coordination
Linda Olson

**Ⓜ Mosby
Great Performance**

Editor: Stephanie Slon

Manuscript Editor: Annette Hall

Production Manager:
Christine Jennings

Art Direction: Nancy Olson

Cover Design: Studio Montage

Illustrations: Joan Orme, Karen Morgan

Design and Layout:
Seventh Generation Design

COLOR PLATES

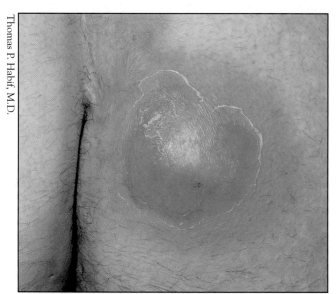

Boil—see text p. 151

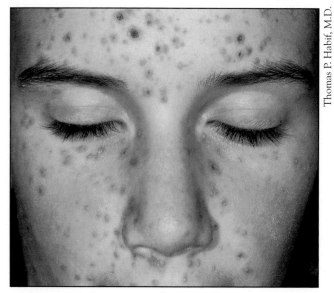

Chicken pox rash—see text p. 152

Three stages of chicken pox rash—see text p. 152

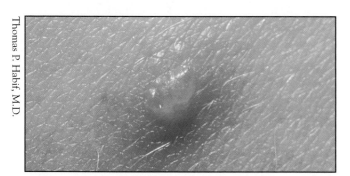

Stage 1—Flat, red marks with central clear blister.

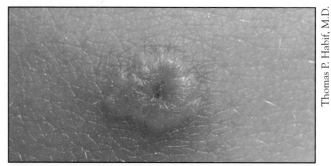

Stage 2—Blister becomes cloudy and depressed in center. Border irregular.

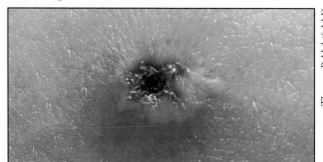

Stage 3—Crust forms in center.

Thomas P. Habif, M.D.

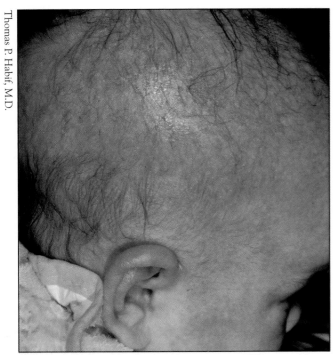

Thomas P. Habif, M.D.

Cradle cap (seborrheic dermatitis)—see text p. 155

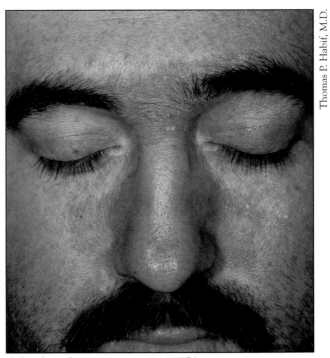

Thomas P. Habif, M.D.

Seborrheic dermatitis—see text p. 156

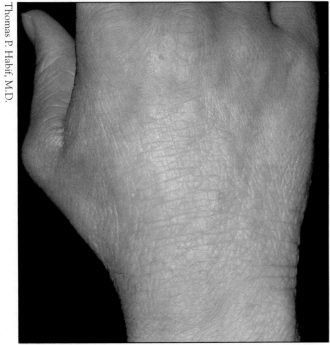

Thomas P. Habif, M.D.

Atopic dermatitis—see text p. 156

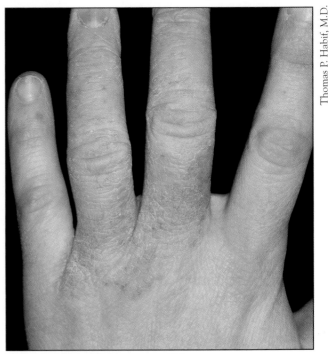

Thomas P. Habif, M.D.

Contact dermatitis—see text p. 156

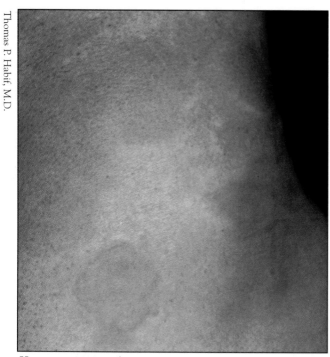

Thomas P. Habif, M.D.

Hives—see text p. 158

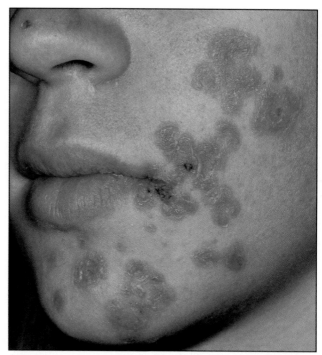

Thomas P. Habif, M.D.

Impetigo—see text p. 160. Red sores ooze honey-colored liquid which dries into thick crust.

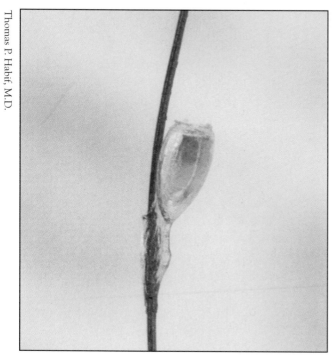

Thomas P. Habif, M.D.

Head lice egg stuck to hair shaft—see text p. 162

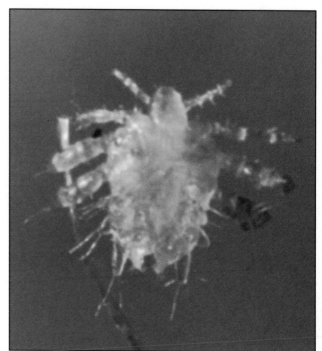

Thomas P. Habif, M.D.

Crab louse—see text p. 162. Has short body and large claws to grasp hair.

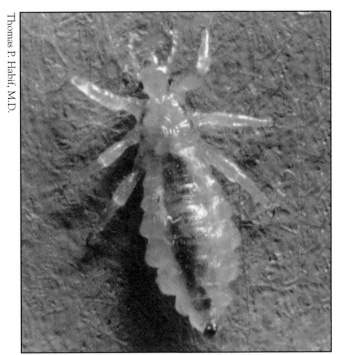

Body louse—*see text p. 162*

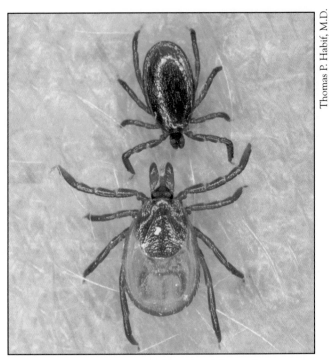

Deer tick *unengorged (top) partly engorged (bottom)*
—see text p. 163

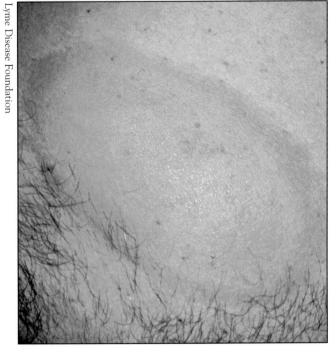

Lyme disease rash—*see text p. 163*

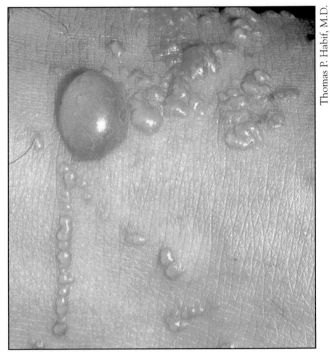

Poison ivy rash—*see text p. 164*

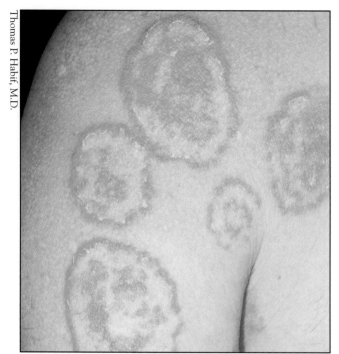

Ringworm fungal skin infection—see text p. 167

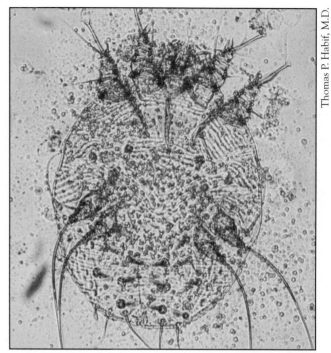

Scabies mite greatly enlarged (40x)—see text p. 168

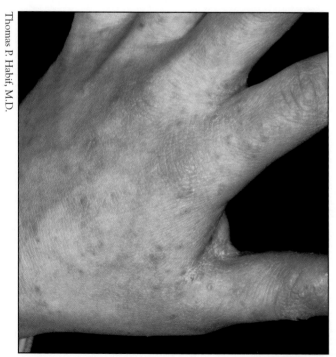

Scabies—see text p. 168. Tiny bumps itch, especially at night.
Burrowing of mites leaves tiny white grooves and tunnels on skin.

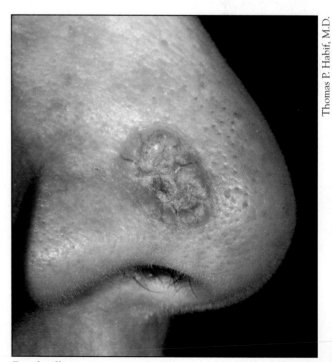

Basal cell cancer—see text p. 169

COLOR PLATES

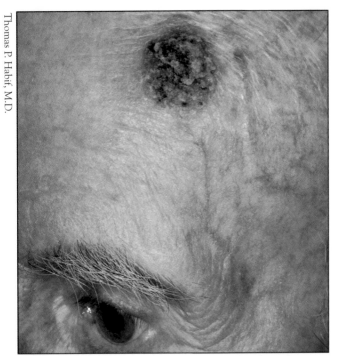

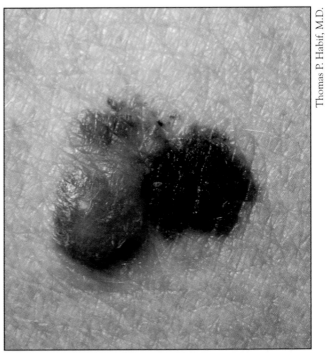

Squamous cell cancer—*see text* p. 169. *Rough scaly surface on reddish base.*

Malignant melanoma—*see text* p. 169. *Mole with uneven border with different colors in the same mole.*

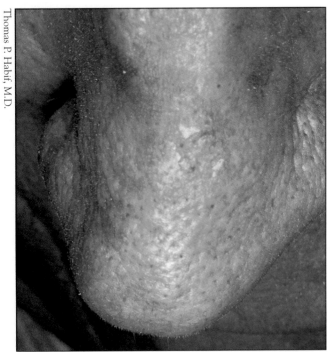

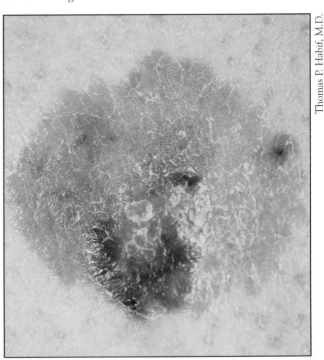

Actinic keratosis—*see text* p. 169. *Red base with dry, yellow-brown scaly area.*

Malignant melanoma—*see text* p. 169. *Later stage.*

MUSCULAR SYSTEM

SKELETAL SYSTEM

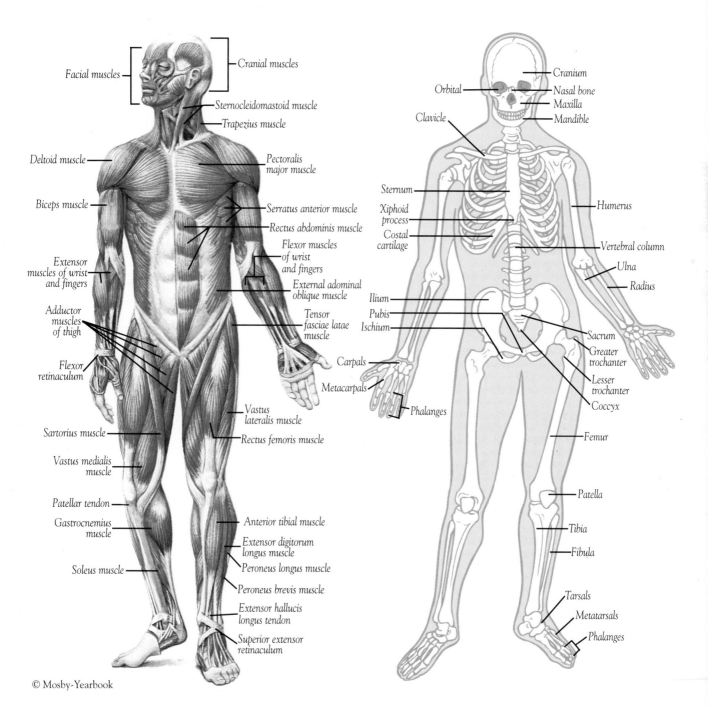

Facial muscles

Cranial muscles

Sternocleidomastoid muscle

Trapezius muscle

Deltoid muscle

Pectoralis major muscle

Biceps muscle

Serratus anterior muscle

Rectus abdominis muscle

Flexor muscles of wrist and fingers

Extensor muscles of wrist and fingers

External adominal oblique muscle

Adductor muscles of thigh

Tensor fasciae latae muscle

Flexor retinaculum

Vastus lateralis muscle

Sartorius muscle

Rectus femoris muscle

Vastus medialis muscle

Patellar tendon

Gastrocnemius muscle

Anterior tibial muscle

Extensor digitorum longus muscle

Peroneus longus muscle

Soleus muscle

Peroneus brevis muscle

Extensor hallucis longus tendon

Superior extensor retinaculum

Orbital

Cranium

Nasal bone

Maxilla

Mandible

Clavicle

Sternum

Humerus

Xiphoid process

Costal cartilage

Vertebral column

Ulna

Radius

Ilium

Pubis

Ischium

Sacrum

Greater trochanter

Carpals

Lesser trochanter

Metacarpals

Coccyx

Phalanges

Femur

Patella

Tibia

Fibula

Tarsals

Metatarsals

Phalanges

© Mosby-Yearbook

FRONT VIEW

COLOR PLATES

MUSCULAR SYSTEM

SKELETAL SYSTEM

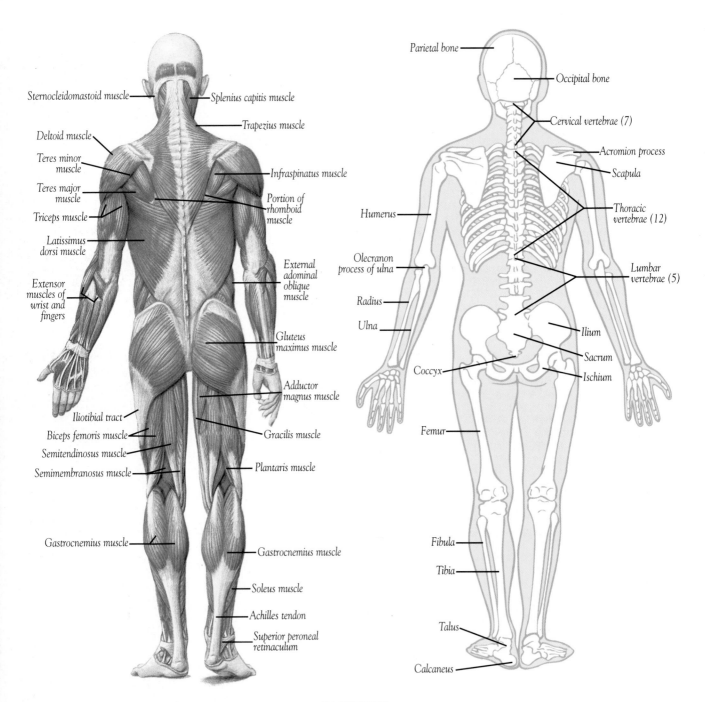

Sternocleidomastoid muscle

Splenius capitis muscle

Trapezius muscle

Deltoid muscle

Teres minor muscle

Teres major muscle

Infraspinatus muscle

Triceps muscle

Portion of rhomboid muscle

Latissimus dorsi muscle

External adominal oblique muscle

Extensor muscles of wrist and fingers

Gluteus maximus muscle

Adductor magnus muscle

Iliotibial tract

Biceps femoris muscle

Gracilis muscle

Semitendinosus muscle

Semimembranosus muscle

Plantaris muscle

Gastrocnemius muscle

Gastrocnemius muscle

Soleus muscle

Achilles tendon

Superior peroneal retinaculum

Parietal bone

Occipital bone

Cervical vertebrae (7)

Acromion process

Scapula

Humerus

Thoracic vertebrae (12)

Olecranon process of ulna

Radius

Lumbar vertebrae (5)

Ulna

Ilium

Coccyx

Sacrum

Ischium

Femur

Fibula

Tibia

Talus

Calcaneus

BACK VIEW